50 - ADMISSION TEST SERIES (NVB)

ISBN 0-8373-5050-6



# NVB

# NATIONAL VETERINARY BOARDS

By Jack Rudman

*Administered by the*

*NATIONAL BOARD OF VETERINARY MEDICAL EXAMINERS (NBVME) of the AMERICAN VETERINARY MEDICAL ASSOCIATION (AVMA)*

## MAJOR AREAS

- Anatomy
- Physiological Chemistry
- Physiology
- Pathology
- Pharmacology and Therapeutics
- Bacteriology
- Parisitology
- Hygiene
- Physical Diagnosis
- Medicine
- Surgery

NLC

NATIONAL LEARNING CORPORATION

212 MICHAEL DRIVE SYOSSET, N.Y. 11791 (516) 921-8888

**National Learning Corporation**

212 Michael Drive, Syosset, New York 11791
(516) 921-8888

PRINTED IN THE UNITED STATES OF AMERICA

# PASSBOOK®

## NOTICE



NATIONAL LEARNING CORPORATION
212 Michael Drive
Syosset, New York 11791

Inquiries re licensing agreements should be addressed to:
The President
National Learning Corporation
212 Michael Drive
Syosset, New York 11791

# PASSBOOK SERIES®

The *PASSBOOK SERIES®* has been created to prepare applicants and candidates for the ultimate academic battlefield – the examination room.

At some time in our lives, each and every one of us may be required to take an examination – for validation, matriculation, admission, qualification, registration, certification, or licensure.

Based on the assumption that every applicant or candidate has met the basic formal educational standards, has taken the required number of courses, and read the necessary texts, the *PASSBOOK SERIES®* furnishes the one special preparation which may assure passing with confidence, instead of failing with insecurity. Examination questions – together with answers – are furnished as the basic vehicle for study so that the mysteries of the examination and its compounding difficulties may be eliminated or diminished by a sure method.

This book is meant to help you pass your examination provided that you qualify and are serious in your objective.

The entire field is reviewed through the huge store of content information which is succinctly presented through a provocative and challenging approach – the question-and-answer method.

A climate of success is established by furnishing the correct answers at the end of each test.

You soon learn to recognize types of questions, forms of questions, and patterns of questioning. You may even begin to anticipate expected outcomes.

You perceive that many questions are repeated or adapted so that you gain acute insights, which may enable you to score many sure points.

You learn how to confront new questions, or types of questions, and to attack them confidently and work out the correct answers.

You note objectives and emphases, and recognize pitfalls and dangers, so that you may make positive educational adjustments.

Moreover, you are kept fully informed in relation to new concepts, methods, practices, and directions in the field.

You discover that you are actually taking the examination all the time: you are preparing for the examination by "taking" an examination, not by reading extraneous and/or supererogatory textbooks.

In short, this PASSBOOK®, used directedly, should be an important factor in helping you to pass your test.

# National Veterinary Boards (NVB)

NATIONAL BOARD VETERINARY MEDICAL LICENSING EXAMINATION (NVBME) (NBE)

I. WHAT ARE THE PURPOSES OF THE EXAMINATION?

The goals of the National Licensing Examination program are to:

- Maintain a high quality of professional practice of veterinary medicine through the formulation of national standards inherent in national examination development
- Assist state boards of examiners in discharging their responsibilities
- Measure the professional competence of veterinarians who have graduated from an accredited program of study
- Increase the mobility of practicing veterinarians
- Contribute to the development of the profession through improved definition of the knowledge and judgment required for professional practice

II. HOW IS THE NATIONAL EXAMINATION CONSTRUCTED?

The licensing examination is developed under the direction of the Examination Committee of the National Board of Veterinary Medical Examiners (NBVME) of the American Veterinary Medical Association in collaboration with the Professional Examination Service (PES). These examinations have been used by state examining boards since 1954.

III. WHAT DOES THE NATIONAL EXAMINATION COVER?

Part I - Consists of 200 questions in Preclinical Sciences (160 questions) and other practice areas (40 questions).
The Preclinical Sciences section includes questions covering
Anatomy (24 questions);
Physiology (28 questions);
Disease Processes (32 questions);
Etiology Agents (20 questions);
Pharmacology (18 questions);
Toxicology (16 questions); and
Immunology (12 questions.
The other practice areas section includes questions covering:
Public Health/Preventive Medicine (32 questions; and
Jurisprudence (8 questions).

Part II- Consists of 200 questions in Clinical Science, including
Diagnostics (48 questions);
Therapeutics (40 questions);
Medicine (48 questions);
Surgery (40 questions); and
Animal Production (24 questions).

For better organization and comprehension, due to the scope and complexity of the examination, we have divided the subject areas into 3 parts and published 3 separate books, as well as a combined abridged edition.

Part I - Anatomy, Physiological Chemistry, Physiology, and Pathology
II - Pharmacology and Therapeutics, Bacteriology, Parasitology, and Hygiene (including Meat and Milk Hygiene)
III - Physical Diagnosis, Medicine, and Surgery

BOVINE: Reproduction, Mastitis, Abortion, Ketosis, Rabies, Milk Fever, Displaced Abomasum, Scabies, Anaplasmosis, Clostridial Infections, Leptospirosis, Orthopedic Problems, Johne's Disease, Toxicosis, Cecal_Torsion, Anthrax, Antibiotics in Feed, Nutrition, Leukemia, Internal and External Parasites, Respiratory Disease, Bovine Viral Diarrhea, Pink Eye, Squamous Cell Carcinoma, Polioencephalomalacia, Rumen Disease, Cardiovascular Disease, Neurologic Disease, Liver Disease, Infectious Disease, Cecal Disease, Renal Disease, Bacterial and Viral Gastroenteritis, and Calfhood Diseases.

CANINE: Canine Distemper, Gastric Dilatation-Torsion, Shock and Fluid Therapy, Heartworm Disease, Internal and External Parasites, Food Allergies, Endocrine without Hypoadrenocorticism, Pyometra, Alopecia, Bacterial Infections, Fungal Infections M. canis and Nocardia, Autoimmune Dermatoses, Parvovirus Infection, Malignant Lymphoma, Diabetes Mellitus, Seizure Disorders, Endocrine Diseases, AIHA, Atopy, Allergic Dermatitis, Rabies, Kidney Failure, Reproduction, Nutrition, Ophthalmic Conditions, Respiratory Disease, Cardiomyopathies, Orthopedic Problems, Toxicosis, Hepatic Disease.

EQUINE: Equine Infectious Anemia, Tetanus Vaccination, Orthopedic Problems, Internal and External Parasites, Azoturia, Restraint, Laceration Repair, Reproduction, Strangles, Abortion, Dentistry, Lameness, Purpura, Respiratory Disease, Aneuyrism, Ophthalmic Conditions, Influenza, Dermal Conditions, Sarcoid, Diarrhea, Pediatrics, Nutrition, Colic, Toxicosis, Shock and Fluid Therapy, Foal Disease, Myopathies, Laminitis, Navicular Disease, Diarrhea, Anesthesia/Sedation (Local and General), Neurological Disease, Liver Disease, Viral and Bacterial Gastrointestinal Disease, Renal Diseases, Endocrine Diseases, and Neoplastic Diseases.

PORCINE: Haemophilus Infections, Transmissible Gastroenteritis, Colibacillosis, Mycoplasmal Pneumonia, Coccidiosis, Chronic Pneumonia, Swine Dysentery, Parvovirus Infections, Pseudorabies, Mange, Salmonellosis, Hog Cholera, Nutrition, Internal and External Parasites, Rhinitis, Erysipelas, Antibiotics in Feed, African Swine Fever, Reproduction, Abortion, Swine Herd Management, Rotavirus Infections, Mastitis/Metritis/Agalactia Syndrome.

FELINE: Leukemia, Feline Urological Syndrome, Panleukopenia, Respiratory Disease Complex, Feline Infectious Peritonitis, Cardiomyopathies, Eosinophilic Skin Diseases, Anemia, Gastrointestinal Diseases, Diabetes Mellitus, Seizure Disorders, Internal and External Parasites, Hepatic Disease, Foreign Bodies, Toxoplasmosis, Endocrine Diseases, Asthma, Kidney Failure, Ophthalmic Conditions, Nutrition, Shock and Fluid

Address all inquiries to:

NBVME
National Board of Veterinary Medical Examiners
American Veterinary Medical Association
930 North Meacham Road
Schaumburg, Illinois 60172

## IV. SAMPLE QUESTIONS AND ANSWERS

Directions: Each question or incomplete statement is followed by several suggested answers or completions. Select the one that *BEST* answers the question or completes the statement. *PRINT THE LETTER OF THE CORRECT ANSWER IN THE SPACE AT THE RIGHT.*

1. Protrusion of the eyeball in the dog may be the result of abscessation of the — 1.____
   A. mandibular lymph node   B. zygomatic salivary gland
   C. submaxillary salivary gland
   D. medial retropharyngeal lymph node
   E. mandibular salivary gland

2. A previously healthy puppy begins vomiting when it is first given solid food. There is no fever and, if it is immediately returned to a liquid diet, no further vomiting occurs. — 2.____

   The congenital anomaly of the cardiovascular system that will cause such symptoms is
   A. dextrorotation of the aorta
   B. subaortic septal defect
   C. persistence of the right aortic arch
   D. patent foramen ovale
   E. patent ductus arteriosus

3. A serological diagnosis of leptospirosis by the agglutination test requires — 3.____
   A. a high level of antibody in a serum sample taken three weeks after illness
   B. acute and convalescent serum samples to show a significant rise in antibody titer
   C. the demonstration of leptospiras in the blood at the time of illness
   D. the production of illness and death of inoculated guinea pigs
   E. a standardized suspension of heat-killed organisms

4. Vegetative endocarditis may be one of the *chief* lesions found in — 4.____
   A. bovine traumatic gastritis
   B. swine erysipelas
   C. equine viral arteritis
   D. hog cholera
   E. canine toxoplasmosis

5. In intussusception in the bovine, one of the *most* characteristic combinations of symptoms is: 5.___
   A. Partial anorexia, but a marked thirst whenever water is presented
   B. A depressed attitude at the onset followed by hyper-excitability which may become maniacal one to two days before death
   C. A fever ranging from 104° to 106° F., but a normal pulse rate until shortly before death
   D. A diminution in size of the left abdominal region with a bloated distention of the right when viewed from behind
   E. A tar-like, bloody anal discharge, together with complete suppression of bowel evacuation

# KEY (CORRECT ANSWERS)

1. B
2. C
3. B
4. B
5. E

# VETERINARY MEDICINE
## CAREER DESCRIPTIONS

## CONTENTS


| | Page |
|---|---|
| I. Animal Technician | 1 |
| II. Veterinarian | 2 |

# VETERINARY MEDICINE
## ·CAREER DESCRIPTIONS

Veterinarians care for the health of the animal population. Veterinarians are also concerned with preventing and eradicating human diseases transmitted through animals, promoting sound public health practices, and medical research. Because of the demand for veterinary services, career opportunities can be found in private practice, research, or government service.

Veterinarians are often assisted by animal technicians. Animal technicians help veterinarians with the care and handling of animals and perform routine laboratory and office procedures. The need for technicians is growing rapidly, as veterinarians recognize more ways to use their skills.

## I. Animal Technician

### Animal health technician
### Veterinary science technician

Animal technicians play an important part in veterinary medicine by providing assistance to the veterinarian in daily work activities. Technicians trained in such areas as animal care and handling, principls of normal and abnormal life processes, and in laboratory and clinical procedures are qualified to assume many of the routine tasks performed by veterinarians.

Working under the direction of practicing veterinarians, animal technicians gather and record information regarding cases, prepare animal patients for examination, and ready instruments and equipment for use. In addition, technicians collect various specimens; perform standardized laboratory tests; and assist veterinarians in diagnostic, medical, and surgical procedures by preparing medications and applying dressings.

Animal technicians work primarily in veterinary clinics and animal research laboratories. However, these technicians are also employed by drug and feed manufacturers; breeders of laboratory animals; zoos; meat packing companies; medical, dental, and veterinary schools; hospitals; and the public health agencies of city, State, and Federal governments. Technicians employed in situations other than veterinary practice work under the supervision of a scientist or senior technologist and, in addition to the duties previously mentioned, may feed and care for animals and inspect product carcasses. For the most part, animal technicians work regular hours in pleasant surroundings and under favorable working conditions. However, it is important to note that animal technicians risk being physically injured by certain animals and are exposed to animal diseases which may be communicable.

### Job Requirements

Most animal technicians complete a 2-year program leading to an associate's degree from a community college offering a training program accredited by the American Veterinary Medical Association. Typically, the training programs cover 2 academic years of college level study and require completion of general courses in biology, chemistry, communications, mathematics, economics, and business management, as well as specific courses covering such subjects as physiology, nutrition, microbiology, parasitology, animal care, laboratory procedures, clinical techniques, radiology, toxicology, ethics, and client relations. Practical experience with live animals and field experience under actual working conditions are important parts of most programs.

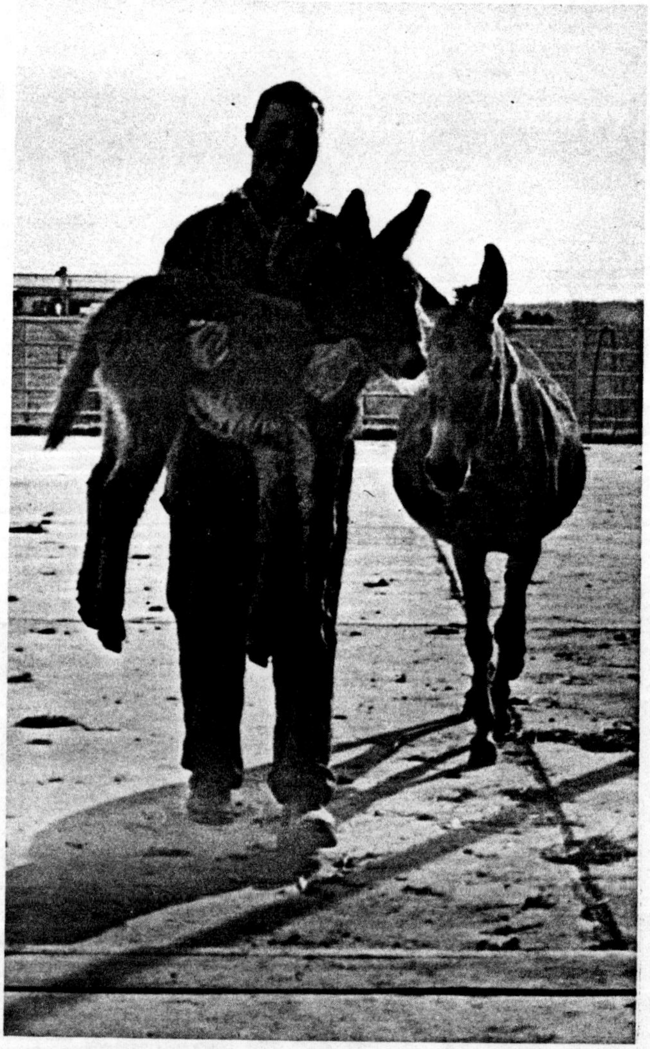

A high school diploma or equivalency certificate evaluated on an individual basis is required by most community colleges offering an associate degree in animal technology. Also considered in the selection of candidates are aptitudes, interests, and the ability to profit from the courses offered. Generally, a strong background in high school science courses, mathematics, and English is most useful to college candidates. In some cases, individuals without formal educational credentials enter this field through on-the-job training in the basic levels of animal care. However, they have considerably less opportunity to attain supervisory or advanced positions and are encouraged to engage in continuing education in this field.

A number of States have recently established certification programs for animal technicians, and several more probably will do so in coming years. Programs vary from State to State, with some established by veterinary medical examining boards and others by State veterinary medical associations. Some require formal education in an accredited program, while others accept on-the-job training. Some issue licenses to those who meet requirements, while others issue certificates or simply register qualified technicians.

One of the professional groups which provides certification in this field is the Animal Technicians Certification Board sponsored by the American Association for Laboratory Animal Science. The board provides examinations and a registry for technicians who are eligible and employed in laboratory animal facilities. The following certification titles used by this organization are based on levels of competency and are not job classifications.

- Assistant Laboratory Animal Technician. This is a first-level position and involves the basic care of animals. Candidates for this classification examination must have 1 full year of work experience and have successfully completed an approved course for assistant technician.
- Laboratory Animal Technician. This is the second level of certification and requires 3 years of employment in laboratory animal technology. Graduation from a 2-year laboratory animal technology school may be substituted for 2 years of experience.
- Laboratory Animal Technologist. This is the third level of competency, and requires 6 years of experience. Credit is allowed when the candidate has completed biological and laboratory animal courses. This worker is qualified to perform high-level tasks, such as training subordinates and assisting with research experiments.

## Opportunities

Employment opportunities for animal technicians appear to be good as veterinarians continue to recognize more ways to use qualified technical assistants. The survey of accredited animal technician training programs conducted by the American Veterinary Medical Association (AVMA) revealed that graduates of these programs have excellent job prospects. Continued prosperity is expected to bring more pets into homes, while the need for protection may increase the number of watchdogs used in homes and businesses. In rural areas, the need for animal technicians is expected to increase along with the population as more animals are bred for use as food. The increasing number of animals used for riding and racing also will require medical care and treatment. There are approximately 30,000 veterinarians in this country actively engaged in some form of professional activity. The AVMA estimates that approximately one animal technical is needed for each veterinarian.

Experience and continuing education are necessary to advance in this field. For technicians or assistants who begin with on-the-job training, completing a formal degree program should enhance advancement. In some laboratories employing a number of technicians, advancement to positions with considerable supervisory responsibility is possible for qualified individuals.

---

For further information, contact:
American Association for Laboratory Animal Science
American Veterinary Medical Association

# II.

## Veterinarian

The care of farm animals and pets is a practice as old as civilization itself. In the past, people lived in close association with animals and soon realized that, like human beings, they were subject to many ills, making them unfit for food, work, or companionship. Practical experience taught people that animals could transmit disease to humans. In older civilizations, the same "medicine man" treated both animals and human beings.

Today, veterinarians have the responsibility for animal health care, and are key figures in general disease prevention programs.

Veterinarians are important to farmers, pet owners, and other animal owners. Untreated bovine disease can ruin a diary farmer, and the loss of a beloved pet can be a very traumatic experience to its owner. But veterinary medicine is just as important to people who don't own animals. When they buy milk, meat, poultry, and eggs, consumers benefit from the veterinarian's services—from efforts to keep food-producing animals in good health and from inspection of foods of animal origin.

Humans also benefit from veterinarians' work in controlling animal diseases which spread to human beings. Rabies, brucellosis, and the form of food poisoning known as salmonellosis are among these diseases.

A majority of veterinarians—an estimated 76 percent—go into private practice. Veterinarians in private practice strive to prevent disease and other health problems by examining their animal patients, immunizing them against diseases, and advising owners on ways to keep pets and livestock healthy. The practitioners diagnose and treat animal patients and frequently require the use of laboratory tests, X-rays, and specialized equipment. Treatment involves a number of procedures such as administering emergency lifesaving measures, prescribing medication, setting fractures, performing surgery, or advising patients' owners on feeding and care. Rural veterinarians generally practice with cows, horses, swine, or poultry. Veterinarians living in cities or large towns usually treat only household pets but may also care for farm animals. A small number of veterinarians specialize in zoo and circus animals or in animals that are raised commercially for their fur.

Veterinarians who begin private practice in a farming area must count on investing several thousand dollars in drugs, instruments, and an automobile, in order to provide needed treatment and reach patients.

Rural veterinarians who develop large practices sometimes build clinics or hospitals where animals can be brought for treatment and surgery, but many practice from offices and travel to their patients. They make use of many modern methods of communication and transportation. It is not at all unusual for rural veterinarians to keep in touch with the office by radiotelephone or to fly a plane.

In addition to working with animal patients, rural veterinarians also teach farmers and their families about diseases that farm animals can transmit to people and show them how to protect themselves. Brucellosis, for example, may attack a farmer who is not careful in handling infected cattle; and ringworm in cattle, horses, or smaller pets may spread to the entire family if strict precautions aren't taken.

Rural veterinarians frequently combine private practice with part-time work for Federal, State, or local government. This public service may be concerned with control and eradication of animal diseases or it may involve the inspection of foods of animal origin, such as meat and poultry.

Veterinarians in private practice in cities usually work only with household pets, although they too may do some work for local health departments. City veterinarians usually have a fully equipped animal hospital for their patients—a fact which makes this an expensive specialty for the beginner. Anyone planning to go into such practice should study the community very carefully before making the investment. Often it is better to associate with an established practitioner, as an assistant or junior partner.

Veterinarians fit easily into the public health field, having been trained to consider diseases as they affect animals in groups. Prevention rather than treatment is stressed—and prevention is the keystone of public health.

Many veterinarians work directly in the public health field—for the Federal Government, State, or local agencies, and international groups. For example, the Agricultural Research Service of the U.S. Department of Agriculture has a full-time staff of veterinarians to inspect meat in packing plants and to work throughout the country on the control and eradication of animal diseases. Other veterinarians in this Department super-

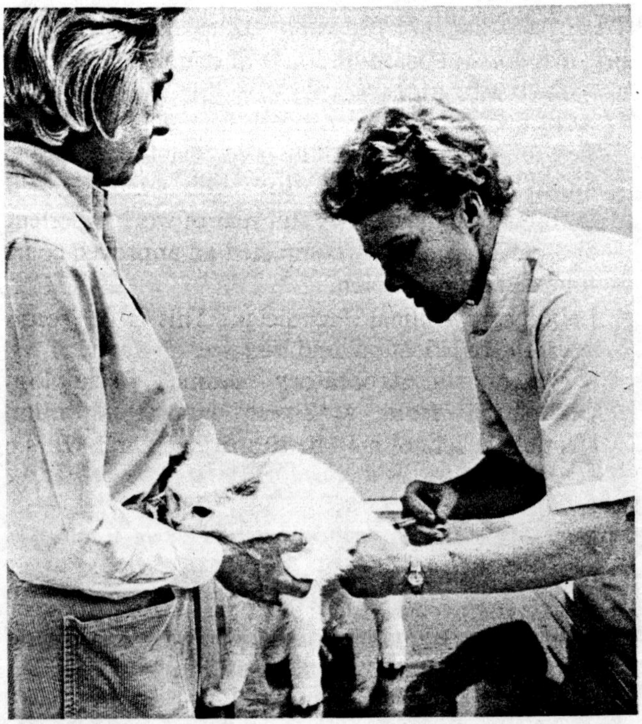

vise stockyards, inspect poultry, and enforce the quarantine regulations, and other laws affecting the import and export of animals and animal products. They also do research work and supervise the licensing of firms manufacturing serums and vaccines for animals. The U.S. Food and Drug Administration also employs veterinarians to help protect consumers of animal food products by assuring the safety and quality of drugs used to treat animals.

A veterinary public health section has been organized in the U.S. Public Health Service. Individuals working in this section develop programs for controlling animal diseases that affect public health, help the States establish veterinary public health programs, and serve as consultants in other Public Health Service activities. Other functions of veterinarians within the Public Health Service are to collect and evaluate statistical data on human illnesses caused by animals, to study the effects of air pollution on animals, and to conduct basic research on chronic and communicable diseases.

Veterinarians employed by State and local health departments cooperate with private practitioners and Federal field workers to control disease among animals and also to protect human health. Some counties and many cities employ veterinarians to see that meats and dairy products are wholesome and that they are sold in clean surroundings. In other instances, veterinarians supervise the production of biologicals—serums, antitoxins—used in the prevention and treatment of disease in human beings.

Internationally, veterinarians are on the central and regional staffs of the World Health Organization and the Food and Agriculture Organization of the United Nations. During the years following World War II, veterinarians worked with the United Nations Relief and Rehabilitation Administration to help war-torn countries build up their supply of food animals. Today they work with the U.S. Foreign Operations Administration to provide economic and technical aid to underdeveloped countries.

Veterinarians interested in a public health career need special training in addition to education in veterinary medicine. It is recommended that after a year or two of practical experience individuals enroll for a program of postgraduate study in an accredited school of public health. Specialized courses will help in understanding how comprehensive health programs are developed and how veterinary medicine can contribute to such programs. This postgraduate work leads to a master's degree—usually Master of Public Health.

Today a new responsibility for veterinarians is membership on the radiological health team in various health administrations. Training courses in radiology and its health aspects are now given to all veterinary officers of the U.S. Armed Forces and also to veterinarians who work in State and local health departments. Veterinarians are likewise playing an important role in civil defense programs—studying how to protect both man and animals against atomic, biological, and chemical warfare.

Progress in veterinary medicine has been greatly influenced by the veterinary activities of the U.S. armed forces. Today commissioned officers of the veterinary corps of the Army and the Air Force work to protect our military personnel stationed in all parts of the world. During World Wars I and II and the Korean and Vietnam conflicts, they were largely responsible for the low incidence of food poisoning and food-borne disease among our troops.

As members of the medical department, veterinary officers cooperate with colleagues—physicians, dentists, nurses, or other specialists—on problems affecting the health of the Armed Forces, in training and in the field, at home and abroad. Veterinary officers have an obligation to protect the Government's pocketbook by rejecting substandard food products and by developing effective ways of preparing, producing, and serving foods. Often these officers, as members of the medical team, work on newly recognized diseases of animals and man and provide medical care to animals used for guard duty and other purposes.

Some veterinarians go into teaching in schools of veterinary medicine, public health, or medicine. Others are employed by firms which produce or sell biological and pharmaceutical products for animal and human use. In industrial fields, veterinarians are employed on a consultant basis.

Whether entering private practice or taking salaried posts, veterinarians are entering a profession with high standards of service.

Veterinarians in private practice usually set their own appointment hours, although emergency services and heavy caseloads may cause irregular work hours. Those working in large animal or mixed animal practices frequently work outdoors, often under difficult weather conditions, and veterinarians always risk injury or exposure to transmittable disease.

## Job Requirements

Anyone planning to become a veterinarian should count on a minimum of 6 years of schooling after graduation from high school. Candidates must complete 2 or 3 years of preveterinary college courses which include basic language arts, social sciences, humanities, mathematics, and biological and physical sciences prior to entry into a college of veterinary medicine. Candidates then enter an approved college of veterinary medicine, which gives a 4-year course leading to the degree of Doctor of Veterinary Medicine (DVM).

Although only 2 or 3 years of college are required, it is best to have a full 4 years of college work, with a bachelor's degree. The extra years give the student a broader cultural background—and mean that the student has more to offer the profession and the community to be served. Also, competition is keen for entry to schools of veterinary medicine; other things being equal, the college graduate has a better chance of acceptance.

Before entering college, prospective veterinary students should write to veterinary schools and ask about entrance requirements. Since these vary from school to school, it is necessary to have this information before planning college studies. Usually, emphasis is placed on inorganic and organic chemistry, biochemistry, zoology, botany, physics, English composition, and speech.

There are 21 accredited colleges of veterinary medicine in the United States and Canada offering a 4-year professional program leading to a Doctor of Veterinary Medicine degree (DVM). During the first phase, preclinical sciences including anatomy, physiology, pathology, pharmacology, and microbiology are emphasized. Most of the students' time is spent in classroom and laboratory study. The second phase of professional study is largely clinical. During much of this time, students work with animal patients and deal with owners who use the school's clinical services. In some areas of the country, States which do not have veterinary schools of their own cooperate on a regional basis with schools in other States. This helps to equalize opportunities for studying veterinary medicine. Chances of admission in times of crowding are best for students with high scholastic averages. The Council on Education of the American Veterinary Medical Association is the accrediting agency for programs in veterinary medical education.

A license is required for the practice of veterinary medicine in all States and the District of Columbia. To obtain a license, an applicant must be a graduate of an accredited veterinary school and pass a State board examination. A number of State veterinary medical associations have established academies of veterinary practice to encourage and improve continuing education, and the licensing boards of several States have legislated continuing education requirements for relicensure. Veterinarians are not required to complete an internship before going into practice. Even so, many internship and residency programs do exist, and increasing numbers of veterinarians are taking advantage of them. A number of nonpractice positions in government do not require a license, although many veterinarians taking these jobs do have licenses. Licenses granted by one State are not necessarily recognized in others. Therefore, veterinarians must check local rulings before starting practice in another State.

## Opportunities

The employment outlook for veterinarians is favorable, and studies by governmental groups and the National Academy of Sciences have concluded that the demand for veterinary medical services is expected to exceed the supply over the next several years. Unfortunately, there are not enough facilities or teachers available to provide the necessary education; however, all existing colleges of veterinary medicine have recently expanded their teaching programs, and several States are developing plans for establishing new medical schools.

Many opportunities for continuing professional and advanced formal education are available to veterinarians who wish to take advantage of them. Advancement in salaried fields of endeavor such as teaching, research, regulatory work, public health, and military service is particularly enhanced by additional academic work.

---

For further information, contact:
American Veterinary Medical Association

# HOW TO TAKE A TEST

You have studied hard, long, and conscientiously.

With your official admission card in hand, and your heart pounding, you have been admitted to the examination room.

You note that there are several hundred other applicants in the examination room waiting to take the same test.

They all appear to be equally well prepared.

You know that nothing but your best effort will suffice. The "moment of truth" is at hand: you now have to demonstrate objectively, in writing, your knowledge of content and your understanding of subject matter.

You are fighting the most important battle of your life -- to pass and/or score high on an examination which will determine your career and provide the economic basis for your livelihood.

What extra, special things should you know and should you do in taking the examination?

## BEFORE THE TEST

### YOUR PHYSICAL CONDITION IS IMPORTANT

If you are not well, you can't do your best work on tests. If you are half asleep, you can't do your best either. Here are some tips:

1. Get about the same amount of sleep you usually get. Don't stay up all night before the test, either partying or worrying -- DON'T DO IT.
2. If you wear glasses, be sure to wear them when you go to take the test. This goes for hearing aids, too.
3. If you have any physical problems that may keep you from doing your best, be sure to tell the person giving the test. If you are sick or in poor health, you really cannot do your best on any test. You can always come back and take the test some other time.

## AT THE TEST

### EXAMINATION TECHNIQUES

1. Read the *general* instructions carefully. These are usually printed on the first page of the examination booklet. As a rule, these instructions refer to the timing of the examination; the fact that you should not start work until the signal and must stop work at a signal, etc. If there are any *special* instructions, such as a choice of questions to be answered, make sure that you note this instruction carefully.

2. When you are ready to start work on the examination, that is as soon as the signal has been given, read the instructions to each question booklet, underline any key words or phrases, such as *least, best, outline, describe,* and the like. In this way you will tend to answer as requested rather than discover on reviewing your paper that you *listed without describing,* that you selected the *worst* choice rather than the *best* choice, etc.

3. If the examination is of the objective or so-called multiple-choice type, that is, each question will also give a series of possible answers: A,B,C, or D, and you are called upon to select the best answer and write the letter next to that answer on your answer paper, it is advisable to start answering each question in turn. There may be anywhere from 50 to 100 such questions in the three or four hours allotted and you can see how much time would be taken if you read through all the questions before beginning to answer any. Furthermore, if you come across a question or a group of questions which you know would be difficult to answer, it would undoubtedly affect your handling of all the other questions.

4. If the examination is of the essay-type and contains but a few questions, it is a moot point as to whether you should read all the questions before starting to answer any one. Of course if you are given a choice, say five out of seven and the like, then it is essential to read all the questions so you can eliminate the two which are most difficult. If, however, you are asked to answer all the questions, there may be danger in trying to answer the easiest one first because you may find that you will spend too much time on it. The best technique is to answer the first question, then proceed to the second, etc.

5. Time your answers. Before the examination begins, write down the time it started, then add the time allowed for the examination and write down the time it must be completed, then divide the time available somewhat as follows:
   a. If 3 1/2 hours are allowed, that would be 210 minutes. If you have 80 objective-type questions, that would be an average of about 2 1/2 minutes per question. Allow yourself no more than 2 minutes per question, or a total of 160 minutes, which will permit about 50 minutes to review.
   b. If for the time allotment of 210 minutes, there are 7 essay questions to answer, that would average about 30 minutes a question. Give yourself only 25 minutes per question so that you have about 35 minutes to review.

6. The most important instruction is *to read each question* and make sure you know what is wanted. The second most important instruction is to *time yourself properly* so that you answer every question. The third most important instruction is to *answer every question.* Guess if you have to but include something for each question. Remember that you will receive no credit for a blank and will probably receive some credit if you write something in answer to an essay question. If you guess a letter, say "B" for a multiple-choice question, you may have guessed right. If you leave a blank as the answer to a multiple-choice question, the examiners may respect your feelings but it will not add a point to your score.
7. Suggestions
   a. Objective-Type Questions
      (1) Examine the question booklet for proper sequence of pages and questions.
      (2) Read all instructions carefully.
      (3) Skip any question which seems too difficult; return to it after all other questions have been answered.
      (4) Apportion your time properly; do not spend too much time on any single question or group of questions.
      (5) Note and underline key words -- *all, most, fewest, least, best, worst, same, opposite.*
      (6) Pay particular attention to negatives.
      (7) Note unusual option, e.g., unduly long, short, complex, different or similar in content to the body of the question.
      (8) Observe the use of "hedging" words - *probably, may, most likely, etc.*
      (9) Make sure that your answer is put next to the same number as the question.
      10) Do not second guess unless you have good reason to believe the second answer is definitely more correct.
      (11) Cross out original answer if you decide another answer is more accurate; do not erase.
      (12) Answer all questions; guess unless instructed otherwise.
      (13) Leave time for review.

   b. Essay-Type Questions
      (1) Read each question carefully.
      (2) Determine exactly what is wanted. Underline key words or phrases.
      (3) Decide on outline or paragraph answer.
      (4) Include many different points and elements unless asked to develop any one or two points or elements.
      (5) Show impartiality by giving pros and cons unless directed to select one side only.
      (6) Make and write down any assumptions you find necessary to answer the question.
      (7) Watch your English, grammar, punctuation, choice of words.
      (8) Time your answers; don't crowd material.

8. Answering the Essay Question

Most essay questions can be answered by framing the specific response around several key words or ideas. Here are a few such key words or ideas:

M's: manpower, materials, methods, money, management

P's: purpose, program, policy, plan, procedure, practice, problems, pitfalls, personnel, public relations

a. Six basic steps in handling problems:

(1) preliminary plan and background development
(2) collect information, data and facts
(3) analyze and interpret information, data and facts
(4) analyze and develop solutions as well as make recommendations
(5) prepare report and sell recommendations
(6) install recommendations and follow up effectiveness

b. Pitfalls to Avoid

(1 *Taking things for granted*

A statement of the situation does not necessarily imply that each of the elements is necessarily true; for example, a complaint may be invalid and biased so that all that can be taken for granted is that a complaint has been registered.

(2) *Considering only one side of a situation*

Wherever possible, indicate several alternatives and then point out the reasons you selected the best one.

(3) *Failing to indicate follow up*

Whenever your answer indicates action on your part, make certain that you will take proper follow-up action to see how successful your recommendations, procedures, or actions turn out to be.

(4) *Taking too long in answering any single question*

Remember to time your answers properly.

# EXAMINATION SECTION

# EXAMINATION SECTION

# TEST 1

DIRECTIONS:
Each question or incomplete statement is followed by several suggested answers or completions. Select the one that *BEST* answers the question or completes the statement. *PRINT THE LETTER OF THE CORRECT ANSWER IN THE SPACE AT THE RIGHT.*

1. The location of the bifurcation of the trachea on a lateral radiograph is to be found  1. ...
   A. in the 5th rib space
   B. in the 3rd rib space
   C. just above the hyoid lymph nodes
   D. in the intermediate zone of the lung
   E. in a descending angle of $15^{o}$ to $30^{o}$
2. 90% of the flexor of the equine carpus occurs between the following joints. The  2. ...
   A. radio carpal
   B. carpo-metacarpal
   C. radio-carpal and the intercarpal
   D. intercarpal and the carpo-metacarpal
   E. radio-carpal and the metacarpal
3. The annular recess of the vagina of the mare around the terminal portion of the uterus is called the  3. ...
   A. external osteum of the cervix
   B. cervix
   C. fornix vaginae
   D. cervical canal
   E. canal of Fontana
4. An incision in the left paralumbar fossa of a cow reveals the  4. ...
   A. supraomental recess with intestines
   B. caudal blind sac or rumen
   C. caudal flexure of the duodenum
   D. flexor carpi ulnaris
   E. quadriceps femoris
5. The opening of the nasolacrimal duct in the horse is located in the  5. ...
   A. dorsal meatus
   B. middle meatus
   C. ventral nasal cavity at the mucocutaneous junction
   D. pharynx
   E. depressor labii inferioris
6. Bovine chronic fat necrosis is caused by pancreatic  6. ...
   A. necrosis
   B. stones
   C. duct inflammation
   D. anomaly
   E. None of the above
7. The microscopic lesion of infectious canine hepatitis is caused by  7. ...

A. an increase of kumpfer cells and cytoplasmic inclusions
B. vacuolization of the liver cells
C. extramedullary hemopoeisis in the liver
D. focal liver-cell necrosis with intranuclear inclusions
E. bile duct proliferation

8. In bovine clinical listeriosis, micro-abscesses are found in the 8. ..
A. brain
B. kidney
C. subcutaneous tissues
D. spleen
E. mammary glands

9. A definitive diagnosis of equine encephalomyelitis can be made by 9. ..
A. a perivascular cuffing of the brain cells
B. making micro-abcesses in the brain
C. a finding of cerebral meningitis
D. viral isolation
E. evidence of a decrease in the white blood count

10. In cystic degeneration of the ovaries in cattle, the fluids are found to contain 10. ..
A. glycoprotein, but no estrogen
B. estrogen
C. estrogen, but no glycoprotein
D. less estrogen than normal
E. more estrogen than normal

11. The type of incluse or body in IPV resembles that in 11. ..
A. fowlpox
B. herpes simplex
C. nobius
D. distemper
E. trophic disturbance

12. Congenital cystic kidneys may be observed in 12. ..
A. cattle
B. cats
C. pigs
D. horses
E. dogs

13. A thick-walled abscess in the udder of a cow is caused by 13. ..
A. corynbacterium pyogenes
B. spherophorus necrophorus
C. a streptococcus
D. cutaneous nevus
E. habronema

14. The presence of bacteria in the bloodstream *prior* to the induction of clinical disease is referred to as 14. ..
A. bacteremia
B. pyemis
C. empyemis
D. septicemia
E. endobacteremia

15. A feminizing condition of the dog is caused by a testicular lesion known as 15. ..
A. interstitial cell tumor
B. embryonal carcinoma
C. teratoma
D. sertoli cell tumor
E. seminoma

16. The *MOST* common lesion associated with diabetes mellitus in the dog is 16. ...
   A. amyloidosis
   B. pancreatic atrophy
   C. chronic pancreatis
   D. acute pancreatis
   E. interstitial pancreatis

17. The *LOWEST* serum Ca level is illustrated by 17. ...
   A. nutritional secondary hyperparathyroidism
   B. renal secondary hyperparathyroidism
   C. post-parturient paresis
   D. bilateral parathyroidectomy
   E. post-surgical hypoparathyroidism

18. Compared to the blood plasma, the glomerular filtrate in the proximal convoluted tubule is 18. ...
   A. hypotonic
   B. hypertonic
   C. isotonic
   D. higher in glucose
   E. higher in protein

19. A normal dog has a high BUN because 19. ...
   A. it is readily excited
   B. of its high protein intake
   C. of its excess of fat intake
   D. of its hair ball
   E. of its excess of carbohydrate intake

20. Control of intestinal digestive secretions lies in the 20. ...
   A. vagus
   B. stimulation of mucosa
   C. hormones
   D. absorption of fats
   E. general metabolism or absorption of food

21. Bollinger bodies may be seen in 21. ...
   A. fowlpox
   B. pseudorabies
   C. bluetongue
   D. rinderpest
   E. dirofilaria

22. Osteosarcomas are *MOST* common in ________ animals. 22. ...
   A. canine
   B. bovine
   C. ovine
   D. porcine
   E. equine

23. Fibrous tissue is produced when 23. ...
   A. endothelial cells proliferate and produce fibrous network
   B. collagen is synthesized by fibroblasts
   C. thrombin converts collagen at the chronic infection site
   D. a blood clot hardens on exposure to air
   E. a blood clot softens on exposure to air

24. A period of time that produces an increased number of normal cells is termed 24. ...
   A. anaplasia
   B. neoplasia
   C. hyperplasia
   D. hypoplasia
   E. metaplasia

25. The percentage of feed absorbed is classified as the 25. ...
   A. BMR
   B. N-free extract ration
   C. substrate percentage
   D. respiratory quotient
   E. digestibility coefficient
26. A neoplasm that has three types of primary germ layers (ectoderm, mesoderm, and endoderm) is called 26. ...
   A. teratoma
   B. terabdella
   C. teratology
   D. terbium
   E. terebinth
27. $H_2O$ secreted by the alimentary tract is 27. ...
   A. lost and of no significance
   B. absorbed by waste products
   C. not reabsorbed
   D. conserved
   E. None of the above
28. Seepage of fluid into interstitial tissue, associated with inflammation and swelling, is caused by 28. ...
   A. histamine
   B. lactampoule
   C. lactein
   D. histidin
   E. histozyme
29. Chicken grit which yields higher digestibility is located in the 29. ...
   A. ventriculus
   B. crop
   C. gizzard
   D. proventriculus
   E. ventromyel
30. The hormone which controls pancreatic secretion is 30. ...
   A. enterokinin
   B. gastrin
   C. secretin
   D. pancreozymin
   E. eukinase
31. Secretin is produced in the duodenum, absorbed, and acts on the pancreas; therefore, it can be classified as a (n) 31. ...
   A. exocrine
   B. endocrine
   C. hormone
   D. pancreatin
   E. diamide
32. In a dog, the glomerular filtrate is alkaline; how, then, does the urine become acidic? 32. ...
   A. K+ exchanges with H+
   B. Due to action by bladder bacteria
   C. Na+ exchange with H+
   D. Due to action by Bacteria apii (Brizi)
   E. Caused by Bacteria eta (Dyar)
33. An intestinal hormone 33. ...
   A. is not a true hormone
   B. does not come from the endocrine gland
   C. derives from intestinal mucosa
   D. appears along with the digestive juices
   E. controls the rate of secretion of the digestive juices

34. A double external os to the cervix uteri in a cow is due to lack of fusion of the 34. ...
   A. metanephric
   B. mesanephric
   C. müellerian
   D. urogenital sinus
   E. ducts of Gartner

35. Persistent dribbling of urine in a one-week-old foal is *most likely* due to a patent 35. ...
   A. metanephric duct
   B. mesonephric duct
   C. urachus
   D. urogenital
   E. allantois

36. If a small probe can be passed throught the ductus arteriosus in a two-week-old calf, the *most likely* explanation is: 36. ...
   A. Failure of the smooth muscle in the tunica media to contract fully
   B. Incomplete development of internal connective tissue
   C. Pulmonary hypertension
   D. Development of an abcess
   E. Clinically patent ductus arteriosus

37. The foramen ovale is an opening through the 37. ...
   A. septum, primary and secondary
   B. interventricular septum
   C. endocardial cushion on the right A-V valve
   D. septum obturator in atria
   E. septum intermusculare

38. $CO_2$ in the blood is carried *mainly* as 38. ...
   A. carbamyl groups
   B. dissolved $CO_2$
   C. bicarbonate ions
   D. carboxyhemoglobin
   E. carbonic acid

39. One component of the blood is always at a constant level and from it blood determination can be made at any time; it is 39. ...
   A. glucose
   B. calcium
   C. fat
   D. alcohol
   E. amino acid (protein)

40. The bulbar surface of the 3rd eyelid of the *dog* contains a tissue type which is often inflamed and swollen; it is __________ tissue. 40. ...
   A. epithelial
   B. lymphoid
   C. glandular
   D. lepidic
   E. muccid

41. A functional Beta cell tumor in the dog would be *most likely* to result in 41. ...
   A. diabetic coma
   B. diabetes insipitus
   C. Cushing's disease
   D. hypoglycemic seizures
   E. glucosuria

42. The epithelium lining the trachea is *BEST* described as 42. ....
  A. stratified squamous
  B. stratified columnar
  C. pseudostratified ciliated columnar
  D. simple cuboidal
  E. simple squamous

43. The circulating blood cell that *most closely* approaches the macrophage in function is the 43. ....
  A. lymphocyte
  B. neutrophil
  C. eosinophil
  D. basophil
  E. monocyte

44. The reason a dog's eyes shine at night when a light is shown on them is because of the tapetum lucidum. This is a component of the 44. ....
  A. iris
  B. lens
  C. retina
  D. choroid
  E. sclera

45. A bitch or mare should be attended during parturition to prevent suffocation of the newborn in the fetal membranes because 45. ....
  A. they have epithelial chorial placentation
  B. they do not have discoid placentas
  C. the amnion is not connected to the chorion
  D. the ammion is connected to the chorion
  E. the neonate is exceptionally weak

46. During exercise, motor impulses from higher brain centers when passing to skeletal muscles increase respiration and cardiac output by 46. ....
  A. increasing vagal tone
  B. stimulating respiratory centers and inhibiting cardio-inhibitory centers.
  C. stimulating the brain-ridge reflex
  D. increasing lactic acid release to the brain stem
  E. increasing $O_2$ utilization of the medulla

47. If the dorsal roots of the spinal nerves to the hind leg are cut and then the peripheral ends are stimulated, there is 47. ....
  A. no result
  B. movement
  C. pain
  D. motor and secretory activity
  E. danger of tetany

48. The term recruitment as applied to skeletal muscle refers to an increase in the 48. ....
  A. number of ATP molecules available to the muscle fibers
  B. motor unit threshold stimulation
  C. number of motor units activated
  D. refractory period of the motor neuron
  E. frequency of each active motor unit disc

49. Acetylcholine does not mediate the impulses at the 49. ....
  A. sympathetic postganglion nerve endings
  B. parasympathetic postganglion nerve endings
  C. autonomic ganglion
  D. secretory fiber at the exocrine and endocrine glands
  E. motor nerve endings at the skeletal muscle

50\. Mucous is secreted by the renal pelvis and the proximal uretus in *which* species? The 50. ...

A. pig
B. horse
C. dog
D. ruminant
E. cat

---

# KEY (CORRECT ANSWERS)

| | | | | |
|---|---|---|---|---|
| 1. B | 11. B | 21. A | 31. C | 41. D |
| 2. A | 12. C | 22. A | 32. C | 42. C |
| 3. C | 13. A | 23. B | 33. C | 43. E |
| 4. B | 14. A | 24. C | 34. C | 44. D |
| 5. C | 15. D | 25. E | 35. C | 45. C |
| 6. E | 16. D | 26. A | 36. A | 46. B |
| 7. D | 17. D | 27. D | 37. D | 47. A |
| 8. A | 18. C | 28. A | 38. C | 48. C |
| 9. D | 19. B | 29. A | 39. E | 49. A |
| 10. D | 20. B | 30. C | 40. B | 50. B |

---

# TEST 2

DIRECTIONS:
Each question or incomplete statement is followed by several suggested answers or completions. Select the one that BEST answers the question or completes the statement. *PRINT THE LETTER OF THE CORRECT ANSWER IN THE SPACE AT THE RIGHT.*

1. Salt poisoning shows as a microscopic lesion in 1. ...
   A. eosinophilic meningitis
   B. fatty necrosis of the liver
   C. micro-abcesses of the lymph nodes
   D. swelling of the Kupfer cells with intracytoplasmic inclusions
   E. all of the above
2. Vacuolation of neuronal cytoplasm is characteristic of 2. ...
   A. distemper
   B. listeriosis
   C. dropsy
   D. lead intoxication
   E. rabies
3. Polioencephalomalacia, a disturbance of thiamine metabolism, is found in *which* of the following groupings? 3. ...
   A. cow, horse, goat
   B. cow, swine, horse
   C. monkey, dog, swine
   D. cow, horse, dog
   E. sheep, pig, goat
4. A budding yeast-like fungus is 4. ...
   A. actinomycosis
   B. coccidiodomycosis
   C. cryptococcosis
   D. blastomycosis
   E. meloidiasis
5. *Which* of the following conditions is *most likely* to result in embolic pneumonia? 5. ...
   A. Inhalant of mineral oil
   B. Pulmonary neoplasm
   C. Septic mastitis
   D. Stricture of the esophogus
   E. Blennenteritis
6. *How* does digested fat *alter* the fatty deposits in bovine species (saturated or unsaturated)? 6. ...
   A. Marked alterations - absorbed fatty acids are unchanged by ruminal flora or metabolism
   B. Relatively insensitive - saturated fatty acids are oxidized by rumen flora
   C. Relatively insensitive - unsaturated fatty acids are hydrogenated by rumen flora
   D. Relatively insensitive - saturated fatty acids are oxidized by metabolism
   E. Relatively insensitive - unsaturated fatty acids are hydrogenated by metabolism
7. The EKG wave exemplifying repolarization of the cardiac muscle is: 7. ...

A. Q
B. R
C. S
D. T
E. P

8. Blood pressure is *primarily* controlled via the  8. ...
   A. arterioles
   B. venous return
   C. capillaries
   D. heart rate
   E. pulse beat

9. Starling's law explains:  9. ...
   A. Increase in blood pressure with vaso-constriction
   B. Slowing with vagal increase
   C. Acceleration with sympathetic increase
   D. Increase in heart rate with epinephrine
   E. Increase in CO with exercise

10. An accumulation of epitheloid cells in the intestinal submucosa of cattle is seen in *which* of the following diseases?  10. ...
   A. BUD
   B. Winter dysentery
   C. Johne's disease (enteritis chronica pseudotuberculosa bovis)
   D. Colibacillosis
   E. Salmonillosis

11. Canine black tongue, a reproducible nutritional disease with gastro-intestinal lesions, is caused by a deficiency in the diet of  11. ...
   A. pyridoxine
   B. niacin
   C. pantothenic acid
   D. riboflavin
   E. thiamine

12. The lesions seen in a dog that has died of diabetes mellitus would be:  12. ...
   A. Fatty liver with pancreatic atrophy
   B. Liver degeneration with fatty pancreas
   C. Liver degeneration with normal pancreas
   D. Fatty liver with hydrophic degeneration of the pancreas
   E. Fatty liver with normal pancreas

13. A disease of high mortality in chickens of less than three weeks, marked by prostration, white diarrhea, and death, is  13. ...
   A. salmonella typhumurium
   B. colibacillosis
   C. salmonella pullorum
   D. staphylococcus
   E. salmonella

14. Shortening of the villi (villous atrophy) is characteristic of transmissible gastroenteritis and is *BEST* shown in the  14. ...
   A. duodenum
   B. large intestine
   C. cecum
   D. colon
   E. jejunum and the ileun

15. *Which* phase of the electocardiogram represents the re-polarization phase of the ventricals?  15. ...
   A. QRS complex

B. P wave
C. ST segment
D. P-r interval
E. T wave

16. The *MOST* effective way to treat ventricular fibrillation in the dog is 16. B..
A. intracardiac epinephrine
B. direct electrical impulses
C. cardiac massage
D. sodium bicarbonate injected into the heart
E. indirect electrical impulses

17. Experimental hypertension can be produced by partial occlusion of one renal artery. The proposed mechanisim is: 17. E..
A. Release of erythropoietin from the juxtaglomerular cells
B. Back-up pressure in the aorta
C. Release of adrenal epinephrine
D. Neurologic reflex vasoconstriction
E. Renin release

18. Sinus arrhythmia is caused by 18. A..
A. vagal tone
B. lack of contractibility of a ventricle
C. decreased blood Ca concentration
D. decreased blood K+ concentration
E. increased P-R interval

19. The mechanism of lymph formation is caused by 19. B..
A. the death of cells within the capillaries
B. leakage from the capillaries reabsorbed from interstitial spaces
C. Na+-K+ pump, creating an osmotic gradient
D. lymph node secretion
E. the nascence of cells within the capillaries

20. The cranial rumenal papilla 20. D B..
A. separates the reticulum from the central cranial sac of the rumen
B. separates the reticulum from the cranial sac of the rumen
C. connects the rumen and the reticulum
D. separates the caudal dorsal blind sac from the cranial sac of the rumen
E. connects the reticulum and the cranial sac of the rumen

21. The spleen is visualized on VD radiograph as a triangular mass 21. C..
A. caudal to the right kidney
B. caudal to the left kidney
C. caudal to the fundus of the stomach
D. cranial to the fundus of the stomach
E. cranial to the right kidney

22. The pulse may be taken from the major artery of the digit in the equine metatarsus 22. D A..
A. medial to the long digital extensor
B. medial on the metatarsus
C. lateral in the proximal third of the great metatarsal bone
D. lateral between the suspensory and the deep digital flexors
E. medial between the suspensory and the deep digital flexors

23. The progress of blood from the vena cava to the aorta is: 23. ...
   A. Left atrium-right ventricle-pulmonary artery-pulmonary vein-right atrium-left ventricle
   B. Right atrium-left ventricle-pulmonary artery-pulmonary vein-left atrium-right ventricle
   C. Right atrium-left ventricle-pulmonary vein-pulmonary artery-left atrium-left ventricle
   D. Left atrium-left ventricle-pulmonary artery-pulmonary vein-right atrium-right ventricle
   E. Right atrium-right ventricle-pulmonary artery-pulmonary vein-left atrium-left ventricle

24. The long plantar ligament which is often inflamed in "curb" is associated with the ________ joint. 24. ...
   A. tarsal
   B. stifle
   C. hock
   D. pastern
   E. coffin

25. Incision into the left paralumbar fossa in the cow will penetrate the 25. ...
   A. gravid uterus
   B. duodenum
   C. caudal dorsal blind sac of the rumen
   D. cranial dorsal blind sac of the rumen
   E. uterus acollis

26. The descending colon in the dog may be palpated in the 26. ...
   A. right dorsal abdomen
   B. left dorsal abdomen
   C. left ventral abdomen
   D. ventral midline
   E. right ventral abdomen

27. The brain excretes $NH_3$ as 27. ...
   A. urea
   B. glutamine
   C. glutamate
   D. arginine
   E. alanine

28. To acidify urine, use 28. ...
   A. NaOH
   B. Na Cl
   C. Na proprionate
   D. $CH_3COOH$
   E. $NH_4CL$

29. The reaction of urine in a suckling calf is 29. ...
   A. acid
   B. alkaline
   C. isoelectric
   D. neutral
   E. electric

30. The hormone in water regulation that acts to change the permeability of distal tubule cells is 30. ...
   A. vasopressin
   B. oxytocin
   C. corticotropin
   D. prednisone
   E. cortisone

31. *What is least likely* to change in urine from day to day? 31. ...
   A. $NH_3$
   B. Na
   C. Creatinine
   D. Water
   E. None of the above

32. Glucose is *MOST* necessary in the ________ tissue. 32. ...
   A. skeletal muscle
   B. brain
   C. liver
   D. cardiac muscle
   E. biventer muscle

33. In the bovine, hypomagnesemia will induce tetany when the magnesium drops *below* 33. ...
   A. 1 mg/100 ml
   B. 3 mg/100 ml
   C. 5 mg/100 ml
   D. 10 mg/100 ml
   E. 12 mg/100 ml

34. The cell which produces a substance that forms fibrin is the ________ cell. 34. ...
   A. mast
   B. hepatocyte
   C. fibroblast
   D. lymphocyte
   E. neutrophil

35. The virus that causes myocarditis is: 35. ...
   A. Rinderpest
   B. FMD
   C. Bovine malignant catarrah
   D. Vesicular stomatitis
   E. Unorganized virus

36. A patent foramen ovale is common at necropsy on the 36. ...
   A. foal
   B. calve
   C. pig
   D. kid
   E. lamb

37. Aortic rupture is of *economic* concern in 37. ...
   A. sheep
   B. chickens
   C. turkeys
   D. cattle
   E. dogs

38. On exercise, cardiac output increases as a result of 38. ...
   A. greater heart-rate increase plus stroke-volume increase
   B. greater stroke-volume increase plus heart-rate increase
   C. equal heart-rate increase plus stroke-volume increase
   D. stroke-volume increase *only*
   E. heart-rate increase *only*

39. Continuous heart murmur is indicative of 39. ...
   A. PDA
   B. mitral insufficiency
   C. tricuspid insufficiency
   D. patent foramen oval
   E. patent deep digital flexor

40. SA node action 40. ...
   A. excites the ventricular fibers
   B. initiates heart contractions
   C. excites the atrial fibers
   D. stimulates the AV node
   E. depresses the pterygoideus medialis

41. Active transport in the newborn is effected through 41. ...
   A. pinocytosis
   B. phagocytosis
   C. osmosis, diuresis, diffusion
   D. simple diffusion
   E. differential permeability

42. Mastocytoma in the dog 42. ...
   A. is seen in young dogs *only*
   B. has a predilection for skin, head, and neck
   C. is characterized by metachromatic cytophillic granules
   D. is seen in cocker spaniels *only*
   E. results in mastochondroma

43. Practical laboratory tests most useful in the diagnosis of hypoadrenalcorticism are: 43. ...
   A. BUN, serum Ca, serum P
   B. BUN, serum Na, serum P
   C. BUN, lactic dehydrogenase, alkaline phosphatase
   D. BUN, serum lipase, serum Ca
   E. BUN, serum Ca1 serum P

44. Of the following species, embryonal nephroma is *MOST* common in 44. ...
   A. swine
   B. horses
   C. dogs
   D. cattle
   E. sheep

45. A cow exposed to the IPV virus will produce inclusions *MOST* resembling 45. ...
   A. pox virus
   B. rabies
   C. distemper
   D. herpes simplex
   E. myxoma

46. The *preferred* method of tissue preservation for chemical analysis is 46. ...
   A. freezing
   B. alcohol fixation
   C. drying
   D. formalin fixation
   E. heating

47. A *marked INCREASE* in urine urobilinogen could result from 47. ...
   A. obstructive icterus
   B. hemolytic icterus
   C. toxic icterus
   D. pyelonephritis
   E. hemorrhagic enteritis

48. Sweating occurs whether the skin is hot and flushed or cold and clammy because of 48. ...
   A. sweat stored in the gland
   B. the excitement of sweat centers
   C. a specific sweating hormone
   D. the filtration of sweat from the blood
   E. the filtration of sweat from the abdomen

49. A urine index of intestinal putrefaction is 49. A ...
   A. indican
   B. scalal
   C. mercaptoethanol
   D. urobilinemia
   E. urobilinuria

50. During exercise, motor impulses from the higher brain centers when passing to skeletal muscles increase respiration and cardiac output by 50. B ..
   A. increasing vagal tone
   B. stimulating respiratory centers and inhibiting cardio-inhibitory centers.
   C. arousing the Bainbridge reflex
   D. increasing lactic acid release to the brain stem
   E. increasing oxygen utilization of the medulla

# KEY (CORRECT ANSWERS)

| | | | | | | | | | |
|---|---|---|---|---|---|---|---|---|---|
| 1. | A | 11. | B | 21. | C | 31. | C | 41. | A |
| 2. | C | 12. | A | 22. | D | 32. | B | 42. | C |
| 3. | E | 13. | C | 23. | E | 33. | A | 43. | B |
| 4. | D | 14. | E | 24. | A | 34. | B | 44. | A |
| 5. | C | 15. | E | 25. | C | 35. | B | 45. | D |
| 6. | C | 16. | B | 26. | B | 36. | B | 46. | A |
| 7. | D | 17. | E | 27. | B | 37. | C | 47. | B |
| 8. | A | 18. | A | 28. | E | 38. | E | 48. | B |
| 9. | E | 19. | B | 29. | A | 39. | A | 49. | A |
| 10. | C | 20. | D | 30. | A | 40. | C | 50. | B |

# EXAMINATION SECTION

## TEST 1

DIRECTIONS: Each question or incomplete statement is followed by several suggested answers or completions. Select the one that BEST answers the question or completes the statement. *PRINT THE LETTER OF THE CORRECT ANSWER IN THE SPACE AT THE RIGHT.*

1. The foramen ovale goes through the septum 1.____
   A. primum
   B. spurium
   C. primum *and* the septum secundum
   D. atriorum
   E. pectiniform

2. In the ruminant, ketosis is a clinical syndrome of many diseases. A *true* statement may be: 2.____
   A. It is easily differentiated from a DA by analyzing blood and plasma ketones
   B. Ovine ketosis occurs in the last trimester of pregnancy
   C. Subclinical ketosis is insidious and not important
   D. Ketosis occurs 2-4 weeks post-partum and may be fatal if not treated
   E. Secondary ketosis is easily treated and, therefore, is not important

3. The basal border of the lung in a medium-sized horse extends from 3.____
   A. along the apical and diaphragmatic lobes
   B. the sixth costochrondal cartilage to the dorsal part of the sixteenth rib
   C. the fifth costochrondal cartilage to within five centimeters of the tuber coxa
   D. the olecranon to the intercostal space of the eighteenth rib
   E. the caudal, dorsally in a convex arc

4. In the middle one-third of the neck, the relationship of of the esophagus to the trachea is 4.____
   A. ventral to the trachea
   B. to the right side of the trachea
   C. dorsal-lateral to the right
   D. dorsal-lateral to the left
   E. to the left

5. In a blood smear stained with Wright's stain, a leucocyte having a relatively large dark nucleus with sparse pale blue cytoplasm, would, *most likely*, be a 5.____
   A. basophil B. eosinophil C. heterophil
   D. monocyte E. lymphocyte

6. Hemoglobinuria is a common finding in cattle disease conditions. *WHICH* of the following does NOT have hemoglobinuria? 6.____
   A. Texas Cattle Fever B. anaplasmosis
   C. Raynaud's Disease D. Clostridium hemolyticum
   E. Winckel's Disease

7. The fluid in the hepatic sinusoids is 7. A
   A. blood B. lymph C. chyme D. chyle E. bile

8. Since articular cartilage is avascular, the chondrocytes 8. D
   *must* receive their nutrients from the
   A. metaphysical-epiphysical arteries
   B. vessels in the Haversian canal
   C. vessels in Volkmann's canals
   D. synovial fluid
   E. nutrient artery

9. Birefringent crystals are seen in the kidney tubules, 9. B
   but no inflammatory response is present in
   A. glomerular damage with alkaloid casts
   B. ethylene glycol toxicity with Ca oxalate crystals
   C. overdose of sulfa drug
   D. obstruction with normal urine components precipitated
   E. cystitis

10. Fatty liver may be seen in a dog with 10. D
    A. ICH
    B. distemper
    C. ethylene glycol poisoning
    D. diabetes mellitus
    E. cystalgia

11. In diabetes insipidus, the specific gravity of the 11. A
    urine is
    A. less than 1.005 B. 1.010-1.015
    C. 1.020-1.025 D. 1.030-1.035
    E. greater than 1.050

12. Pyometra in a bitch is likely to be the sequela 12. A
    A. of hormone imbalance, with resultant damage to the endometrium
    B. of infection that came up the tract from a cystitis with crystals
    C. following retained placentation after whelping
    D. of infection that started as a peritonitis and passed down the Fallopian tubes
    E. from copulation

13. *What* condition would be expected following surgical 13. B
    ablation of the cloacal bursa in birds?
    A. Inability to reject grafts
    B. Marked impairment of delayed hypersensitivity
    C. Excessive gamma globulin
    D. Deficiency in plasma cells
    E. Insufficient gamma globulin

14. In a vaginal smear of the bitch in estrum, the diagnostic 14. C
    cell-type is
    A. rbc
    B. leutenizing cell
    C. keratinized epithelial cell
    D. neutrophil
    E. bacteria

15. The esophageal portion of the stomach in the horse 15.____
A. is lined with many glands that secrete pepsin
B. contains many fundic glands
C. contains many cardiac glands
D. contains stratified squamous
E. is composed of glandular epithelium

16. In the metacarpal region of the dog, proximal to the metacarpal pad, is the largest artery of the foreleg. It is superficial and covered only by the skin, fascia, *and* the 16.____
A. superficial digital flexor
B. deep digital flexor
C. interosseous
D. intermaxillary
E. intermesoblastic

17. The species with a functional renal-hepatic system is the 17.____
A. hare
B. cow
C. rat
D. chicken
E. dog

18. In the pig, the cranial vena cava in the region of the thoracic inlet lies 18.____
A. dorsal to the esophagus, trachea, and bicarotid trunk
B. ventral to the trachea with the bicarotid trunk between
C. ventral to the esophagus and bicarotid trunk, and dorsal to the trachea
D. ventral to the trachea and dorsal to the bicarotid trunk
E. midway between the esophagus on the left and the trachea on the right

19. In the ox, the *minimum* number of serous membranes through which a nail must pass from the fundus of the reticulum to the myocardium is 19.____
A. 2
B. 3
C. 4
D. 5
E. 6

20. A part of the chicken's anatomy *not* found in mammals is the 20.____
A. larynx
B. hyoid apparatus
C. metanephric kidney
D. nasopharynx
E. syrinx

21. The guttural pouch of the horse is a diverticulum of the 21.____
A. inner ear
B. recensus epitympanicus
C. eustachian tube
D. wall of the pharynx
E. larynx

22. The posterior chamber of the eye of the horse is between the 22.____
A. lens and the vitreous
B. lens and the retina
C. iris and the lens
D. cornea and the iris
E. pupil and the retina

23. When incising the skin of the right paralumbar fossa of the cow, if the surgeon is too zealous, he may incise the 23.____
   A. duodenum
   B. dorsal sac of the rumen
   C. gallbladder
   D. spleen
   E. superior occipital fossae

24. All of the following structures go through the inguinal ring EXCEPT the 24.____
   A. genitofemoral nerve
   B. internal pudendal artery
   C. external pudendal artery
   D. testicular artery
   E. ductus deferens

25. The percentage of iron in the hemoglobin molecule is 25.____
   A. .34%  B. .49%  C. .68%  D. .94%  E. 1.23%

26. Intracellular respiration is catalyzed by enzymes found in 26.____
   A. mitochondria
   B. nucleus
   C. ribosomes
   D. endoplasmic reticulum
   E. cytoplasm

27. Glycogenolysis is produced by injecting 27.____
   A. insulin
   B. glucose
   C. ACTH
   D. invert sugar
   E. parasympathomimetic drugs

28. Injection of epinephrin causes 28.____
   A. glycogenolysis
   B. gluconeogenesis
   C. glygenesis
   D. glyconeogenesis
   E. glycolysis

29. Feeding of high levels of protein causes 29.____
   A. glycogenolysis
   B. gluconeogenesis
   C. glycogenesis
   D. glyconeogenesis
   E. glycolysis

30. The *primary* energy source for ruminants is 30.____
   A. acetate
   B. propionate
   C. citrate
   D. glucose
   E. proteins

31. The surface tumor *most readily* transplanted in domestic animals is the 31.____
   A. myeloma
   B. lymphocytoma
   C. papilloma
   D. mastocytoma
   E. venereal tumor

32. *Erysipelothrix insidiosa* causes skin lesions in swine and man, which, although similar, differ in certain respects. A correct characterization of such a lesion, among the following, is: 32.____
   A. A wound infection in a dog
   B. Rhomboid shape in swine
   C. Primarily on the abdomen of man
   D. Primarily on the back of man
   E. Sloughing in man

33. Phylloerythrins are photodynamic substances producing a photosensitizing dermatitis of domestic animals. They are derived from 33.____
   A. xanthophylls  B. porphyrins  C. chlorophylls
   D. phenothiazine  E. hemoglobin

34. Icterus associated with an elevated indirect-reacting serum bilirubin and an increased urinary urobilinogen is probably due to 34.____
   A. biliary obstruction  B. hepatocellular damage
   C. toxic hepatitis  D. hemolytic process
   E. viral hepatitis

35. Glucose absorption in the small intestine takes place by means of 35.____
   A. active transport  B. passive absorption
   C. indirect passage  D. active absorption
   E. osmosis

36. The enterogastrone function 36.____
   A. increases stomach motility
   B. decreases stomach motility
   C. decreases stomach secretion
   D. increases stomach secretion
   E. increases stomach motility *and* decreases stomach secretion

37. The *primary* site of bacterial digestion in the horse is the 37.____
   A. cecum  B. fetlock  C. loin  D. pastern  E. gaskin

38. Rumen protozoa are reduced by a(n) 38.____
   A. increase in fiber  B. decrease in pH
   C. overwhelming quantity of bacteria
   D. decrease in fiber  E. increase in pH

39. Increased gluconeogenesis is *primarily* the effect of 39.____
   A. insulin  B. glucogen  C. thyroxin
   D. ACTH  E. growth hormone

40. Increased thermogenesis is due to 40.____
   A. thyroxin  B. insulin  C. ACTH
   D. thyroprotein  E. thyroidectin

41. The organ of gluconeogenesis is the 41.____
   A. spleen  B. brain  C. liver
   D. heart  E. kidney

42. Rapid change in ventricular pressure is due to the 42.____
   A. affect of atria on the ventricles
   B. conduction through the A-V node to the ventricle
   C. affect of returning venous flow on the ventricle
   D. contractility of the ventricle
   E. distension of the ventricle

43. A horse has been gored in the thorax by a bull in pasture. He has bilateral pneumothorax. He is hypoxic and will die if he cannot meet the demands for 43.____
   A. vital capacity B. inspiratory volume
   C. tidal volume D. residual volume
   E. inspiratory reserve

44. An animal has damaged its lungs. The resultant pulmonary edema can best be assessed by measuring the 44.____
   A. vital capacity B. tidal volume
   C. residual volume D. expiratory reserve
   E. inspiratory reserve

45. The atmospheric p02 at sea level is 45.____
   A. 20 B. 80 C. 95 D. 104 E. 159

46. The fluid in the subarachnoid space communicates with that in the ventricles via the 46.____
   A. foramen magnum B. foramen of Soemmering
   C. foramen of Monro D. mesencephalic aqueduct
   E. central canal of the spinal cord

47. The lung of the chicken differs from that of mammals in that 47.____
   A. there are no layers interposed between the alveoli and the blood
   B. gaseous exchange occurs only at inspiration
   C. air passes through the lung into the air sac where most of the gaseous exchange occurs
   D. gaseous exchange occurs only at expiration
   E. air sacs are present and they increase pulmonary ventilation and tidal volume and facilitate an exchange of gases in the parabronchi in both inspiration and expiration

48. The nerve fibers to the respiratory centers from the lung are 48.____
   A. totally inhibitory to inspiration
   B. totally stimulatory to inspiration
   C. totally inhibitory to expiration
   D. totally stimulatory to expiration
   E. may be both inhibitory or stimulatory to respiration

49. The area most sensitive to $CO_2$ levels in plasma is located in the 49.____
   A. lung B. carotid body
   C. medulla oblongata D. aortic body
   E. cerebellum

50. The amount of oxygen that can combine with one gm. of hemoglobin is ______ ml. 50.____
   A. 1.0 B. 1.36 C. 2.3 D. 5.4 E. 10.3

# KEY (CORRECT ANSWERS)

| | | |
|---|---|---|
| 1. C | 11. A | 21. C |
| 2. B | 12. A | 22. C |
| 3. B | 13. B | 23. A |
| 4. E | 14. C | 24. B |
| 5. E | 15. D | 25. A |
| 6. B | 16. A | 26. A |
| 7. A | 17. D | 27. C |
| 8. D | 18. B | 28. A |
| 9. B | 19. D | 29. B |
| 10. D | 20. E | 30. D |

| | |
|---|---|
| 31. E | 41. C |
| 32. B | 42. D |
| 33. C | 43. C |
| 34. D | 44. A |
| 35. A | 45. E |
| 36. C | 46. D |
| 37. A | 47. E |
| 38. B | 48. E |
| 39. B | 49. C |
| 40. A | 50. B |

# TEST 2

DIRECTIONS: Each question or incomplete statement is followed by several suggested answers or completions. Select the one that BEST answers the question or completes the statement. *PRINT THE LETTER OF THE CORRECT ANSWER IN THE SPACE AT THE RIGHT.*

1. Collapse of the lungs in the normal thorax is due to 1.____
   A. relaxation of external intercostal muscles and diaphragm
   B. continuous absorption of fluid from the interpleural space
   C. elastic recoil and surface tension of the fluid lining the alveolar spaces
   D. the fact that there is a lower oxygen partial pressure in the alveoli than in the atmosphere
   E. intra-alveolar pressure and pulmonary capillary pressure

2. Injection of estradiol into a castrated female rat causes 2.____
   A. decornification of vaginal epithelial cells
   B. no change in the vaginal smear
   C. many leukocytes in the vaginal smear
   D. erythrocytes in the vaginal smear
   E. cornification of vaginal epithelial cells

3. Pseudo-pregnancy occurs in the bitch because 3.____
   A. pet animals are kept in an unnatural environment
   B. there is a rapid decrease in luteolysin in the dog
   C. corpora lutea persists for 30 to 60 days in the dog
   D. the dog has low levels of estrogen
   E. the dog has high levels of LH

4. The hormone directly responsible for preparation of the uterine mucosa for implantation is 4.____
   A. LH B. FSH C. estradiol
   D. progesterone E. prolactin

5. In spermiogenesis,the acrosome of the mature spermatozoon is formed from 5.____
   A. the lipid membrane B. Golgi apparatus
   C. endoplasmic reticulum D. the nucleus
   E. mitochondria

6. Biologic tests for pregnancy are very useful in humans, but not in animals because of lack of, or low levels of, chorionic gonadotropins. However, biologic tests are useful in the mare because of 6.____
   A. high levels of these hormones in the urine
   B. secretion of progesterone from the placenta
   C. secretion of gonadotropins from the pituitary and the adrenal cortex during pregnancy
   D. the presence of gonadotropins in the plasma from day 55 to day 145 of gestation
   E. interaction of progesterone with gonadotropins secreted from the adrenal cortex

7. Steatorrhea is a manifestation of — 7. ____
   A. acinar degeneration
   B. low fat diet
   C. hyperfunction of the gall bladder
   D. high protein diet
   E. kidney necrosis

8. The area of the canine digestive tract LEAST susceptible to inflammation is the — 8. ____
   A. oral cavity
   B. esophagus
   C. stomach
   D. small intestine
   E. colon

9. A tumor associated with tympanic dilation of the rumen in cattle is — 9. ____
   A. leiomyosarcoma
   B. lymphosarcoma
   C. liver cell tumor
   D. abomasal carcinoma
   E. adromal carcinoma

10. Intestinal emphysema, with gas bubbles occurring below the serosa, is seen at postmortem *most commonly* in — 10. ____
    A. sheep
    B. cattle
    C. swine
    D. the horse
    E. the chicken

11. Oral papilloma tumors are seen *most commonly* in the — 11. ____
    A. cow
    B. sheep
    C. dog
    D. horse
    E. chicken

12. Liver infarcts are *most commonly* seen in — 12. ____
    A. bacillary hemoglobinuria
    B. brisket disease
    C. leontiasis
    D. Horner's disease
    E. serpigo

13. Media hypertrophy, interna fibrosis, and arteriosclerosis of pulmonary arteries are caused by — 13. ____
    A. distemper
    B. Ehrlich's anemia
    C. chronic failure of the left ventricle
    D. chronic failure of the right ventricle
    E. egols

14. Changes in the rbc seen with hemolytic anemia from chemical agents arise from — 14. ____
    A. amylaceous bodies
    B. reticulocytosis
    C. bigeminal bodies
    D. basophilic stipling
    E. Heinz bodies

15. Cardiac rhabdomyoma is *most frequently* seen in the — 15. ____
    A. lamb
    B. calve
    C. foal
    D. piglet
    E. kid

16. Acute pericarditis can cause, *most frequently*, the sequela — 16. ____
    A. aortic stenosis
    B. fibrinous pericarditis
    C. hydropericardium
    D. mural thrombosis
    E. adhesive pericarditis

17. In toxic aplastic anemia, the rbc's show 17.____
A. no change B. poikilocytosis C. anisocytosis
D. periblepsia E. lithotresis

18. Clinically, a sertoli cell tumor exhibits 18.____
A. virilism B. polyuria C. feminizing
D. no signs E. lithoxyduria

19. Steroids act as anti-inflammatory agents due to 19.____
A. stabilization of the lysosomal membrane
B. lithonephria
C. lithoprisy
D. nosophthoria
E. flexing of the lysosomal membrane

20. The condition with the lowest calcium in the blood is 20.____
A. renal secondary hyperparathyroidism
B. post-parturient paresis
C. bilateral parathyroidectomy
D. nutritional secondary hyperparathyroidism
E. nutritional primary hyperparathyroidism

21. Hyperplasia of the parathyroid is caused by 21.____
A. chronic interstitial nephritis
B. chronic interstitial hepatitis
C. diet
D. chronic enteritis
E. hematolysis

22. Goitrogens work by means of 22.____
A. stimulation of the thyroid
B. stimulation of the pituitary
C. stimulation of the pituitary, thyroid, and adrenal
D. decreased thyroxin, which results in increased TSH
E. increased thyroxin, which results in decreased TSH

23. Traumatic perforation of the liver (excluding external puncture) is *most common* in 23.____
A. the cow B. the horse C. the chicken
D. the goat E. sheep

24. *What* organism is the *most common* cause of a purulent lesion in the brain of farm animals? 24.____
A. Listeria B. Salmonella
C. Pasturella D. Hemophilus-like organisms
E. Toxoplasma

25. The cells in the gastric mucosa which form the precursors of hydrochloric acid are _____ cells. 25.____
A. poeth B. mucus neck C. chef
D. parietal E. argenti nitras fusus

26. The sebaceous glands of the skin are classified as 26.____
A. endocrine B. apocrine C. holocrine
D. merocrine E. hypocrine

27. Bile is drained from the liver cells by 27.___A___
 A. the small canaliculi B. the hepatic sinusoids
 C. small hepatic veins D. lymphatics
 E. small intercellular spaces

28. In *what* species are hemal lymphnodes BEST developed? In the 28.___D___
 A. horse B. pig C. dog D. cow E. chicken

29. *How many* bands are there in the large colon of the horse at the pelvic flexure? 29.___A___
 A. One B. Two C. Three D. Four E. Five

30. The medial retropharyngeal lymph node of the cow drains the 30.___A___
 A. floor of mouth, tongue pharynx, hard palate, soft palate, rectus capitus, verticlis muscle
 B. muzzle and lips
 C. muscles of eyelids and cheek
 D. muscles of cheek
 E. hock and withers

31. Under normal conditions of health, *which* has the HIGHEST level of protein? 31.___B___
 A. Serum B. Plasma C. Urine
 D. CSF E. Pleural fluid

32. The *most common* site for neoplasm of the intestines in a dog is the 32.___D___
 A. duodenum B. jejunum C. colon
 D. rectum E. cecum

33. In an aged dog with a tumor of the distal radius, the *most likely* place to see evidence of metastasis on X-ray is the 33.___D___
 A. elbow B. mediastinal lymph node
 C. forelimb D. lung
 E. liver

34. Leucopenia is *most commonly* seen with 34.___A___
 A. hog cholera B. anthrax
 C. IBR D. circumscribed peritonitis
 E. equine influenza

35. A horse has an intermittent bilateral nasal discharge, which is evident principally when the horse lowers its head, and a unilateral pharyngeal swelling. The *most likely* cause is 35.___A___
 A. infection of the guttural pouch
 B. sinusitis from an infected tooth
 C. chronic pharyngitis
 D. distemper
 E. rhinosporidiosis

36. A dog has complete loss of the right optic nerve. The result of shining a light in the right eye *only* is 36.____
   A. normal vision but no pupillary response in either eye
   B. loss of vision in the right eye with loss of pupillary response in the right eye only
   C. loss of vision in the right eye with loss of pupillary response in the left eye only
   D. loss of vision in the right eye with loss of pupillary response in both eyes
   E. loss of vision in the right eye with normal pupillary response in both eyes

37. A cow appears with bilateraly distended jugulars and submandibular edema. The *most likely* cause is 37.____
   A. actinobacillosis
   B. snake bite
   C. traumatic pericarditis
   D. intestinal parasitism
   E. diastematia

38. Primary pyodermas in the dog are caused by 38.____
   A. streptococcus
   B. staphylococcus
   C. corynebacterium pyogenes
   D. proteus vulgaris
   E. distemper virus

39. A dermatophyte isolated from the ring worm of a cat that is transmissable to man is the 39.____
   A. microspyrum gypseum
   B. tricophytom verticosun
   C. microsporum canis
   D. tricophyton mentagraphytes
   E. microsporon furfur

40. Exocrine sweat glands in the dog are 40.____
   A. associated with the hair follicles
   B. in the foot pad
   C. found only in the flank
   D. in the perineal region
   E. ductless glands found in the epidermis

41. The lesion in diabetes insipidus produces 41.____
   A. beta islet cells
   B. pituitarycytes and neurohypophysis
   C. acidiphils from adenohypophysis
   D. a small quantity of normal urine of high specific gravity
   E. a nutritional disease

42. The effective method of differentiating pyometra, ascites, ruptured bladder, etc., is through 42.____
   A. paracentesis
   B. deep palpitation
   C. finger ballottement
   D. surgical incision
   E. all the the above

43. A case was presented of several cows *acutely* dead in a dairy herd. A postmortem revealed septicemia, large spleen, hemolyzed blood, petechial hemorrhages. What is the proper diagnosis? 43.____
   A. Anthrax
   B. Hemorrhagic septicemia
   C. Malignant edema
   D. Bracken Fern
   E. Pott's aneurysm

44. The *only positive* indication of pregnancy in the Bovine upon rectal palpations is 44.____
   A. membranes slip, amniotic vesicle, fetus
   B. hard substance in uterus
   C. Cl on ipsilateral ovary
   D. enlargement of both horns
   E. soft substance in uterus

45. There are signs of polydypsia- polyuria in a female dog. *Which one* of the following diseases should NOT be in the DX? 45.____
   A. Diabetes mellitus
   B. CIN
   C. Urolithiasis
   D. Pyometra
   E. Cushings

46. Non-inherited cerebellar hypoplasia in the Bovine calf is caused by 46.____
   A. IBR
   B. BVD
   C. Lepto
   D. Bovine enzootic pleuropneumonia
   E. Haplodermitis

47. One of the signs of Bracken Fern poison in cattle which is not evidential is: 47.____
   A. Decreased prothrombin
   B. Hypothiaminosis
   C. Laryngeal edema
   D. Petechial hemorrhage
   E. Intestinal hemorrhage

48. The fresh froth blood from both nostrils is *most likely* caused by 48.____
   A. nasal hemorrhage
   B. pulmonary hemorrhage
   C. hepatization of lung
   D. pulmonary congestion and edema
   E. upper respiratory infection

49. The most frequent cause of purulent pericarditis in the cow is 49.____
   A. foreign body traumatism
   B. congenital heart disease
   C. allergic reaction due to streptococcus infection
   D. blepharosymphysis
   E. craniorrhachisis

50. Congestive heart failure involves a complex interaction between heart, kidney, adrenal cortex, and pituitary resulting in 50.____
   A. *increased* Na reabsorption *plus increased* water reabsorption
   B. *increased* Na reabsorption *plus decreased* water reabsorption

C. *decreased* K reabsorption *plus decreased* water reabsorption
D. *increased* K reabsorption *plus increased* $H_2O$ reabsorption
E. *decreased* Na reabsorption *plus decreased* $H_2O$ reabsorption

# KEY (CORRECT ANSWERS)

| | | | | |
|---|---|---|---|---|
| 1. C | 11. C | 21. C | 31. B | 41. B |
| 2. E | 12. A | 22. D | 32. D | 42. A |
| 3. C | 13. C | 23. A | 33. D | 43. A |
| 4. D | 14. E | 24. A | 34. A | 44. A |
| 5. B | 15. D | 25. D | 35. A | 45. C |
| 6. D | 16. B | 26. C | 36. D | 46. B |
| 7. A | 17. A | 27. A | 37. C | 47. B |
| 8. B | 18. C | 28. D | 38. B | 48. B |
| 9. B | 19. A | 29. A | 39. C | 49. A |
| 10. C | 20. C | 30. A | 40. B | 50. A |

# EXAMINATION SECTION

DIRECTIONS: Each question or incomplete statement is followed by several suggested answers or completions. Select the one that BEST answers the question or completes the statement. *PRINT THE LETTER OF THE CORRECT ANSWER IN THE SPACE AT THE RIGHT.*

1. All of the following organs are drained by the portal vein EXCEPT the 1. ____
   A. spleen B. stomach C. liver
   D. intestines E. pancreas

2. An adrenal as well as an hepatic portal system would be found in 2. ____
   A. dog and cat B. ox, goat, sheep C. hoofed animals
   D. horse, mule, donkey E. chicken, duck, turkey

3. In the non-ruminant, *which* species has the HIGHEST percentage of non-glandular stomachs? 3. ____
   A. Primates B. Dog C. Cat D. Monkey E. Pig

4. In a cross-section of skeletal muscle, *where* are the nuclei? 4. ____
   A. Under the sarcolemma
   B. Located in the center with few at the periphery
   C. Few in the ends of the skeletal muscle
   D. Above the sarcolemma
   E. Many in the ends of the sarcolemma

5. *Which* ligament is involved in the condition of horses called "Curb"? The ____________ ligament. 5. ____
   A. collateral B. plantar C. suspensory
   D. inferior check E. cernean

6. The function of the pectineus, often associated with the condition of hip dysplasia in the dog, is to 6. ____
   A. extend the stifle B. flex the hip
   C. adduct the hip D. extend the hip
   E. abduct the hip

7. The mesotendon is defined as a 7. ____
   A. section through the middle of the tendon
   B. lining of the synovial sheath
   C. fibrous tissue over a joint on which the tendon rides
   D. synovial living of a bursa over which the tendon rides
   E. synovial membrane connecting the inner and outer parts of the synovial sheath

8. Secretion of an acid urine is due to compensation for 8. ____
   A. salt deficiency B. salt intoxication
   C. chronic vomiting D. chronic diarrhea
   E. chronic dehydration

9. The secretion of urine of omnivores and carnivores is — 9. ____
A. $pH_2$ B. $pH_{10}$ C. of high titratable acidity
D. of low titratable acidity E. ventral

10. The pH of the urine of a calf on milk is — 10. ____
A. acid B. base C. neutral D. alkalosic
E. acidosic

11. In recent years, the temperature for pasteurization of milk has been raised because of — 11. ____
A. heat-resistant coliforms B. staphlococci
C. anthrax D. carbuncles E. anthracoid

12. The TB test is an example of — 12. ____
A. Arthus Rx B. Strauss Rx C. cell-mediated immunity
D. anaphylaxis E. antipraxia

13. The cell of the gastric mucose that produces precursors of hydrochloric acid is the — 13. ____
A. parietal B. paneth C. chief D. mucose
E. argentaffin

14. The function of the sustenacular cells of Sertoli is to — 14. ____
A. produce estrogen B. produce testosterone
C. produce sperm D. support and nourish sperm cells
E. form the connective-tissue framework of the testes

15. The location of the cellular tapetum lucidum in dogs is in the — 15. ____
A. choroid B. retina C. lamini fusca
D. ciliary body E. vitreous humor

16. Hexose sugars are absorbed in the SI by a process of — 16. ____
A. imbibition B. chelation C. diffusion
D. filtration E. active transport

17. *Which* of the following terms refers to the HIGHEST glycemic level? ____________ level. — 17. ____
A. Post-absorptive blood-sugar B. Fasting blood sugar
C. Normal blood sugar D. Renal threshold
E. Liver threshold

18. *What* is the total number of large calories per gram of the three major foodstuffs? — 18. ____

| | FAT | PROTEIN | CHO |
|---|---|---|---|
| A. | 9 | 4 | 4 |
| B. | 4 | 9 | 4 |
| C. | 4 | 4 | 9 |
| D. | 3 | 4 | 4 |
| E. | 4 | 4 | 8 |

19. *What* is the percent of Fe in Hb? — 19. ____
A. .34 B. .62 C. 1.00 D. .70 E. .50

20. In A.A. metabolism, *which* is the important coenzyme? 20. ___
   A. Pyridoxine   B. Pantothenic   C. Thiamine
   D. Niacin   E. Nicotine

21. The constituent in urine which does *not* vary much daily is 21. ___
   A. Na   B. Creatine   C. Urea   D. $H_2O$
   E. Glycerol

22. A substance used as an anticoagulant which does *not* bind Ca is 22. ___
   A. Heparin   B. EDTA   C. Na oxalate   D. Na fluoride
   E. Duroleum

23. The tissue reaction to certain agents such as Hycobacterium Tuberculosis is characterized by formation of nodules of epithelial cells, with a zone of necrosis in the center. The necrosis is, *most often*, 23. ___
   A. calcareous   B. ischemic   C. hyaline
   D. coagulative   E. caseous

24. Tumors, besides being classified as malignant and benign, are also classified as: 24. ___
   A. Epithelial-connective tissue
   B. Inflammatory-non-inflammatory
   C. Vascular-non-vascular
   D. Neoplastic-metaplastic
   E. Acute-chronic

25. The term that applies to a part or organ that does *not* develop is: 25. ___
   A. Hypoplasia   B. Metaplasia   C. Anaplasia
   D. Atrophy   E. Hypertrophy

26. The condition that does *not* lead to generalized edema is: 26. ___
   A. Arterial hypertension
   B. Chronic general passive hyperemia
   C. Starvation
   D. Tricuspid stenosis
   E. Hypoproternemia

27. The expiratory movement of air is due to the 27. ___
   A. relaxation of inspiratory muscles and the elastic recoil of the lungs
   B. elastic fibers in alveoli
   C. forced contraction of expiratory muscles
   D. forced retraction of inspiratory muscles
   E. rigid fibers in alveoli

28. *What* is the factor that has the *most* profound effect on the movement of gases through body fluids and tissues? The 28. ___
   A. viscosity of fluids   B. competition for available space
   C. distance from the lungs   D. gas solubility
   E. temperature of the body

29. *Which* is the following ratios is used to determine the respiratory quotient? 29. ____

A. $\frac{\text{Vol of } CO_2 \text{ expired}}{\text{Vol of } O_2 \text{ absorbed}}$

B. $\frac{\text{Vol of } O_2 \text{ absorbed}}{\text{Vol of } CO_2 \text{ expired}}$

C. $\frac{\text{Amount of water (vapor) expired}}{\text{Amount of water (vapor) absorbed}}$

D. $\frac{\text{Vol of } N_2 \text{ expired}}{\text{Vol of } N_2 \text{ absorbed}}$

E. $\frac{\text{Vol of } CO_2 \text{ expired}}{\text{Vol of } CO_2 \text{ absorbed}}$

30. In animals that produce urea as a nitrogenous waste, it is produced by the 30. ____
   A. liver
   B. renal tubular cells from carbon dioxide and ammonia
   C. renal tubular cells by an exothermic reaction
   D. proximal convoluted tubule cells of the kidney
   E. distal convoluted tubule cells of the kidney

31. The function of the nerve supply of the kidney has been indicated as 31. ____
   A. limited to the vasomotory control of a vessel of the kidney
   B. important in the regulation of absorption of certain crystalloids
   C. controlling the release of renal hypertensive hormones
   D. functional in conserving baje
   E. controlling water conservation by the distal convoluted tubules

32. The function of the malpighian corpuscle is the 32. ____
   A. absorption of water from urine that has already been excreted
   B. filtration of fluids
   C. absorption of glucose and chloride from excreted urine
   D. concentration of urea
   D. formation of uric acid

33. Touch and adaptation stimulation is rapidly accommodated due to 33. ____
   A. *decreased* blood supply to the receptors
   B. *decreased* rate of formation of sensory impulses by the receptors
   C. *decreased* sensitivity of the receptors
   D. *central* sensory inhibition
   E. *increased* inhibitory activity by interneurons in the spinal cord

34. The known hormones of the anterior pituitary are: 34. ____
   A. Steroids, *and* different from species to species
   B. Proteins, *and* similar in all species, but non-antigenic
   C. Steroids, *and* similar in all species and antigenic
   D. Proteins, *and* similar in all species and antigenic
   E. Steroids, *and* similar in all species and non-antigenic

35. Production of an antihormone by injecting one of the following hormones from another species into a different species would be GREATEST in — 35. B
A. stilbesterol B. TSH C. testosterone
D. estrogen E. cortisone

36. The *PRIMARY* defect in diabetes mellitus is — 36. C
A. increased absorption of glucose from the gut
B. increased gluconeogenesis
C. failure of glucose to pass into tissue cells and increased production of glucose by the liver
D. failure of the Meyerhoff-Embdem pathway
E. decreased protein catabolism

37. Production of *which* of the following hormones is due to production of a hypothalamic inhibiting factor rather than an hypothalamic releasing factor? — 37. E
A. TSH B. ACTH C. Stilbesterol
D. Testosterone E. Prolactin

38. The absence of urobilinogen in a cow showing clinical icterus indicates — 38. ~~C~~ A
A. biliary obstruction B. intestinal parasites
C. hemolytic poison D. anaplasmosis
E. leptospirosis

39. Gram negative, filamentous, red-like organism from smears of encapsulated abscesses of rumen and liver parenchyma, describes — 39. ~~C~~ B
A. salmonella enteritichis B. spherophous necrophorus
C. mycobacterium tuberculosis D. actinomyces bovis
E. actinobacillus lignieresi

40. In the treatment of cows for milk fever with Ca salts, heart block may occur but can be *corrected* with the administration of — 40. A
A. Atropine sulfate B. Sodium bicarbonate
C. Epinephrine D. Sodium ossalinate
E. Sodium phenate

41. *What* treatment would be BEST for a valuable 4-year-old heifer with hygroma of the knee? — 41. ~~B~~ A
A. Extirpation B. Incision and drainage
C. Antiphlogistic pack D. Solarization
E. Jactitation

42. For the diagnosis of navicular disease in a horse, you would block the — 42. A
A. posterior digital B. volar C. anterior digital
D. plantar E. cion

43. *What* structure(s) would be affected in an 8-month old holstein heifer with spastic paresis? — 43. A
A. Superficial flexor and gastrocnemius tendons
B. Deep flexor tendon and gastrocnemius tendons
C. Gastrocnemius tendon
D. Deep flexor tendon
E. Superficial flexor tendon

44. A 7-year-old Fox Terrier injured the right stifle 12 days ago. The terrier still has pain and swllling but will occasionally place weight on it. 44.
The BEST diagnostic procedure to perform is:
A. Inject procaine into the joint, then evaluate
B. Inject the joint with corticosteroid
C. Use short-acting anesthesia and try Paatsama anterior drawer sign
D. Use tranquilizer, and take radiographs in A-P and Lateral views
E. Spread Coster's paste over the joint

45. To perform a posterior digital neurectomy, it is important to know the arrangement of the artery, vein, and nerve at this region of the pastern. 45.
The arrangement from anterior to posterior is:
A. Artery, vein, nerve
B. Nerve, artery, vein
C. Vein, artery, nerve
D. Vein, nerve, artery
E. Nerve, vein, artery

46. The *most common* cause of encephalitis in sheep is: 46.
A. Western encephalitis
B. Toxoplasmosis
C. Listeriosis
D. Gid
E. Malignant catarrhal fever

47. *Most common* cause of formation of metamyoglobulin in cattle is ______________ poisoning. 47.
A. Nitrate
B. Cyanide
C. Wild cherry
D. Methyl alcohol
E. Colchicum autumnale

48. An unarmed tapeworm cyst found in the muscle of a cow is due to exposure to: 48.
A. Taenia saginata
B. Taenia echinococcus
C. Taenie solium
D. Taenia coenurus
E. Tenia thalami

49. A disease found ONLY in chickens is: 49.
A. Infectious larynotracheitis
B. Aspergillosis
C. Infectious bronchitis
D. Chronic respiratory disease
E. Newcastle

50. Certain cardiac anomalies, white muscle disease of calves, and stomach worms in sheep, share the tendency to cause pulmonary 50.
A. osteoarthropathy
B. edema
C. emphysema
D. arteries
E. valves

# KEY (CORRECT ANSWERS)

| | | | | | | | | | |
|---|---|---|---|---|---|---|---|---|---|
| 1. | C | 11. | A | 21. | B | 31. | C | 41. | A |
| 2. | E | 12. | D | 22. | A | 32. | B | 42. | A |
| 3. | E | 13. | A | 23. | E | 33. | B | 43. | A |
| 4. | A | 14. | D | 24. | A | 34. | D | 44. | D |
| 5. | B | 15. | A | 25. | A | 35. | B | 45. | C |
| 6. | C | 16. | E | 26. | C | 36. | C | 46. | C |
| 7. | C | 17. | A | 27. | A | 37. | E | 47. | A |
| 8. | C | 18. | A | 28. | D | 38. | A | 48. | A |
| 9. | C | 19. | A | 29. | A | 39. | B | 49. | C |
| 10. | A | 20. | A | 30. | A | 40. | A | 50. | B |

# EXAMINATION SECTION

# TEST 1

DIRECTIONS: Each question or incomplete statement is followed by several suggested answers or complestions. Select the one that BEST answers the question or completes the statement. *PRINT THE LETTER OF THE CORRECT ANSWER IN THE SPACE AT THE RIGHT.*

1 *What two* infectious diseases cause CNS lesions in the cat? 1. ____
   A. Rabies *and* listeriosis
   B. Rabies *and* leptospirosis
   C. Rabies *and* toxoplasmosis
   D. Toxoplasmosis *and* leptospirosis
   E. Choriomeningitis *and* rabies

2. The finding of stratified squamous epithelium in the bronchi is an example of 2. ____
   A. aplasia B. metaplasia C. anaplasia
   D. neoplasia E. hyperplasia

3. The *main* pulmonary lesion in shipping fever is 3. ____
   A. interstitial pneumonia B. fibrinous lobar pneumonia
   C. pulmonary congestion D. purulent pneumonia
   E. efibroid pneumonia

4. A respiratory disease found *only* in chickens is: 4. ____
   A. laryngotracheitis B. CRD C. newcastle
   D. infectious bronchitis E. septinous disease

5. The MOST common type of pneumonia in domestic animals is __________ pneumonia. 5. ____
   A. bronchial B. interstitial C. gangrenous D. larval
   E. purulent

6. *Which* tumors do NOT produce hormones? 6. ____
   A. Seminona and disgerminoma
   B. Interstitial cell
   C. Basophilic cell and acidophilic cell
   D. Granulosa cell, luteal cell, and thecal cell
   E. Sertoli cell

7. *What* causes the brown discoloration of the lungs in chronic passive congestion? 7. ____
   A. Protein in the edema fluid
   B. Hemosiderin in macrophages
   C. Methemoglobin production from hemoglobin
   D. Fibrous connective tissue from hypoxia
   E. Poorly oxygenated blood in the capillaries

8. In *which* breed is osteosarcoma MOST common? 8. ____
   A. Boston Terrier B. Boxer C. Daschund
   D. Great Dane E. Poodle

9. In cats, juvenile osteoporosis can be caused by a diet deficient in — 9. ____
   A. phosphorous  B. copper  C. Vitamin D
   D. magnesium  E. calcium

10. The casual relationship of a virus to neoplasms has been shown by the fulfillment of Koch's postulates for — 10. ____
    A. Hodgkin's disease  B. Bovine leukemia
    C. Canine malignant lymphoma  D. Mouse leukemia
    E. Feline lymphosarcoma

11. Branches of arteries which supply the rumen are derived from the ________ artery. — 11. ____
    A. splenic  B. hepatic  C. cranial mesenteric
    D. celiac  E. pancreatic

12. The pulse of the horse is taken on the ventral part of the mandible, using *which* artery? — 12. ____
    A. External maxillary  B. Internal maxillary
    C. Sublingual  D. Masseteric  E. Buccinator

13. The celiac artery of the dog supplies *which* organs? The — 13. ____
    A. stomach, liver, spleen, pancreas, and the first part of the duodenum
    B. liver and spleen
    C. stomach and pancreas
    D. liver and pancreas
    E. liver, spleen, pancreas, and all of the duodenum

14. The lymphatic system of the chicken varies with the mammalian in that: — 14. ____
    A. It is the same as the mammalian and has a thoracic duct.
    B. There are only scattered lymph nodes in the muscle.
    C. The lymph vessels do not lie in close proximity to the blood vessels.
    D. There is lymph tissue only in the bursa of F. and a few scattered lymph nodes.
    E. There are no lumph nodes in the chicken.

15. The femoral artery is cranial to *which* muscle? The — 15. ____
    A. sartorius  B. pectinius  C. psoas minor
    D. tensor fascia lata  E. rectus femoris

16. In the calf, *what* is the size relationship of the rumen, reticulum, and omasum to the abomasum? — 16. ____
    A. The rumen, reticulum, and omasum together = the abomasum.
    B. The rumen + $\frac{1}{2}$ reticulum + $\frac{1}{2}$ the omasum = the abomasum.
    C. The rumen + the reticulum + $\frac{1}{2}$ the omasum = the abomasum.
    D. $\frac{1}{2}$ the rumen + $\frac{1}{2}$ the reticulum + $\frac{1}{2}$ the omasum = the abomasum.
    E. The rumen and the reticulum together = $\frac{1}{2}$ the abomasum.

17. *Which* nerve goes through the maxillary foramen of the pyterygopalatine fossa? The ________ nerve. — 17. ____
    A. inframaxillary  B. infratrochlear  C. intercostal
    D. intercostobrachialis  E. infraorbital

18. *Where* is the spleen located in the horse? Along the — 18.
   A. greater curvature of the stomach
   B. lesser curvature of the stomach
   C. greater curvature of the abdomen
   D. lesser curvature of the stomach
   E. None of the above

19. In the cow, *what* is the hard structure lateral and caudal to the plane of the urethral orifices? The [redacted] gland. — 19.
   A. admaxillary  B. acinous  C. conglobate
   D. Huguier's  E. major vestibular

20. The colon of the pig and cow have *what* in common? The [redacted] coils. — 20.
   A. centripetal *and* centrifugal
   B. gland *and* induction
   C. Leiter's *and* primary
   D. resistance *and* secondary
   E. None of the above

21. Papillomatosis is MOST common in the — 21.
   A. dog  B. cow  C. horse  D. chicken  E. pig

22. A white exudate lining the trachea and esophagus of chickens is due to a deficiency of — 22.
   A. Vitamin A  B. Vitamin $B_{12}$  C. Vitamin D
   D. pyroxidine  E. riboflavin

23. Secretin may be called a(n) — 23.
   A. apoenzyme  B. organic catalyst  C. hormone
   D. enzyme  E. callogen

24. A nutritionally important substance absorbed in the large intestine of solipeds is — 24.
   A. fats  B. proteins  C. lower fatty acids
   D. indol  E. colchicine

25. Endopeptidases act on [redacted] linkages. — 25.
   A. intracellular protein  B. arginine-phenylalinine
   C. internal protein  D. guanine-lysine
   E. external lipoid

26. Bile secretion occurs — 26.
   A. continously
   B. as a result of the action of fats in the small intestine
   C. as a result of the action of pancreozymin in the small intestine
   D. as a result of the action of choleystokinin in the small intestine
   E. indirectly as the result of the action of secretin on the pancreas

27. *Which* of the following is neoplastic? — 27.
   A. Papilloma  B. Xanthoma  C. Dermoid cyst
   D. Granuloma  E. Xanthin

28. Unilateral paralysis of the lip indicates — 28. C
    A. paralysis of the trigeminal nerve
    B. paralysis of the maxillary nerve
    C. paralysis of the facial nerve
    D. paralysis of the infraorbital nerve
    E. rabies

29. The cornual nerve in the cow is a branch of the ______ nerve. — 29. E
    A. facial   B. trigeminal   C. glossopharyngeal
    D. first cervical   E. auricular

30. Preganglionic fibers associated with the sympathetic system are components of the — 30. A
    A. thoraco-lumbar NN   B. sacral NN
    C. cervical NN   D. cranial-sacral NN
    E. buccal-cervical NN

31. *Which* nerve runs to the extensors of the forearm? — 31. E
    A. Median   B. Musculocutaneous   C. Axillary
    D. Ulnar   E. Radial

32. *Which* is the artery whose main branches supply rumen? — 32. D
    A. Pudendal   B. Helatic   C. Splenic   D. Celiac
    E. Mesenteric

33. Phlorizin causes glucosuria by — 33. ~~D~~ B
    A. *increasing* the glomerular filtration
    B. *increasing* the glomerular capillary vasodialation
    C. *increasing* tubular resorption
    D. *decreasing* tubular resorption
    E. causing an acute nephrosis

34. Contraction of the bladder is due to *which* parasympathetic neurohormone? — 34. C
    A. Norepinephrine   B. Epinephrine   C. Acetylcholine
    D. Cholocyanin   E. Lecithin

35. *What* is the cause of the normal venous pulse in the cow? — 35. ~~B~~ A
    A. Bulging of the right A-V valve into the atrium
    B. The volume of the atrium being larger than the ventricle
    C. Contraction of the atrium
    D. Insufficiency of the right A-V valve
    E. Stenosis

36. In a spayed female, high levels of *what* hormone are found? — 36. A
    A. FSH   B. LH   C. Progesterone   D. Estrogen
    E. Testosterone

37. The *most common* cause of post-coital pyometra in the cow is: — 37. D
    A. C.pyogenes   B. P.neruginosa   C. Trichinosis
    D. V.fetus   E. Gonoccus

38. The ureters of thc chicken empty into the — 38. ~~B~~ A
    A. urodeum   B. urethra   C. lata fasia   D. propria fascia
    E. anal fascia

39. In the necropsy of swine, lungworms are *most commonly* found in ________ lobe. 39. ____
   A. apical  B. diaphragmatic  C. cardiac
   E. cacuminal  E. intermediate

40. *Which* of the following is actively secreted by the mammalian kidney? 40. ____
   A. NaCl  B. Urea  C. Na hippurate  D. Na
   E. Achilleic acid

41. Blood pressure in the large arteries is propagated by the 41. ____
   A. force of the heart beat
   B. smooth muscle contraction in the wall
   C. elastic fiber content and arrangement
   D. smooth muscle expansion in the wall
   E. rate of the heart beat

42. *What* is the SMALLEST unit of pulmonary absorption in the hen's lung? 42. ____
   A. Alveolar sac  B. Alveolar ducts
   C. Recurrent bronchi  D. Air capillaries
   E. Air sacs

43. The *main* receptor regulating the pressure of $CO_2$ is in the 43. ____
   A. medulla  B. aortic arch  C. carotid body
   D. alveoli  E. anterior hyoid arch

44. *Which* of the following is a tumor? 44. ____
   A. Granuloma  B. Coloboma  C. Papilloma
   D. Corneal dermoid  E. Corium

45. Embryologically, the retina differs from other eye tissues because it is ________ in origin. 45. ____
   A. endodermal  B. ectodermal  C. mesodermal
   D. mesenchymal  E. notochord

46. *Which* of the following blood constituents is constant and may be sampled at any time? 46. ____
   A. Fat  B. Glucose  C. Calcium  D. Plasma
   E. Red corpuscles

47. The action of the gracilis muscle is to 47. ____
   A. extend the stifle joint  B. abduct the front limb
   C. flex the stifle joint  D. adduct the hind limb
   E. flex the hind limb

48. The large muscle that arises from the ligamentum nuchae, $C_2$ to $T_{10}$, and inserts of the spine of the scapula is the 48. ____
   A. latissimus dorsi  B. supraspinatus  C. trapezius
   D. rhomboideus  E. serratus ventralis

49. The distal patellar ligaments of the horse are: 49. ____
   A. Three strong bands connecting the patella with the tibial tuberosity
   B. Two strong bands attaching the patella to the epicondyles of the femur
   C. Three strong bands attaching the patella to the tendon of the quadriceps

D. Three strong bands attaching the patella to the neck of the femur
E. Three strong bands connecting the patella with the tibial tuberosity

50. A nail puncture through the apex of the frog that penetrates the distal inter-phalangeal joint passes through the 50. C
A. laminar corium B. superficial flexor tendon
C. deep flexor tendon D. coronary band
E. periople

# KEY (CORRECT ANSWERS)

| | | | | | | | | | |
|---|---|---|---|---|---|---|---|---|---|
| 1. | C | 11. | D | 21. | B | 31. | E | 41. | |
| 2. | B | 12. | A | 22. | A | 32. | D | 42. | |
| 3. | B | 13. | A | 23. | C | 33. | B ?, D | 43. | A |
| 4. | D | 14. | D | 24. | C | 34. | C | 44. | |
| 5. | A | 15. | B | 25. | C | 35. | A | 45. | |
| 6. | A | 16. | E | 26. | A | 36. | A | 46. | |
| 7. | C | 17. | E | 27. | ~~B~~ A | 37. | D | 47. | |
| 8. | D | 18. | A | 28. | C | 38. | A | 48. | |
| 9. | E | 19. | E | 29. | E | 39. | A | 49. | |
| 10. | D | 20. | A | 30. | A | 40. | B | 50. | |

# TEST 2

32/50

DIRECTIONS: Each question or incomplete statement is followed by several suggested answers or completions. Select the one that BEST answers the question or completes the statement. *PRINT THE LETTER OF THE CORRECT ANSWER IN THE SPACE AT THE RIGHT.*

1. The normal structure of a tendon includes: 1. B
   A. mostly fibroblasts with a collagen stroma
   B. parallel bundles of fibrous tissue or collagen separated by rows of fibroblasts
   C. mostly yellow elastic tissue with fibrous tissue and fibroblasts
   D. vertical bundles of fibrous tissue or collagen separated by rows of fibroblasts
   E. mostly fibroblasts with a fascial stroma

2. The term *diarthrosis* describes an articulation that is 2. ~~C~~ B
   A. rigid with no mobility
   B. covered by a capsule
   C. bone joined by ligaments
   D. bone joined by fibrous tissue
   E. rigid but flexible

3. *Which* of the following passes through the foramen triosseum of the chicken? The 3. A
   A. deep pectoral muscle tendon
   B. ischiatic artery
   C. common carotid artery
   D. vein of the renal portal system
   E. tendon of the biceps femoris

4. An autopsy of a dog with a suspected intracranial lesion revealed a tumor in the third ventricle extending into the sella turcica. 4. A
   *Which* of the following signs would lead to a *probable* diagnosis?
   A. Polyuria and polydipsia
   B. Diabetes mellitus
   C. Ataxia
   D. Muscular tremors
   E. Hemopexia

5. *Why* is NaF added to blood drawn for glucose determinations? It 5. C
   A. ties up the thromboplastin
   B. adjusts the pH for transit
   C. inhibits glycolysis produced by enzymes in the RBC's
   D. frees the thromboplastin
   E. speeds up glycolisis produced by enzymes in the RBC's

6. Hypoglycemia from partial or complete lack of nutrition is 6. A
   A. a cause of death in newborn pigs
   B. due to pancreatic deficiency in pigs
   C. due to pancreatic deficiency in calves
   D. a cause of early death in foals
   E. a cause of increased liver glycogen stores

7. *Which* is the predominant cell in the alveoli of lungs with gray hepatization? The 7. B
   A. red blood cell
   B. lymphocyte
   C. neutrophil
   D. granulation tissue
   E. proliferating fibroplasts

8. In ventricular fibrillation, the pulse is 8. C
A. slow and irregular B. fast and irregular
C. absent D. slow and weak
E. fast and weak

9. Sinus arrythmia in the dog is caused by an increase 9. C
A. in serum chloral
B. *and* decrease in serum $HCO_3$
C. *and* decrease in vagal tone
D. *and* decrease in sympathetic activity
E. *and* decrease in activity of the strial node

10. *Which* compound has an acidifying effect on the body? 10. A
A. $NH_4CL$ B. NaCl C. Ammonium oxalate
D. Sodium propionate E. Sodium citrate

11. The HCL in the stomach has a pH of approximately 1. This is equivalent to 0.1N of concentrate. HCl has a specific gravity of 1.10 and an assay of 37%. 11. B ~~C~~
How much concentrated $HC_2$ is needed to make 1 liter of 0.1NHCL?
A. 1 ml B. 10 ml C. 100 ml
D. 1 liter E. 10 liters

12. The molecular weight of chloride is 35.5 . A plasma with a chloride concentration of 3.55 mg/100 ml contains 12. B ~~C~~
A. 1 milliequivalent of chloride per liter
B. 10 milliequivalents of chloride per liter
C. 100 milliequivalents of chloride per liter
D. 1 equivalent of chloride per liter
E. 10 equivalents of chloride per liter

13. In tissue anoxia, erythrocyte production may be stimulated by: 13. C
A. Apoferritin B. Histamine C. Erythropoietin
D. Vitamin $B_{12}$ E. Apocythein

14. In the cow, careless incising of the right paralumbar fossa may result in cutting the 14. B
A. liver B. duodenum C. dorsal sac of the rumen
D. gallbladder E. spleen

15. In a horse which has laryngeal hemiplegia, a muscle which can be externally palpated to be atrophied is the 15. C
A. arytenoideus transversus B. cricoarytenoideus lateralis
C. cricoarytenoideus dorsalis D. vocalis
E. cricothyroideus

16. The cells of the glandular stomach which form the precursors of hydrochloric acid are termed ________ cells. 16. B
A. chief B. parietal C. paneth
D. argentaffin E. mucous neck

17. Cells of the nervous system which are generally believed to be equivalent in function to the reticulo-endothelial cells elsewhere in the body are the ________ cells. 17. B
A. ependymal B. microglial C. astrocyte
D. oligodendrocyte E. neuron

Test 2

18. On slaughter of a bovine, a granulomatous lesion in the thoracic lymph node was seen. A microscopic examination showed a double spherical shaped object.
The condition *most likely* is: 18. ____
   A. Actinymycosis B. Coccidiomycosis
   C. Nocardiosis D. Monialiasis
   E. Aspergillosis

19. A transmissible virus in cattle is 19. ____
   A. carcinoma of the ocular adenoxa
   B. fibro-papilloma on the genitals
   C. neurofibroma
   D. leulenia
   E. duct carcinoma of the mammary gland

20. On autopsy of a dog, no lesions were noted except for a tumorous mass extending from the 3rd ventricle of the brain downward into the sella turcica. 20. ____
Signs manifested by the animal while alive would include
   A. polyurea polydipsea
   B. tremors of the voluntary muscles
   C. cardiac arrythmia
   D. ataxia
   E. agastroneuria

21. Paralysis of the seventh cranial nerve would *not* affect function of *which* of the following? 21. ____
   A. Nasolabialis B. Depressor labii inferioris
   C. Masseter D. Zygomaticus
   E. Levator palpebrae superioris

22. Unilateral paralysis of lips indicates damage to the ________ nerve. 22. ____
   A. trigeminal B. masseter C. facial
   D. lingual E. lesser splanchnic

23. The great crossing of the fibers of the two cerebral hemispheres is called the corpus 23. ____
   A. caudatum B. ciliare C. callosum
   D. luteum E. phacoide

24. The origin of nerve tissue is the 24. ____
   A. endoderm B. mesoderm C. ectoderm
   D. blastoderm E. mesoblast

25. The substance actively secreted by the kidney is: 25. ____
   A. Urea B. Na Hypophosphate
   C. Na Hippurate (Hippuric Acid) D. Na Bicarbonate
   E. Disodium Phosphate

26. Acetylcholine is the chemical mediator in all of the following cells EXCEPT the: 26. ____
   A. Pre-ganglionic sympathetic B. Post-ganglionic sympathetic
   C. Pre-ganglionic parasympathetic
   D. Post-ganglionic parasympathetic
   E. None of the above

27. Urea is actually formed in the 27. B
A. kidney tubules B. liver C. renal epithelium
D. loop of Henle E. occipital notochord

28. Increased secretion of ~~oldosterme~~ aldosterone by the adrenal cortex 28. ~~B~~ C
causes the effect of:
A. Na secretion B. Na retention C. K and Na secretion
D. External secretion E. None of the above

29. The lesion of Nutmeg Liver is a result of chronic passive 29. ~~E~~ A
congestion. In the bovine this is *most often* accompanied
by:
A. Valvular endocarditis of the left A-V valve
B. Abomasal ulcers
C. Traumatic reticulitis
D. Thrombisi of the hypatic artery
E. Parasitic migration into the liver

30. The *most commonly* accepted theory of the kinetics of leu- 30. D
kocytes is that, in inflammation:
A. They flatten against the endothelium and extend their
pseudopods through
B. An antigen-antibody response draws them
C. They pass through weakened vessel walls
D. They are able to pass through due to increased osmotic
pressure in the area
E. They come from punitive cells in the area

31. A genetic reason for prolonged gestation in Guernsey cattle 31. A
is:
A. Adenohypophyseal Hypoplasia B. Hyperpituitanism
C. Hyperadrenal corticalism D. Hyperspasmia
E. Hypersplenotrophy

32. A characteristic of basal cell carcinomas is that they 32. ~~B~~ D
A. usually grow quite large
B. commonly metastasize
C. rarely ulcerate
D. are very sensitive to X-radiation
E. do not arise from the basal cells of the hair follicles

33. Fibrosarcomas and osteosarcomas may be associated with the 33. C
parasite:
A. Ostertagia B. Bacterium violaceus sacchari
C. Spirocirea lupi D. Eimeria
E. Fasciola hepotica

34. Juvenile osteoporosis in tne cat may be induced by a diet 34. E
deficient in
A. phosphorus B. copper C. Vitamin D
D. magnesium E. calcium

35. Failure of an organ or a part to grow to its full size is 35. C
an example of
A. anaplasia B. metaplasia C. hypoplasia
D. hypertrophy E. atrophy

36. The absorption of glucose in the small intestine is 36. D
   A. retarded greatly during insulin deficiencies
   B. dependent upon adequate bile-salt secretion by the liver
   C. largely a process of diffusion across the mucous membrane
   D. accomplished by an active transport mechanism
   E. more rapid than the absorption of galactose

37. The movement of a bolus of food down the esophagus is the result of 37. C
   A. contractions stimulated by the sight and smell of food
   B. a parasympathetic reflex excited by chewing
   C. a stimulus in the upper part of the esophagus due to the act of swallowing
   D. a pressure gradient created by the piston-like action of the tongue during swallowing
   E. facilitation by the phallic phase of gastric activity

38. A nutritionally important substance absorbed in the large intestine of solipeds is: 38. C
   A. Fats B. Proteins C. Lower fatty acids
   D. Indol E. Indoxyl

39. The substance found in the lymphatics during active digestion is 39. D
   A. serum B. plasma C. chyme D. chyle
   E. plasmin

40. A factor that aids in normal inspiration is: 40. C
   A. Contraction of the abdominal muscles
   B. Increased intrapulmonic pressure
   C. Contraction of the diaphragm
   D. Dilation of the bronchioles
   E. Closure of the glottis

41. Intrapulmonary pressure is the same as atmospheric 41. A E
   A. during increased inspiration
   B. during decreased inspiration
   C. during increased expiration
   D. during decreased expiration
   E. when at rest

42. The area MOST sensitive to $CO_2$ is the: 42. C A
   A. Medulla oblongata B. Pulmonary artery
   C. Alveolae D. Carotid sinus
   E. Aortic arch-pressure receptors

43. Aldosterone increases the reabsorption of 43. B
   A. urea B. Na C. H D. K E. Cl

44. From *what* embryonic tissue is the mammary gland derived? 44. D A
   A. Ectoderm B. Endoderm C. Mesenchyme
   D. Mesoderm E. Coelom

45. *Why* do you get four calories of heat per gram of CHO metabolized and concurrently nine calories per gram of fat? 45. ___
   A. The oily nature of fats yields increased heat
   B. Fats "burn" more completely
   C. There is a larger number of carbons and hydrogens in fats as compared to oxygens
   D. There is a larger number of carbons and oxygens in fats as compared to hydrogens
   E. There is a larger number of hydrogens in fats as compared to carbons and oxygens

46. The disease that is *not* transmitted by a tick is 46. ___
   A. typhus B. tick-borne fever of sheep
   C. tick-borne fever of dogs D. heart water
   E. Q fever

47. Infectious or chick bronchitis 47. ___
   A. usually affects all the birds of a young age in the same pen about the same time
   B. is seen in all birds of all ages annually
   C. usually spreads slowly by bird-to-bird contact
   D. affects only the young when numerous ages are gathered together
   E. affects all ages with high mortality

48. The *most commonly* incriminated fungi isolated in bovine abortions are: 48. ___
   A. Apergillosis + histoplasmosis
   B. Mucoromycosis + spirotrichosis
   C. Coccidiomycosis + ascomycete
   D. Mucoromycosis + aspergillosis
   E. Trichophyton + spirotrichosis

49. A yearling bovine is observed with small raised nodules of the gastric mucosa. This is caused by: 49. ___
   A. Oesophagostomum radiatum B. Tricanstrongylus sp
   C. Ostertagia ostertagi D. Hemopexia
   E. Cooperia

50. *What* is the treatment for gastric dilation in a Great Dane? 50. ___
   A. Gastrotomy B. Gastrectomy C. Gastric stimulants
   D. Gastric depression E. Gastric impression

# KEY (CORRECT ANSWERS)

| | | | | |
|---|---|---|---|---|
| 1. B | 11. B | 21. E | 31. A | 41. |
| 2. B | 12. B | 22. C | 32. D | 42. |
| 3. A | 13. C | 23. C | 33. C | 43. |
| 4. A | 14. B | 24. C | 34. E | 44. |
| 5. C | 15. C | 25. C | 35. C | 45. |
| 6. A | 16. B | 26. B | 36. D | 46. |
| 7. B | 17. B | 27. B | 37. C | 47. |
| 8. C | 18. B | 28. B | 38. C | 48. |
| 9. C | 19. B | 29. C | 39. D | 49. |
| 10. A | 20. A | 30. A | 40. C | 50. |

# EXAMINATION SECTION

## TEST 1

DIRECTIONS: Each question or incomplete statement is followed by several suggested answers or completions. Select the one that BEST answers the question or completes the statement. *PRINT THE LETTER OF THE CORRECT ANSWER IN THE SPACE AT THE RIGHT.*

1. For the GREATEST public protection, the BEST way to take care of ornithosis infection in adult turkey flocks is to 1._____
   A. provide 5% malathion dust and burning febrile turkeys
   B. test with hemagglutination inhibition and eliminate positives
   C. test by indirect CF test and eliminate positives
   D. quarantine the flock for 2 weeks
   E. put 400 grams of tetracycline per ton of feed for 3 weeks

2. Genetic information necessary for the reproduction of viruses is carried by the 2._____
   A. virus-related enzymes
   B. protein coat of the virus particle
   C. viruscytes
   D. lipid components
   E. nucleic acid portion of the virus particle

3. Biologic vectors, in which part of the life cycle of the virus is spent are *usually* 3._____
   A. arthropods B. molluscs C. mammals
   D. birds E. fish

4. Kaolin belongs to a class of drugs known as 4._____
   A. demulcents B. astringents C. adsorbants
   D. emulsifiers E. emollients

5. The MAJOR pathway for detoxification of morphine by the liver is 5._____
   A. conjugation with glucosamine
   B. conjugation with glucuronic acid
   C. destruction of the nitrogen ring
   D. acetylation of the phenolic hydroxyl group
   E. N-demethylization at position C-17

6. If a piperazine carbon disulfide complex solution containing 7.5 gm to oz. is used to treat a horse for large strongyles, pinworms and bots, the dose per 100 lbs. of body weight should be __________ fluid ounce(s). 6._____
   A. ½ B. 1 C. 2 D. 3 E. 3 3/4

7. A material that enhances the antigenicity of a substance is called an 7._____
   A. adjuvant B. atopen C. allergen
   D. autogen E. aggressin

8. The sulfa that would be MOST effective in treating an enteritis in a calf is 8.____
   A. sulfamerazine B. sulfamethazine
   C. sulfasoxazole D. phthalysulfathiazole
   E. sulfapyridine

9. One of the drugs for treatment of organic phosphate poisoning in mammals is 9.____
   A. eseine B. carbochol C. physostigmine
   D. pilocorzine E. atropine

10. A solution of protein hydrolosate for intravenous therapy *generally* includes dextrose to 10.____
   A. neutralize the excessive production of ammonia from the rapid utilization of the protein hydrolysate
   B. provide an adequate source of tissue energy in order to conserve the protein hydrolysate for tissue repair
   C. stabilize the solution of protein hydrolysate
   D. *increase* the osmotic pressure of the protein hydrolysate so that the solution diffuses in the tissue more rapidly
   E. delay renal excretion of the protein hydrolysate by blocking renal glomeruli by preferential filtration

11. The MOST common chronic toxic action of streptomycin is 11.____
   A. toxic action on the liver and kidneys
   B. neurotoxic action on the vestibular and auditory mechanisms
   C. interference with wound healing by suppressing fibroblast
   D. incompatibility with urinary phosphates-crystalurie
   E. tendency to cause apastic anemia on prolonged administration

12. The urinary antiseptic action of methanamine is due to the formation of 12.____
   A. formalin B. annomia C. glycol
   D. formaldehyde E. phenol

13. The *usual* and *principal* site of action of atropine is the 13.____
   A. parasympathetic postganglionic synapse or receptor
   B. sympathetic postganglionic synapse or receptor
   C. parasympathetic ganglionic synapse or receptor
   D. sympathetic ganglionic synapse or receptor
   E. somatic motor nerve end plate

14. The antibiotics streptomycin, neomycin, polymycin and bacitracin have the important *common* characteristic of 14.____
   A. being derivatives of molds
   B. primary effectiveness against gram + organisms
   C. primary effectiveness against gram - organisms
   D. similarly intoxic effects on animals
   E. poor absorption from GI tract

15. Following depletion due to hemorrhage, the parenteral fluid of *choice* is — 15. ____
   A. saline
   B. 15% solution of hemoglobin
   C. plasma
   D. whole blood
   E. gelatin solution and 15% acacia

16. Carbachol increases intestinal motility and — 16. ____
   A. bile flow  B. salivation  C. blood pressure
   D. dyspnea  E. mydriasis

17. The molecular weight of chloride is 35.5. A plasma with chloride concentration of 355 mg per 100 ml contains ________ of chloride per liter. — 17. ____
   A. 1 milliequivalent  B. 10 milliequivalent
   C. 100 milliequivalent  D. 1 equivalent
   E. 10 equivalent

18. Phlezern produces diuresis by — 18. ____
   A. inhibiting tubular reabsorption of glucose and sodium
   B. inhibiting tubular reabsorption of sodium
   C. inhibiting tubular reabsorption of glucose
   D. stimulating rèlease of vasopressin
   E. inhibiting release of vasopressin

19. Aspirin in cats is — 19. ____
   A. safe if given with an alkalyzing agent
   B. safe if given with antibiotics or steroids
   C. safe if given at LESS than 10 grains per day
   D. toxic *even* at 5 grains per day
   E. toxic *only* over 15 grains per day

20. A drug contraindicated in acute canine pancreatitis is — 20. ____
   A. prednisolone
   B. penicillin
   C. morphine sulfate
   D. atropine sulfate
   E. meperidine HCl Demeral

21. Phenobarbital is NOT used as a general anesthetic because it — 21. ____
   A. has an action that is too short
   B. has an action that is too long
   C. decreases heart rate more than others
   D. fails to produce unconsciousness
   E. accumulates in fatty tissues

22. The compound that has an acidifying effect on the body is — 22. ____
   A. $NH_4Cl$  B. NaCl
   C. ammonium oxalete  D. sodium propionate
   E. sodium citrate

23. Epinephrine 23. A
   A. does NOT *decrease* HR
   B. *decreases* HR by vagal stimulation
   C. *decreases* HR by coronary artery constriction
   D. *decreases* HR by ischemic of the carotid body
   E. *decreases* HR reflex by increasing blood pressure

24. One of the actions of bishydroxcoumerol is 24. C B
   A. to produce hyperprothrombinemis
   B. to produce hypoprothrombinemis
   C. to decrease prothrombin time
   D. synergistic with vitamin K
   E. to antagonize salysilic acid

25. Anabolic steroids are indicated for 25. D
   A. bitches persistent estrus
   B. sertoli tumor in male dog
   C. dermatitis in a cat
   D. wasting disease in aged dog
   E. nymphomania in cow

---

# KEY (CORRECT ANSWERS)

1. E
2. E
3. A
4. C
5. B

6. B
7. A
8. D
9. E
10. B

11. B
12. A
13. B
14. E
15. D

16. B
17. C
18. C
19. D
20. C

21. B
22. A
23. A
24. B
25. D

# TEST 2

DIRECTIONS: Each question or incomplete statement is followed by several suggested answers or completions. Select the one that BEST answers the question or completes the statement. *PRINT THE LETTER OF THE CORRECT ANSWER IN THE SPACE AT THE RIGHT.*

1. Besides *increasing* intestinal motility, carbamachol may be expected to — 1.____
   A. raise blood pressure
   B. *increase* bile flow
   C. *increase* salivation
   D. pyuria
   E. mydriasis

2. The drug that is contraindicated in acute pancreatitis in the dog is — 2.____
   A. prednisolone
   B. meperidine
   C. penicillin
   D. morphine
   E. atropine

3. Hemophilia in Irish setters is a sex-linked recessive defect affecting males. In this defect, the clotting time is prolonged. This can be *temporarily* alleviated by administering — 3.____
   A. calcium gluconate
   B. serum trypsinase
   C. vitamin K
   D. fibrinogen
   E. thromboplastin

4. In the horse, the acute abdominal pain associated with spasmodic colic can BEST be alleviated by administration of — 4.____
   A. $NaSO_4$
   B. atropine
   C. mineral oil
   D. physostigmiral
   E. lentin

5. The use of aspirin in cats is BEST described as — 5.____
   A. safe if given 10 gr/day for a few days
   B. safe if given in combination with A/3 or cortisone
   C. safe with alkalinizing substances such as $CaCO_3$
   D. toxic *even* in doses of 5 gr/day for a week
   E. toxic in doses of 15 gr/day or MORE over long periods

6. In treating congestive heart failure in dogs, you should — 6.____
   A. balance the electrolytes and *increase* the sodium intake
   B. give IV fluids to combat dehydration
   C. restrict fluid intake to help combat ascites
   D. give a salt-free diet high in animal protein
   E. restrict sodium intake and *increase* sodium excretion

7. Besides *increasing* intestinal motility, carbamachol may be expected to — 7.____
   A. raise blood pressure
   B. *increase* bile flow
   C. *increase* salivation
   D. result in psyuria
   E. result in indriasis

8. The action of nicotine is usually at the ganglia, but with acute intoxication, death is due to — 8.____
   A. inhibition of the S.A. node
   B. increased bronchiola spasms
   C. respiratory failure caused by paralysis of the muscles of respiration
   D. inhibition of A-V node conduction
   E. increased bronchiolar secretions leading to death by drowning animal

9. Arecholine is used for esophageal obstruction because it — 9.____
   A. produces mild tetany of esophageal muscle
   B. produces rhythmic peristalsis
   C. stimulates secretion of saliva which aids passage of food
   D. produces reversed peristalsis which ejects the obstruction
   E. relaxes the esophagus

10. How would you counteract an eye that had just been treated with a local midriotic? — 10.____
   A. Pitrissin
   B. Flurocein
   C. Atropine sulfate
   D. Physostigamine
   E. Cocainehydrochloride

11. A large group of chemicals that have a benzene ring as part of their structure are especially dangerous to animals and man because of their ability to induce — 11.____
   A. disecting aneurysm and aortic rupture
   B. proliferative dermatitis
   C. aplastic anemia
   D. liver infarction and necrosis
   E. peripheral vascular necrosis

12. The calcemic effect obtained by the administration of a massive dose of vitamin D to dairy cows may be expected to last for — 12.____
   A. 30 minutes
   B. approximately 3 hours
   C. 1 or 2 days
   D. 2 weeks
   E. an undetermined length of time

13. Penicillin, streptomycin, and sulfonamides have been determined to be of value in treating — 13.____
   A. coccidoidomycosis
   B. mucormycosis
   C. aspergillosis
   D. histoplasmosis
   E. nocardia

14. Lactic acid that accumulates in the forestomachs following CHO engorgement is neutralized MOST safely by the addition of — 14.____
   A. $NaHCO_3$
   B. $Mg(OH)_2$
   C. electrolytes
   D. $MgSO_4$
   E. oil of turpentine

15. The anesthetic that causes the *greatest* irritation to the respiratory tract of the dog is 15.____ A D
A. pentobarbital sodium B. chloroform
C. fluothane D. ether
E. thropental sodium

16. Administration of Ca I.V. can, in some cases, result in heart block. 16.____ C
It is MOST satisfactorily treated with
A. Na bicarbonate B. epinephrine
C. atropine D. dextrose
E. lactated ringers

17. Given orally, __________ have specific stimulant effects on the large intestine. 17.____ B C
A. lubricant oils B. irritant oils
C. emodin cathartics D. osmotic cathartics
E. hydrophyllic colloids

18. Polaxalene acts in controlling bloat by 18.____ B
A. *increasing* rumen motility
B. *decreasing* froth
C. *increasing* rumen peristalsis
D. *decreasing* gas formation
E. inducing regurgitation

19. Which of the following is NOT cholinergic? 19.____ D
A. Preganglionic sympathetic
B. Preganglionic parasympathetic
C. Somatic
D. Postganglionic sympathetic
E. Postganglionic parasympathetic

20. The addition of DOCA to a dog 20.____ A E
A. *increases* Na excretion and *decreases* K+ excretion
B. *increases* blood glucose
C. *decreases* blood glucose
D. *decreases* circulating eosinophilus
E. *decreases* Na excretion and *increases* K+ excretion

21. A potent, dangerous and sometimes fatal drug interaction can occur when an animal on anticholinesterase treatment is given 21.____ D
A. epinephrine B. penicillin
C. corticosteroids D. succinylcholine
E. phenylbutazone

22. 72 PPM is equivalent to 22.____ A
A. .072 mg/kg B. 7.2 ug/100 ml C. 7.2 ug/mg
D. 72 lb/ton E. 72 mg/kg

23. A toxoid is a(n) 23.____ C
A. bacterin B. specific antitoxin
C. detoxified toxin D. vaccine
E. anaculture

24. You are presented with a comatose dog that consumed an unknown old medication. 24. B
Which of the following would do LEAST harm and MOST good?
A. Activated charcoal
B. 30% $O_2$
C. Saline Cathartic
D. Phenobarbital
E. IV Saline

25. An antibiotic that is NOT potentially nephrotoxic for use in a male cat with cystitis - urethritis - obstruction syndrome is 25. B
A. bacitracin
B. penicillin G.
C. kanamycin
D. gentomycin
E. streptomycin

---

# KEY (CORRECT ANSWERS)

1. C
2. D
3. D
4. B
5. D
6. E
7. C
8. C
9. C
10. D
11. C
12. E
13. E
14. B
15. D
16. C
17. E
18. B
19. D
20. E
21. D
22. A
23. C
24. B
25. B

# TEST 3

DIRECTIONS: Each question or incomplete statement is followed by several suggested answers or completions. Select the one that BEST answers the question or completes the statement. *PRINT THE LETTER OF THE CORRECT ANSWER IN THE SPACE AT THE RIGHT.*

1. A *narcotic* analgesic that can be used safely as a pre-anesthetic agent in cats is 1. _____
   A. chlorpromazine B. meperidine C. morphine
   D. thiopental E. heroin

2. In heart disease accompanied by acute congestive heart failure, epinephrine is 2. _____
   A. a useful cardiac stimulant
   B. dangerous and, with few exceptions, should never be given
   C. effective to initiate ventricular contractions in auricular fibrillation
   D. indicated when edema is severe to *increase* venous return and *decrease* vascular congestion
   E. dangerous because it may cause heart block

3. Which *one* of the following cardiac glycosides requires the *longest* time to exhibit its maximal cardiac effect? 3. _____
   A. Digitoxin B. Digoxin C. Lanatoside C
   D. Ouabain E. Deslanoside

4. One of the *principal* side effects resulting from prolonged therapy with corticosteroids is attributable to excessive retention of 4. _____
   A. potassium B. sodium C. nitrogen
   D. phosphorus E. calcium

5. In horses, nutritional secondary hyperparathyroidism MOST often results from feeding 5. _____
   A. excessive amounts of grain and minimal amounts of legume hay
   B. excessive amounts of grain and minimal amounts of grass hay
   C. corn for the grain portion and alfalfa for the hay portion of the diet
   D. hay ad lib and NOT feeding any grain
   E. a milk replacer supplement to horses who are already on a grain ration containing 14% protein

6. Iron deficiency anemia is *common* in the nursing young of ALL species because 6. _____
   A. *only* elemental iron can be absorbed and divalent iron *only* is available to the nursing young
   B. the iron in milk is chelated and absorption is prevented

C. even though sufficient iron is available, erythropoiesis is inadequate to maintain normal hemoglobin levels
D. rapid neonatal growth *increases* demands for hemoglobin synthesis, but the ability for intestinal absorption of iron has not been developed
E. milk, their *primary* source of nutrients, provides an amount of iron *lower* than the requirement

7. Naturally occurring iso-immune hemolytic anemia (neonatal hemolytic anemia) has been observed MOST frequently in — 7.____
A. horses B. dogs C. cats D. cattle E. sheep

8. Feline infectious anemia is caused by — 8.____
A. ancylostoma caninum
B. hemobartonella felis
C. isospora felis
D. ctenocephalides felis
E. feline distemper virus

9. Which of the following findings is pathognomonic of brucellosis in the mature bovine? — 9.____
A. Lowered milk production, chronic metritis, and temporary infertility in the female
B. Enlargement and abscessation of the genital organs of the male
C. Demonstration of the causative organisms in the outer layer of cells of the chorion expelled after the fetus is aborted
D. History of abortion in the third trimester of pregnancy in several cows in the herd
E. Lymphadenopathy, hygroma, and gonitis with an accumulation of fluid

10. In the United States, the *greatest* number of reported cases of rabies in farm animals occur in — 10.____
A. goats B. cattle C. sheep
D. pigs E. horses

11. Clinical manifestations and herd history are NOT adequate to differentiate vibriosis from — 11.____
A. trichomoniasis
B. mycotic abortion
C. brucellosis
D. enzootic bovine abortion
E. leptospirosis

12. Abortions have occurred in a herd of cows, which have temperatures of 104$^{o}$ to 106$^{o}$, atypical mastitis with a flaccid udder, and coffee or wine-colored urine. The disease which should be suspected is — 12.____
A. brucellosis B. trichomoniasis
C. staphylococcus mastitis D. leptospirosis
E. vibriosis

13. In a herd of calves, death losses have occurred that are attributable to parasitism. The *predominant* parasites being large stomach worms (haemonchus), intestinal hairworms (trichostrongylus), thread-necked strongyles (nematodirus), and lungworms (dictyocaulus). The drug of *choice* for rational treatment to *minimize* further losses is 13.____
   A. levamisole  B. diethylcarbamazine
   C. haloxon  D. thiabendazole
   E. phenothiazine

14. The MOST important aspect of treatment of feline distemper is the 14.____
   A. performance of blood transfusions
   B. maintenance of fluids and electrolytes
   C. administration of penicillin
   D. use of oxygen therapy
   E. administration of antisera

15. The MOST effective and specific treatment for clinical giardiasis in a young puppy is administration of 15.____
   A. bacitracin  B. atabrine
   C. dihydrostreptomycin  D. dismuth subnitrate
   E. sulfadimethoxine

16. The sign that is considered to be pathognomonic for salt poisoning in swine is 16.____
   A. frequent urination
   B. ecchymoses on the pericardium
   C. acute gastritis
   D. eosinophilic meningoencephalitis
   E. subcutaneous edema

17. The MOST effective treatment for salmonellosis in the dog is administration of 17.____
   A. dihydrostreptomycin  B. isoniazid
   C. chloramphenicol  D. hetacillin
   E. erythromycin

18. Cyanosis and a dark chocolate discoloration of blood in sheep or cattle suggest poisoning due to 18.____
   A. nitrates  B. aldrin  C. arsenic
   D. cyanide  E. lead

19. The contagious disease MOST likely to cause diarrhea, NO vomiting, dehydration, a *low* to *high* mortality, and high morbidity in baby pigs is 19.____
   A. colibacillosis
   B. swine erysipelas
   C. salmonellosis
   D. swine dysentery
   E. transmissible gastroenteritis

20. When urea is fed to the ruminant, it becomes particularly important to provide a generous amount of 20.____
   A. fat  B. carbohydrates  C. vitamins
   D. minerals  E. proteins

21. Atropine sulfate, a therapeutic agent used in the treatment of periodic ophthalmia in horses, is useful in 21. D
   A. preventing excessive lacrimation and tear-scalding of the face
   B. reducing the overall tenseness caused by the pain because it relaxes smooth muscle
   C. reducing inflammation and *decreasing* the number of blood-borne spirochetes that cause the condition
   D. preventing adhesions between the iris and the lens
   E. preventing excessive light damage to the internal structures of the eye by constricting the pupil

22. A *high* reticulocyte count in an anemic animal *generally* indicates that the 22. E
   A. disease is caused by a filtrable virus
   B. animal has an iron deficiency anemia
   C. hematopoietic tissues are completely aplastic
   D. proportion of old cells to young cells is in favor of the old cells
   E. hematopoietic tissues are responding by an *increased* erythropoiesis

23. The antibiotic that is MOST likely to induce resistance in initially susceptible bacteria is 23. B
   A. chlortetracycline
   B. streptomycin
   C. penicillin
   D. erythromycin
   E. neomycin

24. Dilation of the pupil will result from the use of 24. C
   A. arecoline
   B. eserine
   C. atropine
   D. lentin
   E. pilocarpine

25. During effective epidural procaine anesthesia, pain is blocked, *usually* without interference with motor function, because 25. C
   A. the sensory neurons are in the dorsal quadrants of the cord and in contact with the strongest concentrations of procaine
   B. procaine is selective for dorsal horn neurons which receive pain impulses
   C. pain fibers are small and/or unmyelinated
   D. motor neurons and their processes are inherently refractory to procaine
   E. the dentate ligaments prevent procaine from coming in contact with the ventral roots of the spinal nerves

---

# KEY (CORRECT ANSWERS)

| | | |
|---|---|---|
| 1. B | 11. A | 21. D |
| 2. B | 12. D | 22. E |
| 3. A | 13. A | 23. B |
| 4. B | 14. A | 24. C |
| 5. B | 15. B | 25. C |
| 6. E | 16. D | |
| 7. A | 17. C | |
| 8. B | 18. A | |
| 9. D | 19. D | |
| 10. B | 20. B | |

---

# EXAMINATION SECTION

# TEST 1

DIRECTIONS: Each question or incomplete statement is followed by several suggested answers or completions. Select the one that BEST answers the question or completes the statement. *PRINT THE LETTER OF THE CORRECT ANSWER IN THE SPACE AT THE RIGHT.*

1. Viruses are satisfactorily cultivated in — 1. ____
   A. chick embryo
   B. egg-glycerin agar
   C. litmus milk
   D. none of the above

2. Once a virus has penetrated the cells of a susceptible host it — 2. ____
   A. cannot be affected by specific Ab
   B. can be affected by Ab which enters the cell by pinocytosis
   C. can be affected by intra-nuclear Ab
   D. can be destroyed by interferon

3. Agglutination of bacteria with homologous antiserum is enhanced by (or occurs with) — 3. ____
   A. incubation at 37°C
   B. complement
   C. conglutinen
   D. reduced $O_2$ tension

4. The nucleic acid structure of an RNA virus contains the soluble antigen of the virus as well as — 4. ____
   A. the type-specific properties of the virus such as hemadsorption and hemagglutination
   B. information for replication of the virus
   C. lipid and protein substances
   D. the measure of the viral invasiveness

5. Leptospirosis can be differentiated from other pathogenic spirochetes by — 5. ____
   A. cultural character
   B. relative pathogenicity for lab animals
   C. morphology
   D. any of the above

6. The organism that moves by flagella is — 6. ____
   A. trypanasoma equipendium
   B. entomoeba histolytica
   C. isopora bigemina
   D. all of the above

7. Bacteria and yeasts are differenciated from molds because they are — 7. ____
   A. saprophytes
   B. multicellular
   C. colored
   D. non-lactose fermenters

8. An obligate anacrobe is one which MUST grow in  8.____
   A. the presence of free oxygen
   B. reduced $O_2$ tension
   C. 10% $CO_2$
   D. 50% $CO_2$

9. The media of choice MOST often used for the cultivation of the gonococcus is  9.____
   A. desoxycholate citrate agar
   B. blood agar
   C. desoxycholate agar
   D. chocolate agar

10. The man who first discovered that VES was caused by a different virus than either FMD or VS was:  10.____
    A. Salmon  B. Meyer  C. Troum  D. Goodpasture

11. The MOST reliable test for detecting leptospira antibodies is  11.____
    A. complement fixation
    B. macroscopic agglutination test
    C. Stoenner test
    D. microscopic agglutination (Lysis test)

12. A positive coagulase test with a culture of staph  12.____
    A. means the organism is *probably* pathogenic
    B. means the organism is *probably* non-pathogenic
    C. is *never* obtained
    D. is *always* obtained

13. Which TB strains affect swine?  13.____
    A. Human  B. Avian and human
    C. Avian, human and bovine  D. Bovine and avian

14. Lactogenic immunity refers to the process of immunizing the dam prior to parturition in an attempt to establish high levels of antibody in the neonate via passive immunity through the colostrum.  14.____
    This is practiced in
    A. bluetongue
    B. ICH
    C. feline viral rhinetracheitis
    D. TGE

15. Anthrax organisms in direct smears that are suitably stained and obtained from recently dead animals appear as  15.____
    A. pairs of gram + rods with spores
    B. chains of gram + rods WITHOUT spores
    C. long gram + filamentous rods WITHOUT spores
    D. chain of gram - rods WITHOUT spores

16. Pasteurella pestis injected into a rabbit will NOT produce 16. ____
   A. bacteriolytic amboceptor  B. hemagglutinin
   C. complement  D. bacteriolysin

17. A pasteurization resistant organism is 17. ____
   A. salmonella typhosa  B. staph
   C. strep  D. corynebacteria

18. The organism that belongs to the class sporozoa is 18. ____
   A. balintidium minutum  B. entomoeba histolytica
   C. plasmodium vivax  D. trypanasoma

19. Coxiella bruneti can BEST be cultured on 19. ____
   A. tryptose broth with .1% dextrose
   B. the yolk sac of embroyonated eggs
   C. any bacteriologic media under anaerobic conditions
   D. noguchis leptospira media

20. A highly contagious viral disease of cattle which is characterized by a rapidly febrile course, inflammation of the mucous membranes, and a mortality of 90-95% is 20. ____
   A. foot and mouth disease  B. virus stomatitis
   C. malignant head catarrh  D. rinderpest

21. Bacilli of typhoid belong to the genus 21. ____
   A. salmonella  B. shigella
   C. clostridium  D. klebsiella

22. Potassium tellurite media is used to isolate 22. ____
   A. diphtheria  B. strep. faecalis
   C. S. schottmuelleri  D. Klebisella pneumoniae

23. The animal in the midwest U.S. with the highest incidence of rabies is the 23. ____
   A. fox  B. coyote  C. skunk  D. bat

24. One test used to identify pneumococci is the ____ test. 24. ____
   A. urease  B. coagulase
   C. bile solubility  D. Albert's

25. Bacteria from the genus salmonella and the genus shigella are generally 25. ____
   A. lactose  B. urease positive
   C. non-lactose fermenters  D. $H_2S$ positive

# KEY (CORRECT ANSWERS)

| | | |
|---|---|---|
| 1. A | 11. D | 21. A |
| 2. A | 12. A | 22. A |
| 3. B | 13. C | 23. C |
| 4. B | 14. D | 24. C |
| 5. C | 15. B | 25. C |
| 6. A | 16. B | |
| 7. B | 17. B | |
| 8. C | 18. C | |
| 9. D | 19. B | |
| 10. C | 20. D | |

# TEST 2

DIRECTIONS: Each question or incomplete statement is followed by several suggested answers or completions. Select the one that BEST answers the question or completes the statement. *PRINT THE LETTER OF THE CORRECT ANSWER IN THE SPACE PROVIDED AT THE RIGHT.*

1. Which of the following is acid-fast? 1.____
   A. Nocardia asteroides B. Actinomyces bovis
   C. Blastomyces D. Brucella absortus

2. An exotoxin is produced by 2.____
   A. C. diphtheria B. E. coli
   C. N. gonorrhea D. B. anthracis

3. In MOST bacterial infections, neutrophilia is evident UNLESS the infection 3.____
   A. is associated with a virus
   B. is immediate and overwhelming
   C. has a short course
   D. none of the above

4. The pathological bacteria which can remain after pasteurization is 4.____
   A. brucella abortus B. B. anthracis
   C. lactobacillus thermophilus D. E. coli

5. The bile solubility test is sometimes used to differentiate between 5.____
   A. staph and strep
   B. pneumococci and strep
   C. strep veridans and staph aureus
   D. any of the above

6. Jensen's Paracolon (salmonella dublin) causes 6.____
   A. severe disease in chicks B. severe disease in ducks
   C. enteritis in calves D. fowl pox

7. The introduction of a pyogenic organism along with Cl. tetani will 7.____
   A. provide suitable environment for Cl. to grow
   B. neutralize the toxin
   C. enhance the toxin
   D. change prototoxin to toxin

8. Equine viral rhinotracheitis differs from other respiratory infections in that 8.____
   A. abortion follows 3 to 4 weeks later
   B. it has an incubation period of 4 to 5 weeks
   C. it has a slow onset - 3 to 4 weeks
   D. the temperature remains near normal until the retrepharyngeal LN ruptures

9. Which of the following bacteria is non-motile? 9.____ A B
   A. C. botulinum B. Shigella paradysenteriae
   C. Aerobacter aerogenes D. Ps. aeruginosa

10. The cause of fowl typhoid is 10.____ C
    A. sal. pullorus B. sal. typhus
    C. sal. gallinarum D. haemophillus gallinarum

11. Generally speaking, viral isolation is based on 11.____ A C
    A. tissue location B. particle size
    C. cultural characteristics D. growth characteristics

12. Members of the genus corynebacterium are (G+ rod) 12.____ A
    A. gram positive pleiomorphic rods with some pathogenic species
    B. gram negative anaerobes
    C. acid-fast
    D. spore-forming

13. Viruses are MOST generally categorized by 13.____ A B
    A. tissues affecting
    B. particle size
    C. pathogenicity
    D. virulence in lab animals

14. Salmonella organisms are lactose 14.____ A
    A. *negative* and indole *negative*
    B. *negative* and salicin *positive*
    C. *positive* and salicin *negative*
    D. *negative* and urea *positive*

15. The agent causing a thick walled abscess in the bovine mammary gland is 15.____ D
    A. staphylococcus aureus
    B. escherichis coli
    C. strep. agalectra
    D. corynebacterium pyogenes

16. The phenomenon of virus inactivation in a virus suspension exposed to ether or chloroform indicates that the virus passes to a(n) 16.____ A C
    A. cell B. capsomere
    C. envelope D. nucleic acid

17. Salmonella typhi is found in milk when 17.____ B
    A. a person with S. typhi contaminates milk *before* pasteurization
    B. a person with S. typhi contaminates milk *after* pasteurization
    C. the cow has mastitis
    D. the bulk tank is contaminated

18. Which of the following is the method of infection for Botulism? 18.____
A. Ingestion of spores
B. Wound infection
C. Ingestion of toxin
D. Wound infection with type C. Clastridium

19. The equine piroplasmosis causative agent is a 19.____
A. virus B. bacterium C. protozoan D. ricksettsia

20. Vibriosis in cows and heifers is primarily manifested as 20.____
A. abortion in the 3rd trimester
B. abortion in the 2nd trimester
C. vaginitis
D. infertility

21. Leptospirosis in cattle, in its clinical manifestations, frequently resembles 21.____
A. vibriosis and listeriosis
B. vibriosis
C. brucellosis, trichomoniasis, and vibriosis
D. brucellosis and listeriosis

22. Defense mechanisms of the animal body are usually activated by a specific 22.____
A. antigen B. opsonin C. reagin D. hemolysin

23. The virus of bluetongue in the U.S. has been isolated 23.____
A. only from sheep
B. east of the Mississippi River
C. only from cattle and sheep
D. from sheep, cattle, bighorn sheep, and white-tailed deer

24. The TB test includes 24.____
A. visual observation for 72 hours
B. palpation for 72 hours
C. recording any abnormalities that might confuse observations
D. all of the above

25. Anaplasmasis in bovines in the United States is caused by anaplasma 25.____
A. bigeminum B. centrale C. parva D. marginale

# KEY (CORRECT ANSWERS)

1. A
2. A
3. B
4. C
5. B

6. C
7. A
8. A
9. B
10. C

11. C
12. A
13. B
14. A
15. D

16. C
17. B
18. C
19. C
20. D

21. C
22. A
23. D
24. D
25. D

# EXAMINATION SECTION

## TEST 1

DIRECTIONS: Each question or incomplete statement is followed by several suggested answers or completions. Select the one that BEST answers the question or completes the statement. *PRINT THE LETTER OF THE CORRECT ANSWER IN THE SPACE AT THE RIGHT.*

1. The MOST widely accepted theory explaining why some viruses produce long lasting immunity is the __________ theory of immunity. 1.____
   A. cellular B. humoral
   C. side chain D. ribosomal

2. Immune tolerance is due to 2.____
   A. exposure to an antigen *before* the development of immune competence
   B. repeated injection of antigen
   C. exposure to large doses of toxic substances
   D. exposure to an antigen during the development of immune competence

3. In the Kingdom Protista, the Eucarions have 3.____
   A. nuclei that are free in the cytoplasm
   B. discrete nuclei within the cytoplasm
   C. chromatin that is NOT contained in the nuclei
   D. NO endoplasmic reticulum

4. Toxoplasma are classified as 4.____
   A. bacteria B. protozoa C. amoeba D. fungi

5. Temperature at which Q fever is killed 5.____
   A. 5-60 B. 60-70 C. 70-80 D. 80-90

6. A TOXOID is a(n) 6.____
   A. bacterin B. anaculture
   C. de-toxified toxin D. anti-serum

7. A tissue culture is useful in primary field isolations of a viral agent because 7.____
   A. cytopathogenic effects permit definite identification
   B. it provides ready availability of a homologous and non-homologous host without antigens
   C. a tissue culture is resistant to non-specific toxins produced by virus
   D. only one species of virus grow in a tissue culture

8. Cyclopropagation is demonstrated by 8.____
   A. human epidemic plague B. leismaniasis
   C. anaplasmosis D. tabanus and anthrax

9. In what area does bluetongue MOSTLY occur? 9.____
A. New England
B. Pacific Northwest
C. West-Southwest
D. South

10. The MOST reliable test for detecting leptospira antibodies is 10.____
A. complement fixation
B. macroscopic agglutination test
C. the Stoenner test
D. microscopic agglutination-lysis test

11. Coils of yellow wavy threads found in sputum are 11.____
A. Dittrich's plugs
B. cotton fibers
C. Curschman's spirals
D. elastic

12. The intermediate host for dipylidium canis is 12.____
A. culex
B. ctenocephalides
C. ticks
D. lice

13. The diagnosis of lepto in cattle should NOT be solely based on 13.____
A. clinical signs and necropsy
B. F.A.
C. injection of guinea pig
D. examination for spirochetes

14. Botulism is unlike other food poisonings in that it has 14.____
A. signs that might NOT be *only* gastrointestinal
B. a *shorter* incubation period
C. a *longer* incubation period
D. toxins NOT killed by cooking

15. A ________ sample should be taken to make a diagnosis of anthrax in swine. 15.____
A. blood
B. bronchial lymph node
C. pharyngeal lymph node
D. kidney

16. The MOST common leptospira in cattle and swine is 16.____
A. icterohemorrhagicum
B. pomona
C. canicola
D. hardjoe

17. Atropine sulfate, a drug used in the treatment of periodic ophthalmia of horses is used to 17.____
A. *decrease* tear production and reduce facial scald
B. *decrease* pain because of relaxation of smooth muscle spasms
C. *decrease* damage to intraocular structures due to light by constricting the pupil
D. prevent adhesion of the iris to the cornea

18. The latent period is an important consideration for 18.____
A. picorna
B. myxo
C. herpes
D. parvo

19. Feline infectious peritonitis shows — 19. ~~A~~ C
    A. enteritis B. anorexia
    C. depression D. leucopenia

20. Relief of a viscid mucus is provided with — 20. D
    A. atropine B. pilocarpine
    C. oxygen D. a steam chamber

21. The MOST irritating anesthetic to the respiratory tract is — 21. B
    A. halothane B. ether
    C. chloroform D. thiopental

22. The BEST chemical disinfectant for premises after viral disease is — 22. ~~D~~ B
    A. cresol and soap B. NaOH
    C. creolin D. phenol

23. A positive serum neutralization test is indicated. This suggests the animal has — 23. A
    A. been infected with an organism in the past
    B. active disease
    C. been vaccinated *over* five years ago
    D. had symptoms in the past

24. The nematode NOT capable of transplacental infection is — 24. ~~A~~ B
    A. strongyloides stercoralis
    B. neoascaris vitulorium
    C. ascaris suum
    D. toxocara canis ~ round

25. Thrush is an infection of mucous membranes caused by — 25. A
    A. candida albicans
    B. aspergillus
    C. blastomyces dermatiditis
    D. streptococcus

26. What type of antibody is produced in viral immunity? — 26. ~~B~~ C
    A. Hemagglutinin - inhibition
    B. Complement - fixation antibody
    C. Neutralizing antibody
    D. Agglutinin antibody

27. The virus type BEST known for its latency is — 27. C
    A. corona B. reo
    C. herpes D. pácorna ~~ona~~ ← PICORNA

28. The M. tuberculosis was discovered by — 28. B
    A. Laennec B. Pasteur
    C. Koch D. Lister

29. Early in a case of typhoid fever, the test that is *most likely* to be positive is the 29.____
A. Widal test B. blood culture
C. Stool culture D. CF test

30. Pneumococci may be distinguished from strep. by 30.____
A. morphology B. staining reaction
C. solubility in bile D. precipitating

31. Cultures for Brucella infections should be cultured in a(n) 31.____
A. atmosphere of 10% $CO_2$ B. normal atmosphere
C. anaerobic atmosphere D. atmosphere of 50% $CO_2$

32. Russel's double sugar agar contains 32.____
A. dextrose and sucrose B. lactose and sucrose
C. dextrose and lactose D. glucose and lactose

33. Shigella paradysenteriae produces 33.____
A. acid and gas from dextrose
B. acid from lactose
C. acid from dextrose
D. base from lactose

34. The spreading type of growth of the proteus group of bacteria may be inhibited through addition to the media of 34.____
A. chloral hydrate B. thioglycollic acid
C. brom-cresol purple D. brom-thymol blue

35. The etiological agent of lymphocytic choriomeningitis is a(n) 35.____
A. anaerobic bacterium B. spirochaete
C. virus D. mite

36. The action of heparin is promptly terminated by 36.____
A. menedione B. methylene blue
C. vitamin $K_1$ D. protamine sulfate

37. Quinidine sulfate is used in heart disease because it 37.____
A. depresses cardiac muscle
B. stimulates cardiac muscle
C. abolishes sympathetic response
D. abolishes parasympathetic response

38. The nerve supplying all the intrinsic muscles of the larynx EXCEPT the cricothyroid muscle is the ________ nerve. 38.____
A. cranial laryngeal B. mylohyoid
C. caudal laryngeal D. glossopharyngeal

39. The MOST common bacterial isolate from uterine infections in the mare is 39.____
A. staph. aureus
B. corynebacterium pyogenes
C. pseudomonas SPP
D. strep. zooepidemicus

40. Which is NOT, so far as is known, a factor causing luteal regression? 40. B
A. Prostaglandins
B. Oxytocin
C. Aging of luteal cells
D. FSH

---

# KEY (CORRECT ANSWERS)

| | | | |
|---|---|---|---|
| 1. A | 11. A | 21. B | 31. A |
| 2. B | 12. B | 22. B | 32. C |
| 3. B | 13. A | 23. A | 33. A |
| 4. B | 14. A | 24. B | 34. A |
| 5. B | 15. C | 25. A | 35. C |
| 6. C | 16. B | 26. C | 36. D |
| 7. A | 17. D | 27. C | 37. A |
| 8. C | 18. C | 28. C | 38. C |
| 9. C | 19. C | 29. B | 39. D |
| 10. D | 20. D | 30. C | 40. B |

# TEST 2

DIRECTIONS: Each question or incomplete statement is followed by several suggested answers or completions. Select the one that BEST answers the question or completes the statement. *PRINT THE LETTER OF THE CORRECT ANSWER IN THE SPACE AT THE RIGHT.*

1. Bluetongue is transmitted by the 1.____
   A. tabanid B. gnat C. tick D. contact

2. The parasite that causes cardiovascular problems in the dog is 2.____
   A. T. canis
   B. strongyloides
   C. dirofilaria immitus
   D. diplydium caninuin

3. A cow is presented for slaughter with cancer. The cow is cachectic and has open abscesses. 3.____
   What should be done with the cow?
   A. Slaughtered and cooked
   B. Condemned, slaughtered, and tanked
   C. Condemn head and pass the rest of the carcass
   D. Sold for treatment

4. Squamous cell carcinoma has spread from the eye to the paratid lymph node in an animal. What should be done with the animal? 4.____
   A. Condemn it
   B. Condemn head and tongue
   C. Condemn head, tongue, and liver
   D. Condemn lungs, spleen, and liver

5. Foodborne disease caused by intoxication is characteristic of 5.____
   A. botulism
   B. salmonella
   C. trichinella
   D. shigella

6. Rancid milk is caused by 6.____
   A. lipase activity
   B. improper cooling
   C. coliform container
   D. *increased* leukocytes

7. A mold that is extremely dangerous to handle as it bursts into spores is 7.____
   A. coccidiodimites
   B. histo
   C. blasto
   D. cryptococcus neoformas

8. Which of the following is NOT suitable to use to concentrate sputum? 8.____
   A. trisodium phosphate
   B. sodium hypochlorite
   C. oxalic acid
   D. citric acid

9. Growth of the more fastidious forms of the Neisseria is enhanced by the addition to the medium of — 9. A
   A. bile
   B. yeast concentrate
   C. p-aminobenzoic acid
   D. lymph

10. To examine a smear for Koch's bacillus, you might do a(n) — 10. C
   A. Gram's stain
   B. .Albert's stain
   C. Ziehl-Neilson stain
   D. any of the above

11. Hemophilus pertussis is BEST isolated on — 11. C
   A. dextrose starch agar
   B. Bordet Gengou media
   C. blood agar
   D. any of the above

12. Klebsiella pneumoniae *closely* resembles — 12. B
   A. diplococcus pneumonia
   B. A. aerogenes
   C. P. aeroginosa
   D. E. coli

13. The term ANTISEPSIS means the process of — 13. B
   A. destruction of bacteria
   B. inhibition of bacterial growth
   C. destruction of the toxins produced by bacteria
   D. promotion of bacterial growth

14. Charcot-leyden crystals are — 14. B
   A. rhomboidal
   B. hexagonal
   C. octagonal
   D. round

15. Bile acts on pneumococci as a(n) — 15. A
   A. solvent
   B. inhibitor
   C. enhancer
   D. activator

16. Bile in media for culturing S. typhosa acts as a(n) — 16. A
   A. enhancer
   B. solvent
   C. inhibitor
   D. activator

17. Group A streptococci are *primarily* pathogenic for — 17. B
   A. cattle
   B. humans
   C. horses
   D. dogs

18. The Freil test is a specific intradermal test for — 18. C
   A. influenza
   B. rabies
   C. lymphogranulor inguinale
   D. scrapie

19. The stain used for Vincent's angina is — 19. B
   A. Gram's
   B. carbol fuchsin
   C. gentian violet
   D. Wright's

20. Fecal contamination of water can be suspected if examination reveals the presence of — 20. A
   A. E. coli
   B. S. typhosa
   C. Shigella dysenteriae
   D. S. aureus

21. A few RBC's seen microscopically will give a benzidine test that is 21.B____
   A. *always* negative
   B. *sometimes* positive
   C. *always* positive
   D. NEVER negative

22. Dittrich's plugs originate in the 22.C____
   A. nophron
   B. alveoli
   C. bronchi
   D. trachea

23. The fluorescent antibody principle is based on 23.A____
   A. conjugation of fluorescine with a specific antibody
   B. fluorescents of particles greater than 2600 A
   C. fluorescents of antigen
   D. conjugation of antigen

24. Members of the genus Nocardia are 24.____
   A. anaerobic
   B. occasionally pathogenic
   C. *completely* harmless to man
   D. viral

25. An abscess in the jowl of swine would MOST probably isolate 25.A____
   A. streptococcus
   B. brucella
   C. brysipilas
   D. trichinella

26. A characteristic of bacillus anthrasis that is of great practical importance to the control of the spread of the disease is that it 26.____
   A. demands gaseous oxygen for the formation of spores
   B. requires anaerobic conditions for growth
   C. can live in near-sterile conditions
   D. is found in the blood stream as chains

27. Complement fixation antigen can BEST be produced in tissue culture rather than from the intact animal because it is 27.C____
   A. obtained easily in large volume
   B. easily concentrated
   C. free of complement fixing antibodies
   D. easily assimilated to the conditions

28. A micron is 28.____
   A. 1/2500 of an inch
   B. 1/100 of a centimeter
   C. 1/1000 of a millimeter
   D. 1/100 of a millimeter

29. The BEST illumination for observing colored objects is 29.____
   A. central illumination with bright light
   B. indirect light with low light
   C. central illumination with low light
   D. direct illumination with low light

30. Magnification for a microscope using a 10X ocular and 1.8 objective is __________ diameters. 30. ____
A. 950 B. 200 C. 450 D. 180

31. The objective of the microscope is BEST cleaned with lens paper moistened with 31. ____
A. xylene
B. alcohol
C. water
D. any lens cleaning fluid

32. The spirochete of relapsing fever is stained MOST conveniently 32. ____
A. with Wright's stain
B. by silver impregnation
C. after taking the RBC's
D. Albert's stain

33. MOST bacteria are 33. ____
A. faculative *anaerobes*
B. faculative *aerobes*
C. obligate *aerobes*
D. obligate *anaerobes*

34. When staph. on blood agar produces a lemon yellow color, they are known as staph. 34. ____
A. aureus
B. albus
C. citreus
D. chloraesius

35. Diphtheriae produces a potent 35. ____
A. exotoxin
B. endotoxin
C. hemolysin
D. enzyme

36. Albert's stain is used to study: 36. ____
A. C. diphtheriae
B. Actinomyces bovis
C. P. malariae
D. Koch's bacillus

37. Paratyphoid B refers to: 37. ____
A. S. paratyphi
B. S. shotmuelleri
C. S. chloraesius
D. None of the above

38. Q fever is caused by a 38. ____
A. fungus
B. virus
C. rickettsiae
D. bacterium

39. It is INCORRECT to say that the virus of T.G.E. of swine 39. ____
A. withstands freezing and chemical sterilization, but not heat sterilization
B. is thought to be host specific as far as producing clinical disease
C. is found in ALL tissues, feces, and vomitus
D. persists for weeks in recovered clinical cases

40. The tissue of CHOICE for examination in suspected mycotic abortion in the bovine is the 40. ____
A. placenta
B. fetal skin
C. fetal liver
D. fetal intestine

41. The bacterium moraxella bovis can often be isolated from a disease of cattle characterized by inflammation of the 41. B
   A. brain and spinal cord
   B. cornea and conjunctiva
   C. kidneys and ureters
   D. trachea and bronchi

42. The opsonic index is a measure of the ability of a test serum to enhance 42. C
   A. precipitation
   B. aggsegation
   C. phagocytosis
   D. bacterolysis

43. A pathogen of animals that stains acid-fast is 43. B
   A. corynebacterium pyogenes
   B. mycobacterium aviun
   C. actenomyces bovis
   D. E. coli

44. Specific infectious pyelonephritis of the cow is caused by 44. D
   A. clostridium septicum
   B. staphylococcus aureus
   C. corynebacterium pyogenes
   D. corynebacterium renal

45. The BEST media for the growth of C. diphtheriae is 45. C
   A. Endo's media
   B. EMB
   C. Leoffler's
   D. egg-glycerin agar

46. Autoclaving culture media 46. B
   A. does NOT change the pH
   B. tends to make it MORE acid
   C. tends to make it MORE alkaline
   D. changes the pH depending on the organism

47. Sucrose may be added to Klinger's Iron Agar for a MORE rapid identification of 47. A
   A. E. coli
   B. salmonella
   C. paracolon group
   D. C. botulinum

48. A coagulase test is indicated upon isolation of 48. A
   A. staph. aureus
   B. staph. albus
   C. staph. citreus
   D. NONE of the above

49. Hansen's bacillus is the *same* as 49. B
   A. T. aeroginosa
   B. M. leprae
   C. listerrela monocytogenes
   D. E. coli

50. Cystine heart agar is used *especially* for the cultivation of 50. B
   A. neisseria
   B. pasteurella tularensis
   C. brucella abortus
   D. aerobacter aerogenes

# KEY (CORRECT ANSWERS)

| | | | | |
|---|---|---|---|---|
| 1. B | 11. C | 21. B | 31. A | 41. B |
| 2. C | 12. B | 22. C | 32. B | 42. C |
| 3. C | 13. B | 23. A | 33. A | 43. B |
| 4. A | 14. B | 24. A | 34. C | 44. D |
| 5. A | 15. A | 25. A | 35. A | 45. C |
| 6. A | 16. A | 26. A | 36. A | 46. B |
| 7. A | 17. B | 27. C | 37. B | 47. A |
| 8. B | 18. C | 28. C | 38. C | 48. A |
| 9. A | 19. B | 29. A | 39. C | 49. B |
| 10. C | 20. A | 30. C | 40. A | 50. B |

# EXAMINATION SECTION

## TEST 1

DIRECTIONS FOR THIS SECTION
Each question or incomplete statement is followed by several suggested answers or completions. Select the one that *BEST* answers the question or completes the statment. *PRINT THE LETTER OF THE CORRECT ANSWER IN THE SPACE AT THE RIGHT.*

1. Neoplasms involving the eye and its appendages in cattle are *most likely* to be caused by — 1. ...
   A. carcinoma
   B. adeno carcinoma
   C. carcinomatodes renis
   D. adenoma destruens
   E. adeonoma simplex
2. *Which* of the following anti-fungal antibiotics can be administered, using a 10-day dose *all at once?* — 2. ...
   A. Nystatin
   B. Griseofulvin
   C. Amphoteracin B
   D. Canicidin
   E. Manycin
3. Chronicity, lack of pruritis, bilateral alopecia, bilateral hyper-pigmentation are *all* important characteristics of — 3. ...
   A. parasitic dermatitis
   B. bacterial infection
   C. allergic skin condition
   D. endocrine imbalance
   E. oidial dermatitis
4. A clinical case of trichophyton equinum in the horse would appear as — 4. ...
   A. raw ulcerated disc-shaped lesions that leave a permanent scar
   B. skin blisters filled with a watery fluid that ruptures and heals
   C. disc-shaped skin-lesions devoid of hair, covered with gray to white scales
   D. all of the above
   E. none of the above
5. A swabbed-on taper-point needle is *best* for intestinal surgery because it — 5. ...
   A. is easily adapted to needle holder
   B. causes less tissue trauma
   C. easily passes through the intestine
   D. can be re-autoclaved easily
   E. easily passes through the kidney
6. Saddle thrombosis in cats is located in — 6. ...
   A. the pulmonary vein
   B. the iliac artery and post aorta
   C. the femoral vein
   D. a unilateral area
   E. a bilateral area
7. Pyloric stenosis is *best* treated by — 7. ...
   A. giving paregoric
   B. incising serosa and muscularis of pylorus
   C. passing a stomach tube
   D. incising mucosa and submucosa
   E. giving acetazolamide

8. Muco-purulent nasal discharge of sheep is a manifestation of — 8. ...
   - A. hypoderma infestation
   - B. gasterophilus
   - C. viral arteritis
   - D. oestrus ovis
   - E. fundus oculi

9. All of the following are threatened complications of traumatic gastritis *except* — 9. ...
   - A. traumatic pleuritis
   - B. metastatic pneumonia
   - C. liver abscess
   - D. gangrenous pneumonia
   - E. pulmonary adenomatosis

10. In considering bovine nasal discharge, one should remember that: — 10. ...
    - A. Copious unilateral discharge is considered pathognomonic for IBR.
    - B. Increased temperature and humidity will physiologically result in an increased bilateral discharge.
    - C. The appearance of coarse foam indicates pulmonary edema.
    - D. Slight mucous discharge is normally seen and the nostrils are licked clean.
    - E. Food material is commonly seen in ruminants and is due to rumination.

11. Ethylene glycol poisoning in a dog can be successfully treated if therapy is started early and the dog is given — 11. ...
    - A. massive doses of isotonic saline
    - B. large doses of ethanal and IP $NCO_3$
    - C. large doses of steroids
    - D. IV Pentobarbital
    - E. all the Gatorade he will drink

12. Equine encephalomyelitis virus attacks *primarily* the — 12. ...
    - A. cerebellum, causing hyperesthesis and atoxia
    - B. cerebrum, causing psychic changes
    - C. hypothalamus, causing hypothernuia, hyperphagia, and diabetes insipidus
    - D. hyperthalamus, causing physical changes
    - E. medulla, causing declining blood pressure and respiratory paralysis

13. If a dog has a dilated left pupil that is unresponsive to light in the left and right eyes, this indicates damage to the — 13. ...
    - A. left optic nerve
    - B. right optic nerve
    - C. left oculomotor
    - D. right oculomotor
    - E. left corviathracic gaglion

14. The lesions of acanthosis nigacans *begin* — 14. ...
    - A. in the axilla
    - B. in the groin
    - C. in the flank
    - D. under the chin
    - E. in the ears

15. Coxofemoral luxation in the dog is *usually* — 15. ...
    - A. anterio-dorsal
    - B. anterio-ventral
    - C. ventral
    - D. posterior dorsal
    - E. posterior

16. The anterior draw sign of cranial cruciate rupture is 16. ...
    - A. hypermotility of the patella
    - B. hyperflexion of the stifle
    - C. cranial gliding of the tibia
    - D. caudal gliding of the tibia
    - E. proximal rotation of the femur

17. Orchectomy is used to treat 17. ...
    - A. anal-gland adenoma
    - B. prostate carcinoma
    - C. adenoma diffusum
    - D. colloid carcinoma
    - E. adenoma sudoriparum

18. At *which time* does vaginal hyperplasia in the bitch occur *MOST* often? 18. ...
    - A. Following copulation
    - B. During estrus
    - C. Following estrus
    - D. Following whelping
    - E. During vaginitis

19. A factor which will limit the future usefulness of a cow with a vaginal prolapse is 19. ...
    - A. recurrence during a subsequent pregnancy
    - B. subsequent metritis
    - C. subsequent vaginitis
    - D. cervical atresia
    - E. subsequent vaginal structure

20. The optimum time for repair of hematoma of a bovine penis is 20. ...
    - A. within 24 hours
    - B. five to seven days past injury
    - C. two hours past injury
    - D. four weeks past injury
    - E. at most convenient time

21. The outstanding characteristics of chronic prostatic hyperplasia in a dog are: 21. ...
    - A. Anorexia, dysuria
    - B. Dysuria, pain on rectal palpation
    - C. Urinary retention and tenesmus
    - D. Urinary retention and perineal
    - E. Constipation and tenesmus

22. *Which* of the following *groups of drugs* is considered to be the *MOST* effective in preparing the bowel for colon surgery? 22. ...
    - A. Oxacillin, streptomycin
    - B. Kanamycin, neomycin, phthalysulfathiazole
    - C. Nitrofurantoin, greasiofuluin, oxytetracycline
    - D. Erythromycin, sulfasoxizole, lincomycin
    - E. Penicillin, amposillin, streptomycin

23. *Which* of the following layers of the small intestine is *strongest* and must be included in sutures in anastamosis to *MINIMIZE* dehiscence? The *tunica* 23. ...
    - A. *vaginalis*
    - B. *mucosa*
    - C. *submucosa*
    - D. *seiosa*
    - E. *muscularis*

24. In the dog, intestinal foreign bodies *MOST* frequently lodge in the 24. ...
    - A. duodenum
    - B. ileum

C. jejunum D. iliolecal valve
E. colon

25. *When* is the *BEST* time to fix a hematoma on a bull's penis? 25. ...
A. Five to seven days, when it is clotted
B. Five to seven days, when it is not clotted
C. One to three days, when it is clotted
D. One to three days, when it is not clotted
E. None of the above

26. In the electrocardiogram, the *P-R interval* is measured from 26. ...
A. beginning P - beginning R
B. beginning P - beginning ORS
C. end P - beginning R
D. end P - beginning ORS
E. beginning P - end R

27. In the equine abdominal cryptorchetic operation, the surgeon sections the testis by 27. ...
A. following an imaginary line from the neck of the bladder to the kidney
B. grasping the testis with his hand
C. forcing the testis into the inguinal ring
D. pushing the fecal balls in the small colon out of the way, leaving only the retained testis
E. following the gubernaculum testis or vas deferens to the retained testis

28. In an intestinal end-to-end anastomosis, the use of an eversion suture pattern results in 28. ...
A. quicker healing
B. postsurgical constriction
C. excellent potency
D. quicker innervation restoration
E. an increase in abscess formation

29. A *true* statement concerning a condition in equines called Lampas is that it 29. ...
A. is a thickening of the hard palate that occurs in old, smooth-mouth horses
B. occurs in horses 8-10 years' old
C. is a disease entity that involves swelling of the soft palate
D. is a physiological thickening of the hard palate in horses
E. occurs in horses 3-5 years' old

30. The *most common* condition resulting in congestive heart failure in the dog is: 30. ...
A. Aortic insufficiency
B. Ventricular septal defect
C. Mitral insufficiency
D. Tricusped insufficiency
E. Pulmonic stenosis

31. If there is complete loss of the right optic nerve and you shine a light in the right eye, the result is: 31. ...
    A. Normal vision but no pupillary response
    B. Loss of vision but normal pupillary in the right eye
    C. Loss of vision with no pupillary in either eye
    D. Loss of vision and left pupillary normal
    E. Loss of vision with left and right pupillary normal

32. A purulent discharge from the nose when the head is lowered in the horse is caused by: 32. ...
    A. Sinusitis
    B. Guttural pouch.
    C. Rhinosporidiosis
    D. Chronic catarrhal sinusitis
    E. Exophthalmic goiter

33. In a dog, auscultation of a PDA is *MOST* noticeable and diagnostic at the: 33. ...
    A. Left 2-3 ICS
    B. Right 2-3 ICS
    C. Left 6-7 ICS
    D. Right 6-7 ICS
    E. Left 7-8 ICS

34. Plasmacytomas produce an abnormal amount or number of 34. ...
    A. spinal fluid
    B. lymph
    C. albumen
    D. plasma
    E. immunoglobulins

35. Dogs exposed to ragweed develop an atopic sensitivity characterized by a(n) ________ reaction. 35. ...
    A. CF
    B. HI
    C. Prauznitzer-Haiyer
    D. hemagglutination
    E. complement - fixation

36. A puppy with tenderness in the region of the stomach, temperature of $104^{o}$, enlarged tonsils, petechiae of the mucous membranes, and a clotting time of 5 minutes, probably has: 36. ...
    A. Distemper
    B. ICH
    C. Foreign body
    D. Leptospirosis
    E. Acute tonsillitis

37. In cattle, acute pulmonary emphysema is *most often* associated with 37. ...
    A. moldy hay
    B. high grain intake
    C. frozen forage
    D. lush pastures in the fall
    E. grazing on mountain ranges

38. A cat is blocked with urinary sand; its *MOST* urgent need is: 38. ...
    A. Feed low ash diet
    B. Give urinary antiseptic
    C. Culture and sensitivity of the urine
    D. Relieve obstruction
    E. Give anal antiseptic

39. A horse shows stupor, uncoordination, spells of aimless walking, drags hind hoof, and has an icterus index of greater than 5. 39. ...
    The *correct* diagnosis is:
    A. Cirrhosis of the liver
    B. Encephalomalacia
    C. Congestion
    D. Hematapostasis
    E. Priapitis

40. Systolic bruits are due to 40. ...
   A. pericarditis
   B. A-V insufficiency
   C. semilunar valve insufficiency
   D. PDA
   E. A-V stenosis

41. *Which* is *NOT* a primary skin lesion? 41. ...
   A. Papule
   B. Macule
   C. Wheal
   D. Excoriation
   E. Pustule

42. The part of the electrocardiogram that is represented by the letter *T* is the 42. ...
   A. isoelectric period
   B. final upward or downward deflection
   C. upward curve corresponding to atrial contraction
   D. ventricular complex
   E. downward deflection

43. Left-sided congestive heart failure is *MOST* commonly characterized by: 43. ...
   A. Systolic murmur, liver congestion, increased heart rate, and ascites
   B. Diastolic murmur, pulmonary congestion, increased heart rate, and cough
   C. Diastolic murmur, sinus arrhythmia, cough, and fatigue
   D. Systolic murmur, sinus arrhythmia, cough, and fatigue
   E. Systolic murmur, pulmonary congestion, increased heart rate, and cough

44. Interdigital cysts are *BEST* treated by: 44. ...
   A. Cauterization
   B. Incision and curretage
   C. Surgical excision
   D. Caustic packs
   E. Icthamol packs

45. With reference to the differential diagnoses of *hemorrhagic colitis* and *idiopathic thrombocytopenia purpura*, they are*BEST* differentiated by the fact that in 45. ...
   A. hemorrhagic colitis there is projectile vomiting
   B. hemorrhagic colitis there is pallor of the mucous membranes
   C. thrombocytopenia purpura, there is subcutaneous and subscleral edema
   D. thrombocytopenia purpura, there are deep ulcers in the gums
   E. None of the above

46. A Woods light can be used to diagnose *what* condition in the dog? 46. ...
   A. Microsporum canis
   B. Trichophyton mentagrophytes
   C. North American blastomycosis
   D. Madurmycosis
   E. Cryptococcus

47. *What* is the name of a substance used to increase the antigenicity of a substance? 47. ...
   A. Complement
   B. Adjuvant

C. Immunoceptor D. Amboceptor
E. Maneb

48\. Hyperkeratosis of the foot pad in dogs is sometimes associated with 48. A...
A. distemper D. I C H
B. lepto E. diastasemia
C. histo

49\. *Which* of the following disorders will cause a *lesion* in the musculature of the ventriculus? 49. A...
A. Se deficiency D. Mycoplasmosis
B. Ulcerative enteritis E. Lepto
C. Histomoniasis

50\. Infectious Bovine Rhinotracheitis has been associated with all of the following *EXCEPT:* 50. ... B
A. Conjunctivitis D. Vaginitis
B. Mammillitis E. None of the above
C. Encephalitis

---

# KEY (CORRECT ANSWERS)

| | | | | |
|---|---|---|---|---|
| 1. A | 11. B | 21. E | 31. C | 41. D |
| 2. B | 12. B | 22. B | 32. B | 42. B |
| 3. D | 13. A | 23. C | 33. A | 43. E |
| 4. C | 14. A | 24. D | 34. E | 44. C |
| 5. B | 15. A | 25. A | 35. C | 45. C |
| 6. B | 16. C | 26. D | 36. B | 46. A |
| 7. B | 17. B | 27. E | 37. D | 47. B |
| 8. D | 18. B | 28. B | 38. D | 48. A |
| 9. E | 19. A | 29. D | 39. A | 49. A |
| 10. D | 20. B | 30. C | 40. B | 50. B |

---

# TEST 2

DIRECTIONS: Each question or incomplete statement is followed by several suggested answers or completions. Select the one that BEST answers the question or completes the statement. *PRINT THE LETTER OF THE CORRECT ANSWER IN THE SPACE AT THE RIGHT.*

1. Black pigment on the brain is normal in the 1. ___
   A. gray horse B. Plymouth Rock chicken
   C. Hampshire sheep D. Gloucester hen
   E. Dorchester donkey

2. Traumatic hepatitis *not* associated with external trauma is MOST common in the 2. ___
   A. cow B. dog C. horse D. cat E. pig

3. *What* causes the brown discoloration of the lungs in chronic passive congestion? 3. ___
   A. Hemosiderin in macrophages B. Protein in edema fluid
   C. Hemoglobin-forming methemoglobin due to blood stasis
   D. Fibrous connective tissue from hypoxia
   E. Poorly oxygenated blood in capillaries

4. A condition that may lead to edema is 4. ___
   A. decreased arterial pressure
   B. increased arterial pressure
   C. decreased colloid osmotic pressure of the tissue fluid
   D. increased colloid osmotic pressure of the serum
   E. decreased colloid osmotic pressure of the serum

5. The diameter of the follicle of the dairy cow at ovulation is about ______ mm. 5. ___
   A. 10-20 B. 1-2 C. 35-40 D. 70-80 E. 20-30

6. Spermatazoa placed at the cervix will reach the oviduct end of the uterus in 6. ___
   A. less than 10 minutes B. more than 1 hour
   C. 4 to 5 hours D. more than 24 hours
   E. at any time

7. The irregular spots on the skin of an aborted calf are 7. ___
   A. fungal colonies B. bacterial
   C. calcium deposits
   D. areas of necrosis from the blood supply
   E. self-generating

8. The *primary* function of the pig allentois is to 8. ___
   A. serve as a toxic filter B. absorb urinary products
   C. act as an antibody antigen filter
   D. convey the blood vessels to the heart
   E. protect the mesoblastic layers

9. The adult remnant of the umbilical vein is the — 9. D
   A. umbilical artery  B. round ligament of the bladder
   C. round ligament of the uterus  D. falciform ligament
   E. round ligament of the fundus

10. The cleavage of the fertilized egg into smaller cells results in — 10. d B
   A. blostophores  B. blastomeres  C. blastocytes
   D. blastoderms  E. blastomyces

11. The intrapulmoaortic pressure within the alveoli and bronchi is equal to the atmospheric pressure in — 11. E
   A. labored expiration  B. labored inspiration
   C. normal expiration  D. normal inspiration
   E. the cessation of breathing (thorax at rest)

12. Abnormally shaped red blood cells are characteristic of — 12. B
   A. anisocytosis  B. poikilocytosis  C. poikilonymy
   D. poikioblastomy  E. pogoniasis

13. The respiration center for the body is located in the — 13. B C
   A. cerebellum  B. cerebrum  C. brain stem
   D. spinal cord  E. neocortex

14. The corneal nerve is a branch of the ________ nerve. — 14. E B
   A. facial  B. trigeminal  C. glossopharyngeal
   D. first cervical  E. auricular

15. The celiac artery of the dog supplies *which* of the following organs? The — 15. E
   A. stomach and liver  B. spleen  C. pancreas
   D. first part of the duodenum  E. all of the above

16. A substance that assists in fat breakdown without catalyzing a chemical reaction is — 16. B A
   A. Na taurocholate  B. intestinal lipase  C. lecithin
   D. bilirubin  E. steapsin

17. The *main* factor in the maintenance of negative intrathoracic pressure is the — 17. C
   A. closure of the glottis after inspiration
   B. dilation of the bronchi
   C. contraction of the diaphragm
   D. pressure of all organs on the diaphragm
   E. dilation of the glottis before expiration

18. The percentage of oxygenation of Hb is — 18. A
   A. dependent on $pO_2$  B. independent of $pCO_2$
   C. dependent on $pN_2$  D. independent of pH
   E. dependent on carbonic anyhydrase

19. In those animals with large amounts of urea as the principal nitrogenous waste product, this urea is formed — 19. A
   A. in the liver where it is split off from arginine
   B. in the PCT
   C. from two molecules of ornithine
   D. in the DCT
   E. solely in the kidney

20. Mammals are able to retain fixed bases in the kidney by the 20. ___
   A. selective filtration of acids by the glomerulus
   B. conversion of Na to ammonium salts in the tubules
   C. formation of chloride by the tubule cells
   D. selective filtration of bases
   E. reabsorption of acid by the glomerulus

21. *One* of the *principal* differences between plasma and the glomerular filtrate is that the glomerular filtrate does NOT contain any appreciable amount of 21. ___
   A. glucose B. creatinase C. protein
   D. $HCO_3$ E. Na

22. Piroplasmosis, a hemaprotozoan, has been reported in 22. ___
   A. Georgia B. California C. Arizona
   D. New Mexico E. Texas

23. When swine have been exposed on infected soils, the soil can BEST be safely treated by 23. ___
   A. prophylactic treatment of the swine
   B. removing the swine from the area
   C. adding lime to the soil
   D. cultivating the soil crops
   E. all of the above

24. The absolute refractory period is ________ the systolic contraction period. 24. ___
   A. 1/30 B. 1/5 C. 1/2 D. 1 1/2 E. the same as

25. An increase in cerebral spinal fluid in a calf or pig is due to a deficiency of 25. ___
   A. Vitamin A B. Vitamin D C. Vitamin C
   D. Vitamin E E. Thiamin

26. The *one* of the following statements which is MOST correct referring to the operation for laryngeal hemiplegia in a horse whereby the entire mucosa is removed from the saccule is: 26. ___
   A. On entering the laryngeal cavity, the saccule is found to be upward and backward.
   B. The incision is through the crico-arytenoid membrane.
   C. The crico-arytenoid membrane is the posterior part of the crico-thyroid membrane.
   D. After opening the larynx, an important step is the insertion of the tracheotomy tube.
   E. After making an incision through the skin and subcutis, the common fascia of omohyoids is exposed.

27. The lesion, "sawdust liver," chronic passive congestion, is often caused in the bovine by 27. ___
   A. negative endocarditis of the left AV valve
   B. traumatic pericarditis
   C. ulcers of the abomasum
   D. embolism of the hepatic artery
   E. telangioectasis

28. Anasarca is caused by — 28. D
   A. excess fluid in the pericardium
   B. excess fluid in the thorax
   C. excess fluid in the scrotal sac
   D. generalized edema of the SQ tissue
   E. excess fluid of the abdominal cavity

29. Mellitus is NOT caused in the dog and horse by — 29. A
   A. hyperfunction of the anterior pituitary
   B. space-occupying lesion of the post pituitary
   C. amyloidosis of the pancreatic islet cells
   D. pancreatic fibrosis
   E. hydropic degeneration of the beta cells

30. The blood capillaries of the epithelium run in with the connective tissue of the — 30. B
   A. stratum corneum
   B. area just below the stratum germinativum
   C. prickle cell layer
   D. stratum granulosum
   E. stratum lucidum

31. In the normal adult, the red blood cells and the granulocytes are formed in the — 31. A
   A. bone marrow *only*   B. spleen and bone marrow
   C. spleen and liver   D. spleen *only*
   E. bone marrow of the vertebrae *only*

32. In the lymph system, the area where the GREATEST number of lymphocytes is found is the — 32. ~~B~~ D
   A. thoracic duct   B. thymus   C. hilus
   D. lymph nodes   E. spleen

33. In renal epithelium, the cells with a brush border and a cytoplasm-staining eosinophilic are found — 33. ~~C~~ D
   A. at the nephren
   B. in the distal convoluted tubules
   C. at the glomerulus
   D. in the proximal convoluted tubules
   E. in the collecting ducts

34. *What* artery is available for the pulse on a horse? The ________ artery. — 34. B
   A. internal maxillary   B. external maxillary
   C. transverse facial   D. angular
   E. articular

35. The action of the gracilis muscle is to — 35. ~~A~~ C
   A. abduct the rear leg   B. extend the stifle
   C. abduct the limb   D. flex the rear leg
   E. reverse the front leg

36. To acidify urine via oral administration, employ — 36. C
   A. NaCl   B. NaOh   C. $NH_4Cl$   D. Na propionate
   E. $CH_3COOH$

37. Equine encephalomyelitis is MOST prevalent in *what* season of the year? The — 37. ~~X~~ D
   A. long day spells   B. winter   C. spring   D. summer   E. fall

38. Iridencleisis is a surgical treatment for glaucoma which involves 38. E C
- A. trephining the corneal scleral junction
- B. exercising part of the iris and removing the lens
- C. establishing a permanent filtering cicatrix
- D. puncturing the anterior chamber to relieve pressure
- E. removal of a wedge-shaped piece of the iris

39. In trephining the post-orbital diverticulum of the frontal sinus of the bovine in empyema, one would trephine 39. D A
- A. medial to the bony ridge, which is the lateral edge of the frontal sinus and 1 1/2 inches posterior to the orbit
- B. where the nasal bones diverge
- C. posterior to a line drawn through the orbits and 1 1/2 inches from the midline
- D. 1 1/2 inches from the midline and just anterior to the posterior limit of the sinus
- E. where the nasal bones converge

40. With guttural pouch infection, the MOST characteristic sign is: 40. B
- A. Diffuse, soft tympanic swelling in the parotid area
- B. Pus draining from the nares when the head is lowered to eat or drink
- C. Frequent coughing
- D. Hard swelling on Stenson's duct
- E. Head tilt to the affected side

41. Enzootic atexia in sheep is due to a deficiency of 41. B D
- A. calcium B. manganese C. iodine D. copper
- E. phosphorus

42. A 7½-month male woolly monkey is unable to stand, and suffers from muscle tremors. An x-ray shows several fractures. The monkey has been fed on an almost all-fruit diet. The prescribed treatment for tremors is 42. B A
- A. sedatives and tranquilizers B. calcium
- C. X-irradiation D. an improved diet E. proteins

43. Plants treated with hormone herbicides cause death in animals because 43. E E
- A. the allergy is due to previous exposure
- B. of the formation of toxic polysaccharides from starches of plants by the plants
- C. of the formation of toxic alkaloids by the plants
- D. of the formation of toxic ph ends by breakdown of the hormone
- E. of the accumulation of nitrites and nitrates in the plants

44. In *what* species is catarrhal enteritis found so commonly that it is almost routine? In the 44. D D
- A. horse B. cat C. cow D. dog E. sheep

45. In a cow which has died from chronic disease, the greatly distended gall bladder that is found is in the absence of obstruction, is interpreted as, 45. A E
- A. loss of muscle tone due to general weakness
- B. overproduction of bile
- C. catarrhal cholicystitis due to toxins
- D. evidence of chronic blood destruction
- E. lack of ejaculation due to the absence of stimulation caused by inactive gut

46. In *which* of the following diseases of cattle are erosions of esophygeal mucosa found? 46. ___
   A. Hyperkeratosis B. Malignant catarrhal fever
   C. BVP D. Winter dysentery E. Vitamin A deficiency

47. Hemorrhagic edematous thickening of the wall of the cecum, rectum, and colon of cattle is characteristic of 47. ___
   A. Eimeria arlongii B. Eimeria zurnii
   C. paratuberculosis D. coccidia
   E. protozoa

48. Hepatic passive congestion, without pulmonary congestion, may be the result of 48. ___
   A. tricuspid insufficiency B. aortic valve stenosis
   C. mitral insufficiency D. cardiac sarcosporidiosis
   E. cardiac dropsy

49. The *minimum* amount of fluid needed for a severely dehydrated animal to replace fluids per pound is ______ ml. 49. ___
   A. 2 B. 4 C. 8 D. 16 E. 32

50. On slaughter of a bovine, a granulomatous lesion in the thoracic lymph node was seen. On microscopic examination, a double spherical-shaped object was demonstrated. The condition is: 50. ___
   A. Actinomycosis B. Coccidiomycosis
   C. Nocardiosis D. Monoblepsia
   E. Aspergillosis

# KEY (CORRECT ANSWERS)

| | | | | | | | | | |
|---|---|---|---|---|---|---|---|---|---|
| 1. | A | 11. | E | 21. | C | 31. | A | 41. | D |
| 2. | A | 12. | B | 22. | E | 32. | D | 42. | A |
| 3. | A | 13. | C | 23. | D | 33. | D | 43. | E |
| 4. | E | 14. | B | 24. | A | 34. | B | 44. | D |
| 5. | A | 15. | E | 25. | A | 35. | C | 45. | A |
| 6. | A | 16. | A | 26. | A | 36. | C | 46. | E |
| 7. | A | 17. | C | 27. | E | 37. | D | 47. | B |
| 8. | B | 18. | A | 28. | D | 38. | C | 48. | A |
| 9. | D | 19. | A | 29. | A | 39. | A | 49. | D |
| 10. | B | 20. | B | 30. | B | 40. | B | 50. | B |

# EXAMINATION SECTION

# TEST 1

DIRECTIONS:

Each question or incomplete statement is followed by several suggested answers or completions. Select the one that *BEST* answers the question or completes the statement. *PRINT THE LETTER OF THE CORRECT ANSWER IN THE SPACE AT THE RIGHT.*

1. Injuries and abnormalities of the teats of cattle are frequent. A condition NEVER considered a congenital abnormality is ______. 1. ...
   A. absence of teats
   B. fissured or cracked teats
   C. imperforate teats
   D. milk fistula
   E. supernumerary teats
2. In intestinal surgery, the type of stitch that coapts the peritoneal surfaces by penetrating the lumen of the gut is known as a ______ suture. 2. ...
   A. lembert
   B. right-angle cushing
   C. Connell
   D. Czerny-Lembert
   E. Parker-Kerr
3. When performing a Caesarean section on the bovine through the right ventral portion of the abdominal wall, the structure that is *MOST* commonly met after one passes through the abdominal wall and peritoneum is the 3. ...
   A. large intestines
   B. great omentum
   C. pregnant uterus
   D. small intestines
   E. spleen
4. The prognosis when there is a fractured splint bone depends upon the 4. ...
   A. soundness of the other paired member
   B. duration of the fracture and its severity
   C. presence of non-union, indicating a poor healing response
   D. degree of desmitis of the suspensory ligament
   E. degree of periosteal proliferation about the callus
5. In bone grafting, the trend is toward 5. ...
   A. applying a massive inlay graft after freshening the bone ends and preparing a bed on each fragment
   B. freshening the bone ends and precision fitting an autogenous bone graft for rigid fixation
   C. applying inlay grafts after freshening the bone ends, then immobilizing with pins
   D. freshening the bone ends and seeding with cancellous bone while providing rigid fixation with pins
   E. freshening the bone ends and seeding with cortical bone chips, then providing rigid fixation with pins

6. The unsoundness of the horse commonly referred to as "thoroughpin" is a 6. ...
   A. chronic distention of the capsule of the tibiotarsal articulation
   B. chronic bursitis between the achilles tendon and the deep digital flexor muscle
   C. chronic synovitis of the tarsal sheath of the deep digital flexor tendon at the hock
   D. chronic distention of the bursa over the os calcis
   E. chronic proliferative inflammation on the medial side of the third row of tarsal bones
7. An occasional upward fixation of the patella in a 4-year-old saddle horse weighing 1,000 pounds can be corrected by 7. ...
   A. extending the leg with ropes until the patella drops into place
   B. extending the leg and forcing the patella ventrally
   C. anesthetizing the colt to the point of relaxation, and replacing the patella
   D. giving a dose of 300 mg. of succinylcholine, and replacing the patella
   E. performing a medial patellar desmotomy
8. Intracapsular fractures of the femoral head in dogs are more serious than extracapsular fractures because the 8. ...
   A. chances of infection are greater
   B. blood supply is destroyed
   C. pain is greater and the muscle atrophy more extensive
   D. nerve damage is more extensive
   E. bone fragments cause arthritis
9. Coxofemoral luxation is fairly common in the 9. ...
   A. dog *and* horse
   B. dog *and* ox
   C. dog *and* cat
   D. dog *and* sheep
   E. sheep *and* ox
10. If a horse falls with his hind legs extended behind him and overextends the hock joint when he gets up, the *most likely* cause is rupture of the 10. ...
    A. medial tendon of the tibialis anterior
    B. common digital extensor tendon at the hock
    C. tendon of the peroneus tertius
    D. soleus muscle
    E. lateral digital extensor tendon
11. To bring about reduction of the elbow joint, the forelimb must be 11. ...
    A. rotated clockwise
    B. held in supination
    C. flexed
    D. extended
    E. abducted
12. Following the excision of an interdigital fibroma, immobolization of the claws is *BEST* effected by 12. ...
    A. plaster cast
    B. rubber electrician's tape

C. clip shoes
D. heavy bandaging
E. wiring the toes

13. When performing a posterior digital neurectomy on a horse with navicular disease, it is necessary to differentiate nerve from blood vessels. The relationship of these structures from an anterior to posterior direction is: 13. ...
A. Nerve, vein, artery
B. Nerve, artery, vein
C. Artery, nerve, vein
D. Artery, vein, nerve
E. Vein, artery, nerve

14. A wound in the equine manus or pes should be bandaged with pressure packs to prevent excessive 14. ...
A. hoof growth B. contamination C. granulation
D. desmorrhexis E. movement

15. One of the *oldest* obstetrical operations is 15. ...
A. ovariectomy B. hysterectomy C. caesarean section
D. embryotomy E. laparotomy

16. In a bull, surgical repair of a ruptured penis should be performed *after* 16. ...
A. 1 - 2 months, to allow formation and contraction of the scar tissue
B. 1 - 2 months, since in 50% of cases an abscess develops, which must be drained and allowed to heal
C. 1 or 2 days, to control hemorrhage
D. 2 - 3 weeks, when organization of the clot has occurred
E. 4 - 10 days, when the clot has formed

17. The agent of choice for treating ovarian cysts is 17. ...
A. thyroxin B. cortisone C. progesterone
D. chorionic gonadotropin E. diethylstilbestrol

18. A persistent and enlarged corpus luteum causes 18. ...
A. pregnancy B. estrum C. anestrus
D. abortion E. nymphomania

19. An indication for cystotomy is the presence of ________ calculi. 19. ...
A. vesicular B. renal C. urethral
D. prostatic E. stag horn

20. A persistent urachus in a foal is treated by 20. ...
A. chemical or heat cautery
B. placement of an indwelling catheter in the bladder
C. amputation of the distal part of the urachus
D. incision of the urachus to provide adequate drainage
E. ligation of the involved ureter

21. A horse is presented with the following symptoms: Mucopurulent discharge from the urethra; swelling and redness of the lips of the urinary meatus; pain during micturition. 21. ...
The *logical* diagnosis would be:
A. Balanoposthitis B. Urethritis C. Pyelonephritis
D. Urocystitis E. Urethral calculus

22. Castration is considered an excellent treatment for prostatic hypertrophy in the dog because it 22. ...
    A. slows the animal's metabolic rate
    B. is safer than prostatectomy
    C. removes sertoli-cell tumors which cause hypertrophy
    D. causes atrophy of the gland
    E. tends to prevent cyst formation in the prostate
23. *What* is the differentiation *between PARAPHIMOSIS* and *PHIMOSIS*? 23. ...
    A. Paraphimosis indicates a congenital absence of the penile bone; phimosis indicates a congenital malformation of the glans penis.
    B. Paraphimosis indicates a neoplasm involving the penis; phimosis indicates a neoplasm involving the prepuce.
    C. Paraphimosis is a condition designated as a rupture of the prostatic sheath with subsequent hemorrhage; phimosis designates a prostatic hypertrophy with marked interference with micturition.
    D. Paraphimosis is a condition in which the penis becomes edematous within the prepuce as a result of inflammation; phimosis designates a condition of prepucial edema associated with prolapse of the penis.
    E. Paraphimosis designates a prolapsing of the penis through the prepuce; phimosis is a morbid contraction of the free extremity of the prepuce in front of the glans penis.
24. Castration of swine by laymen is a common procedure, but due to their lack of knowledge concerning proper technique and cleanliness, they frequently meet with difficulties. The *most common* of these is: 24. ...
    A. Prolapse of the intestines due to failure to recognize an inguinal hernia
    B. Peritonitis due to a general lack of knowledge regarding cleanliness
    C. Hydrocele because of failure to remove a sufficient amount of the tunics
    D. Fatal hemorrhage because of a lack of proper instruments
    E. Scirrhous cord due to failure to remove a sufficient amount of the spermatic cord.
25. During development, misplacement of the bovine testicle sometimes occurs. If such misplacement does take place, the condition *most commonly* found is: 25. ...
    A. Location of the testicle in the inguinal canal
    B. Abdominal cryptorchidism
    C. Location of the testicle outside the peritoneum near the right kidney
    D. An ectopic testicle located subcutaneously alongside the penis
    E. Location of the testicle at the internal inguinal ring
26. *Which one* of the following statements with respect to neoplasms occurring in various parts of the body of the bovine is TRUE? 26. ...
    Those occurring in the
    A. thymus gland are usually carcinomas

B. lungs are usually carcinomas
C. uterus are always carcinomas
D. liver are almost invariably sarcomas
E. rumen are often sarcomas

27. The *difference* between *SARCOMAS* and *CARCINOMAS* is *CORRECTLY* expressed in the statement that sarcomas 27. ...
A. metastasize via lymphatics, carcinomas via the blood stream
B. spread by direct invasion, carcinomas by metastasis
C. develop at an early age, carcinomas in later life
D. originate from internal structures, carcinomas from skin
E. arise from connective tissue, carcinomas from epithelium

28. Peri-anal adenomas are *most commonly* found near the anus, but occasionally they are located 28. ...
A. *on* the dorsal surface of the tail
B. *on* the scrotum and *in* the inguinal region
C. *in* the perineal region
D. *along* the sacrum and *along* the hips
E. *on* the inner surfaces of the thighs

29. Both pathologists and clinicans regard the neoplasm lymphocytoma (leukemia) as one of the most important diseases of the bovine. Under certain conditions, this disease may be confused with 29. ...
A. caseous lymphadenitis
B. any disease which causes digestive disturbances
C. blackleg
D. goiter
E. tuberculosis

30. The seminoma is a testicular neoplasm that 30. ...
A. causes the dog to have sexual attractiveness for other males
B. secretes estrogenic hormones producing hyperestrogenism in males
C. has no known endocrine effect
D. produces androgens that have little effect on mature male animals
E. usually occurs in an undescended testicle

31. *Which one* of the following precautions should you take to protect yourself from the destructive effects of the x-ray during fluoroscopy? 31. ...
A. Wear lead apron and lead golves
B. Stand behind the control panel
C. Wear a film badge that will warn you against excess radiation
D. Wear fluoroscopic goggles
E. Wear heavy clothing

32. The structure with the *LEAST* sensitivity to radiation is the 32. ...
A. hemopoietic system
B. skeletal system
C. nervous system
D. skin
E. gastro-intestinal system

33. In radiography on a heavily muscled leg, 30 cm. in diameter, secondary film radiation can *BEST* be controlled by 33. ...
   A. a long cone
   B. 2 mm. of aluminum at the port of the x-ray tube
   C. a lysholm grid
   D. a reciprocating bucky grid
   E. long target-to-film distance

34. Sr-90 applicators can be used for treating carcinoma of the cornea of cattle without producing cataracts because they 34. ...
   A. require short exposure time
   B. do not produce back scatter
   C. emit a gamma ray
   D. give a high energy ray
   E. emit a beta ray

35. The radiographic view of the stifle joint that shows anterior and posterior subluxation of the tibia in horses and cattle *BEST* is the 35. ...
   A. lateral with the tube tilted at a 45-degree angle
   B. anterior-posterior
   C. oblique
   D. posterior-anterior
   E. lateral

36. The *MOST* outstanding symptoms of renal rickets are: 36. ...
   A. Pathological fractures
   B. Subperiosteal and cutaneous hemorrhages
   C. Respiratory abnormalities and swellings of the long bones
   D. Acidosis and uremia
   E. Ricketic rosary, lameness, and joint swelling

37. Of the following treatments for prostatic hyperplasia in the dog, the *one* which is *NOT* effective is 37. ...
   A. prostatalgia
   B. prostatectomy
   C. subtotal prostatectomy
   D. gonadectomy
   E. prostatic massage

38. The *MOST* frequent indication for caesarean section in the ewe is: 38. ...
   A. Incomplete dilation of the cervix
   B. Inadequate exercise due to confinement
   C. Immature ewes
   D. Hypoglycemic ketonuria
   E. None of the above

39. An *essential* amino acid is 39. ...
   A. leucine  B. methionine  C. cystine
   D. norleucine  E. tyrosine

40. The frequent complication of parturient paresis in cows is 40. ...
   A. milk fever  B. acetonemia  C. acalcemia
   D. hypocalcemia  E. acelosis

41. Pneumoperitoneum is used to diagnose 41. ...
   A. cystitis  B. liver neoplasm  C. bladder neoplasm
   D. intestinal foreign body  E. abdominal neoplasm

42. Of the neoplasms listed below, *which* are *MOST* frequently causes of swelling of the maxillary bones in horses? 42. ...
    A. Osteoma B. Rhabdomyoma C. Lymphoma
    D. Lipoma E. Fibrosarcoma

43. Actinobacillosis lagnersci in the horse are characterized by? 43. ...
    A. lymphangitis and lymphanditis of the lower legs
    B. ulcerative lymphangitis of the lower legs causing a positive T.B. test
    C. lesions of the tongue and, occasionally, the pharyngeal lymph nodes
    D. bony lesions of the mandible and maxilla that are painless
    E. bony lesions of the mandible and maxilla that are painful

44. Neoplasms of the hematopoietic system, adenocarcinomas in general, neoplasms of the skeletal system, malignant melanomas and neoplasms of the skin are sensitive to radiation. 44. ...
    Neoplasms of the skin would be listed in order of *decreasing* sensitivity as
    A. first B. second C. third
    D. fourth E. fifth

45. An animal displays laryngospasm under anesthesia. *What* should be done? 45. ...
    A. Resect the soft palate B. Deepen the anesthesia
    C. Intubate D. Do a tracheotomy E. Use atropine

46. After doing a castration in a horse, the tunics should be trimmed to 46. ...
    A. prevent schirrhous cord
    B. prevent stallion-like behavior
    C. prevent hydrocele
    D. prevent ill effects
    E. prevent closure of the wound

47. The agglutination-lysis test is used for the detection of 47. ...
    A. lepto B. brucellosis C. trichinellosis
    D. rabies E. acariasis

48. *Most* cases of Aspergillosis are due to Aspergillus 48. ...
    A. auricularis B. fumigatus C. glaucus
    D. keratitis E. mucoroides

49. The clinical syndrome of lead poisoning in cattle, especially calves, consists of 49. ...
    A. a severe affection of the central nervous system
    B. prolonged affection of the intestinal tract with blood-flicked stools
    C. prolonged affection of the respiratory tract, including occasional epistaxis
    D. laryngeal and nasal discharge
    E. severe hyperkeratosis and emaciation

50. Chiggers are 50. ...
    A. adult ticks B. adult mites C. larval mites
    D. larval ticks E. biting lice

# KEY (CORRECT ANSWERS)

| | | | | | | | | | |
|---|---|---|---|---|---|---|---|---|---|
| 1. | B | 11. | C | 21. | B | 31. | A | 41. | C |
| 2. | C | 12. | E | 22. | D | 32. | C | 42. | E |
| 3. | B | 13. | E | 23. | E | 33. | D | 43. | C |
| 4. | D | 14. | C | 24. | E | 34. | E | 44. | C |
| 5. | D | 15. | C | 25. | D | 35. | E | 45. | C |
| 6. | C | 16. | E | 26. | D | 36. | A | 46. | C |
| 7. | E | 17. | D | 27. | E | 37. | A | 47. | A |
| 8. | B | 18. | C | 28. | A | 38. | A | 48. | B |
| 9. | B | 19. | A | 29. | E | 39. | B | 49. | A |
| 10. | C | 20. | A | 30. | C | 40. | B | 50. | C |

# TEST 2

DIRECTIONS:
Each question or incomplete statement is followed by several suggested answers or completions. Select the one that *BEST* answers the question or completes the statement. *PRINT THE LETTER OF THE CORRECT ANSWER IN THE SPACE AT THE RIGHT.*

1. Louping ill of sheep has been shown to be transmitted by — 1. ...
   A. fleas
   B. lice
   C. mosquitos
   D. ticks
   E. mites
2. On ante-mortem examination, a swine is found to have a temperature of $104^{o}$. The animal is depressed and has red erythematous over the hams, inguinal and axilla. — 2. ...
   The *final* disposition of this animal would be:
   A. Condemn and tank
   B. Hold as suspect; disposition on post-mortem examination
   C. Treat with erysipilas antiserum; slaughter on recovery
   D. Pass for cooked products
   E. Do not pass for cooked products
3. A kennel owner has had an outbreak of leptospirosis. The organism has been positively identified as lepto-canicola. — 3. ...
   The *most likely* source of this infection is
   A. cats
   B. dogs
   C. horses
   D. cows
   E. mice
4. Anthrax in the USA is *commonly* transmitted by — 4. ...
   A. water
   B. wind
   C. trees
   D. fruit
   E. soil
5. Milking-machine disinfection is achieved through the application of — 5. ...
   A. $H_2O_2$
   B. tincture of iodine
   C. Na hypochloride
   D. boric acid
   E. saturated cresols
6. In fractures of the distal third of the femur, the proximal end of the distal fragment is displaced — 6. ...
   A. laterally
   B. medially
   C. caudally
   D. cranially
   E. with long axis rotation
7. Before fresh pork can leave an inspected establishment, it — 7. ...
   A. need not be treated in any way to kill trichina
   B. must be heated to an internal temperature of $137^{o}$
   C. must be heated to an internal temperature of $145^{o}$
   D. can be used only for processed products
   E. must bear recommended cooking instructions

8. Anthrax organisms in direct smears, suitably stained, obtained from recently dead animals, appear as: 8. ...
   A. Pairs of gram + rods with spores
   B. Chains of gram + rods without spores
   C. Long gram + filamentous rods without spores
   D. Long gram - filaments with spores
   E. Chains of gram - rods without spores

9. Administration of Ca I.V. in cases can result in heart block. It is *MOST* satisfactorily treated with 9. ...
   A. Na bicarbonate
   B. epinephrine
   C. atropine
   D. dextrose
   E. lactated ringers

10. Periodic worming of dogs, cooking of vegetables, and sanitary practices will limit the spread of 10. ...
    A. echinococcosis
    B. ascariasis
    C. cinetica
    D. exocardia
    E. hyperemesis

11. The *PRIMARY* lesion of avian TB is found in the 11. ...
    A. lungs
    B. liver
    C. spleen
    D. air sacs
    E. intestines

12. Neoplasm that is *most common* in gray and white horses and often becomes malignant is termed 12. ...
    A. blastoma
    B. chondroma
    C. gloma
    D. enblastoma
    E. melanoblastoma

13. The treatment of a horse with bots is best performed in 13. ...
    A. midwinter
    B. early fall
    C. early spring
    D. early summer
    E. midsummer

14. As a result of fatigue, a "March" fracture of the equine occurs. *Which* long bone is *MOST* frequently affected? 14. ...
    A. 1st phalanx
    B. 2nd phalanx
    C. 3rd phalanx
    D. 3rd metacarpal
    E. Radius

15. The *principal* cause of ruptured bladder in a foal is: 15. ...
    A. Straining from impacted meconium
    B. Pressure exerted by mare at birth or full bladder
    C. Penis doubled over constricted ureter
    D. Debris impacting urethral diverticulum
    E. Constricted prepuce

16. In dogs, osteosarcoma originatesin the: 16. ...
    A. Draphysis - involving the epiphysis and the adjacent bone
    B. Epyphysis - and spreads to the joint and adjacent bones
    C. Metaphysis - spreading along the diaphysis toward the opposite epiphysis
    D. Pericosteum - spreading through the cortex and along the medullary canal
    E. Metaphysis - rapidly involving the epiphysis and the articular cartilage

17. The *appropriate* restraint for rumenotomy is — 17. ...
   A. epidural
   B. general anesthesia
   C. local anesthesia
   D. nose lead
   E. ruptio

18. Which parasite *DOES NOT* migrate through the lungs and/or the liver? — 18. ...
   A. Strongyloides stercoralis
   B. Toxocara leonina
   C. Toxascaris
   D. Ascarides
   E. Ascaris mystax

19. Allergic rhinitis in cattle is treated with — 19. ...
   A. oil of eucalyptus
   B. atropine
   C. sulfas
   D. antihistamines
   E. resacetin

20. Prevention of disease in animals by the use of biologics is *NOT* practiced against — 20. ...
   A. salmonella pullorum
   B. bacillus anthracis
   C. clost. tetani
   D. past. multocida
   E. brucella abortus

21. If, in treating a cow with ferrous sulfate for iron deficiency anemia, the cow doesn't improve, you should — 21. ...
   A. add mb to the diet
   B. increase the dose
   C. slow passage through the gut by atropine
   D. increase energy in the diet
   E. increase essential A.A.

22. In dogs, the vitamin rendered unabsorbable or unusable when raw egg white is fed, is — 22. ...
   A. vitamin A
   B. thiamine
   C. riboflavin
   D. niacin
   E. biotin

23. A cow shows the following signs: abscess of the udder; the connective tissue capsule is flawed with a thick yellow discharge and small yellow granules. The diagnosis is: — 23. ...
   A. Botryomycosis
   B. Actinomycosis
   C. Streptoccosis
   D. TB
   E. Brucella

24. Of the following, the *BEST* viral disinfectant is — 24. ...
   A. lye
   B. Ca (OH)2
   C. phenol
   D. disinfectin
   E. carbolic acid

25. The specimen to submit for anthrax diagnosis in swine is: — 25. ...
   A. Blood
   B. Spleen
   C. Tail
   D. Pharyngeal L.N.
   E. Mediastinal L.N.

26. Leptospirosis can be differentiated from other pathogenic spirochetes by its — 26. ...
   A. cultural character (serological tests)
   B. relative pathogenicity for laboratory animals
   C. morphology

D. morphometry
E. morphosis

27. The *proper* therapy for a cow suffering from dyspnea and bloat due to the injection of tetanus antitoxin is  27. . . .
A. atropine
B. amphetamine
C. promethazine HCl
D. aminopyrine
E. caffeine

28. A well-conditioned cow had an antemortem of 104° and was listless. There was a finding of TB in the lungs and a mediastinal L.N. The disposition should be:  28. . . .
A. Retain the carcass
B. Inspect and pass
C. For cooking only
D. Condemn
E. Inject with atabrine

29. The *most common* tumor found in the cat is:  29. . . .
A. Tubular
B. Squamous
C. Cylindrical
D. Glandular
E. Lympho

30. Tumors are *most commonly* seen on bulls' penises which  30. . . .
A. are used on range breeding
B. have been long-used at stud
C. have been used in natural service
D. are from one to three years' old
E. have been used in cows with granular vaginitis

31. The *most significant* chemical sign of infectious feline enteritis is:  31. . . .
A. Depression
B. Increased temperature
C. Inappetence
D. Appetence
E. Leukopenia

32. The *most common* time for equine encephalomyelites is:  32. . . .
A. Long dry spell
B. Summer
C. Winter
D. Spring
E. Fall

33. To *decrease* the incidence of urea toxicity in ruminants, make certain that  33. . . .
A. there is adequate $H_2O$ during and after feeding
B. no more than 1/3 of the protein supplement in the diet is in the form of urea
C. in cattle on full feed of high-grain, finishing diet, urea does not make up more than 95% of the diet
D. no more than 1/3 of the energy requirement is supplied by urea
E. $NH_4CL$ in the amount of .5% is added to the urea

34. The laboratory reports that a pasteurized milk sample has a coliform count which exceeds acceptable limits. The *most likely* cause is:  34. . . .
A. Contaminated $H_2O$ supply
B. Improper barterícidal cleaning of utensils
C. A toilet was stopped up and overflowed.
D. Improper time-temperature relation
E. Loose-fitting cooler cover

35. A *useful* indicator regarding the state of the bovine udder is: 35. ...
    A. Phosphatase content of milk
    B. Sediment content
    C. Leukocyte count
    D. Rancidity
    E. Water content
36. The invasion of extraintestinal abdominal organs, brain, lungs, and eyes of children infected with the larvae of *Toxacara canis* is known as: 36. ...
    A. Cercaria dermatitis
    B. Rhabditic dermatitis
    C. Hepatitis cysticercosa
    D. Creeping eruption
    E. Visceral larvae migrans
37. *Which* of the following factors producing disease in an overpopulated area does NOT increase with the increase in the disease? 37. ...
    A. Virulence of the virus
    B. Dosage of viral infection
    C. Frequency of exposure
    D. Velocity of spread
    E. None of the above
38. *Which* of the following is now considered to be *MOST* heat-resistant and is *MOST LIKELY* found in pasteurized milk? 38. ...
    A. Rickettsia burnetta
    B. Salmonella typhosa
    C. Brucella sp
    D. Bacilli aerophilus
    E. Bacilli of Flocca
39. In order to reduce routine plate on pasteurized milk at the plant, the action would be directed at: 39. ...
    A. Cooling and refrigeration
    B. Cleaning and sanitizing utensils
    C. Clipping and cleaning udder
    D. Containing and defining
    E. Compensating and decomposing
40. The *most common* source of microsporum gypsum is 40. ...
    A. cattle
    B. soil
    C. rodents
    D. cats
    E. dogs
41. The *most common* ringworm in cats is 41. ...
    A. microsporum canis
    B. microsporum gypsum
    C. Tricophyton flocculosum
    D. tinea amiantaces
    E. tinea barbae
42. The transplacental route is relatively *more* important than the colostral route in the transfer of maternal antibodies in the 42. ...
    A. cow
    B. human
    C. horse
    D. cat
    E. dog
43. *Which* of the following factors influences the frequency of infection at different seasons of the year? 43. ...
    A. Dosage
    B. Vector
    C. Vehicle
    D. Water
    E. Weather

44. The suture material of choice in teat laceration is — 44. . . .
   A. any non-capillary suture
   B. chronic gut
   C. any capillary suture
   D. #3 chronic gut
   E. #3 cat gut

45. The *ideal* time to castrate male swine is — 45. . . .
   A. at birth
   B. at two weeks
   C. at two months
   D. during weaning
   E. at any time within a year

46. The urine of a cat with cystitis or urolithisis is — 46. . . .
   A. *usually* acidic
   B. *usually* alkaline
   C. *always* alkaline
   D. *always* acidic
   E. bloody

47. In a distal 1/3 fx of the humerus, the proximal end of the distal fragment is displaced — 47. . . .
   A. cranially
   B. caudally
   C. laterally
   D. medially
   E. rotated counter-clockwise

48. In reducing an elbow luxation of a dog, one should place the elbow in — 48. . . .
   A. extreme flexion
   B. extreme extension
   C. adduction
   D. normal standing position
   E. medial rotation

49. A common injury of the intra-carpal articulation of the horse is — 49. . . .
   A. fx of the proximal end of the ulnar carpal
   B. fx of the 4th carpal bone
   C. chip fx of the distal end of the radial carpal
   D. chip fx of the accessory carpal
   E. chip fx of the distal radius

50. HPO is frequently associated with chronic lung lesions but the *most characteristic* signs are: — 50. . . .
   A. Cachexia, vomiting, weight loss
   B. Broncho-pneumonia
   C. Hypertrophic lesions of the long bones
   D. Nasal discharge, coughing
   E. Vomiting, nasal discharge, fibroid pneumonia

# KEY (CORRECT ANSWERS)

| | | | | | | | | | |
|---|---|---|---|---|---|---|---|---|---|
| 1. | D | 11. | E | 21. | A | 31. | E | 41. | A |
| 2. | B | 12. | E | 22. | E | 32. | B | 42. | B |
| 3. | B | 13. | B | 23. | C | 33. | B | 43. | B |
| 4. | E | 14. | D | 24. | A | 34. | C | 44. | A |
| 5. | C | 15. | B | 25. | D | 35. | C | 45. | C |
| 6. | C | 16. | C | 26. | A | 36. | E | 46. | B |
| 7. | E | 17. | A | 27. | B | 37. | B | 47. | A |
| 8. | B | 18. | B | 28. | D | 38. | A | 48. | A |
| 9. | B | 19. | C | 29. | E | 39. | A | 49. | E |
| 10. | B | 20. | A | 30. | D | 40. | E | 50. | C |

# EXAMINATION SECTION

# TEST 1

DIRECTIONS:
Each question or incomplete statement is followed by several suggested answers or completions. Select the one that *BEST* answers the question or completes the statement. *PRINT THE LETTER OF THE CORRECT ANSWER IN THE SPACE AT THE RIGHT.*

1. *One* characteristic sign of glaucoma that is NOT found in acute iritis is: 1. ...
   A. Loss of mobility of the iris
   B. A constricted pupil
   C. Mucopurulent secretion
   D. Acute pain
   E. A grossly dilated pupil
2. *Which one* of the following skin lesions may be inherited by animals via recessive genes that follow the Mendelian pattern? 2. ...
   A. Hyperkeratosis
   B. Parakeratosis
   C. Alopecia
   D. Bursatti
   E. Skin tumors
3. Traumatic gastritis in the bovine can *easily* be mistaken for primary indigestion because these two conditions 3. ...
   A. have many signs in common
   B. most commonly affect "greedy eaters"
   C. occur only in adults
   D. are practically identical in their seasonal occurrence
   E. produce the same initial rise in temperature
4. Chronic bloating in mature cattle is *MOST* suggestive of 4. ...
   A. impaction of the abomasum
   B. compression stenosis of the esophagus
   C. atony of the rumen
   D. acute indigestion
   E. intussusception
5. *Which* of the following statements *BEST* describes the situation when there is an anterior dorsal luxation of the coxofemoral joint in a dog? 5. ...
   A. The luxated leg is shorter when the dog is placed on his back and the legs are brought together and extended by holding them up over his body.
   B. When the dog stands, he holds the affected leg in such a manner that the stifle and foot are rotated medially and the back is abducted.
   C. A finger will be displaced if, with the dog lying on his sound side, it is pressed gently into the muscular notch between the tuber ischii and the trochanter major, and the leg is rotated posteriorly on its long axis.
   D. The luxated leg is shorter when, with the dog on his back, the legs are brought together, held over his body, and extended anteriorly.

E. The luxated leg is longer when, with the dog lying on his sound side, the legs are brought together and extended posteriorly.

6. The second, or diastolic, heart sound is caused *PRIMARILY* by the 6. ...
   A. contraction of the auricles
   B. closure of the semilunar valves
   C. closure of the a-v valves
   D. contraction of the ventricular musculature
   E. vibration of the chordae tendineae
7. Acute myocarditis is *BEST* diagnosed by 7. ...
   A. roentgenography
   B. palpation
   C. auscultation
   D. encephaloscopy
   E. electrocardiography
8. Eversion of the bladder in the mare is *easily* diagnosed by 8. ...
   A. passing a catheter into the urethra and observing its course
   B. inspecting for the distended sac-like appearance of the urine-filled bladder
   C. inspecting for the characteristic serosal surface of the bladder
   D. inspecting for the presence of the two ureteral openings near the neck of the bladder
   E. aspirating the distended sac and observing whether or not urine is present.
9. In establishing a positive clinical diagnosis of infectious keratitis in a group of cattle, and differentiating it from other causes of keratitis such as trauma and milignant catarrhal fever, *one* of the *MOST* reliable factors to consider is the 9. ...
   A. number of individuals affected in a given outbreak
   B. time of year and type of climate and environment
   C. age and breed of the individuals involved
   D. characteristic pink cast to the cornea and conjunctiva
   E. complete absence of general symptoms such as anorexia, fever, or rise in pulse rate.
10. The "Mallein Test" and the "Straus Reaction" are useful for the recognition of 10. ...
    A. cholera
    B. anthrax
    C. leprosy
    D. glanders
    E. dengue
11. The *MOST* striking clinical sign of malignant lymphoma is 11. ...
    A. acute course and rapid termination
    B. generalized lymph node enlargement
    C. weight loss to the point of emaciation
    D. palpable masses in the abdominal cavity
    E. cachexia with chronic cough
12. In dogs, symptoms of hyperemia, anxiety, restlessness, whimpering, and elevated temperature followed by collapse and clonic spasms are considered pathognomonic for 12. ...
    A. epilepsy

B. eclampsia
C. strychnine poisoning
D. tetanus
E. encephalitis

13. Following a traumatic injury, the escape of frothy blood from the nose is a symptom of 13. ...
A. a systemic anthrax infection
B. rupture of the aorta
C. degeneration of a malignant neoplasm of the larynx
D. rupture of the pulmonary artery
E. laceration of the lung

14. In the control of psoroptic mange in cattle, it is *important* to know that: 14. ...
A. Stall beds, mangers, partitions, etc., should be thoroughly sprayed as part of the life cycle of the parasite that occurs off the host.
B. Only high pressure spraying or rubbing with a stiff brush while in the dip is satisfactory, because part of the life cycle of the parasite is spent deeply imbedded in the skin.
C. In general, as is the case with many bacteria, drying is the most effective enemy against the parasite while off the host.
D. While other mange parasites complete two or more cycles per year, the slow-growing psoroptes has only one; consequently only one treatment, preferably in December, is necessary for its control.
E. The interval between sprayings or dippings should be 10-12 days because of the rapidity of the complete cycle.

15. A peculiar thickening of the lymphatic vessels of the limbs in the region of the shoulder, tarsus, and fetlocks of bovines 15. ...
A. is undesirable since the carcass is automatically condemned as unfit for human consumption
B. seems to cause reaction to tuberculin and is officially termed "skin tuberculosis"
C. contains acid-fast rods identical with the tubercle bacillus
D. frequently ruptures, and thus predisposes to an undesirable series of Corynebacterium pyogenes abscesses
E. can be relieved by symptomatic treatment

16. Gross enlargement of the body lymph glands associated with anemia and an increased white blood cell count indicates: 16. ...
A. Anaplasmosis
B. Infection by ostertagia
C. Malignant lymphoma
D. Broken fern posioning
E. Copper deficiency

17. A cat shows symptoms of cyanosis, hunching up, and inactivity; a standing chest x-ray of the animal reveals a prominent fluid line. 17. ...
The fluid, aspirated by thoracocentesis, is quickly identified as an exudate because it

A. has a specific gravity less than 1.010
B. has no tendency to clot
C. has a glucose content greater than its plasma content
D. contains white blood cells in abundance
E. reveals no red blood cells

18. A client presents a 5-year-old male English pointer dog for examination because his animal has been "slowed down" in the field for the past 3 months. The animal is an excellent field trial dog which the owner has had in trials all over the United States. The animal eats well and seems fairly alert, but he shows early fatigability when he is worked. There has been a 5% weight loss in the past two months. 18. ...

The preliminary physical examination of this animal does not reveal any abnormalities. The blood urea nitrogen is 15 mg. per 100 ml.; fecal flotation examination reveals three toxocara canis ova.

Following are the detailed findings of this examination:

| URINALYSIS | | HEMOGRAM | |
|---|---|---|---|
| Color | yellow | Hemoglobin | 13 gm.% |
| Turbidity | cloudy | Hematocrit | 38% |
| Spec. grav. | 1.020 | rbc | 6,8000,000 |
| pH | 5.6 | wbc | 13,000 |
| Sugar | neg. | Differential cell count: | |
| Acetone | neg. | lymphocytes | 23% |
| Occult blood | neg. | granulocytes | 75% |
| Bilirubin | neg. | pmn | 49% |
| Albumin | neg. trace | stab | 7% |
| Microscopic exam: | | juvenile | 0% |
| wbc | 5/hpf | basophil | 1% |
| rbc | 2/hpf | eosinophil | 18% |
| crystals | oxolates | monocytes | 2% |
| epi. cells | 2/hpf | | |
| casts | none | | |
| bacteria | none | | |

The *MOST* logical diagnosis of this animal's basic problem is:

A. Early acute interstitial nephritis
B. Heartworm infection
C. Roundworm infection
D. Inadequate nutrition
E. Old age

19. In horses, the neoplasm that *MOST* commonly affects the non-pigmented areas of the skin of the eye, penis, and vulva is 19. ...

A. squamous-cell carcinoma
B. lymphosarcoma
C. adenocarcinoma
D. mast-cell carcinoma
E. papilloma

20. During the stable feeding period, several of a herd of cattle were affected. Soft swellings appeared in several parts of the body; the mucosae were pale; some deaths had occurred. A change in diet was indicated. 20. ...
   This condition would be diagnosed as
   A. vitamin A deficiency
   B. sweet clover disease
   C. blackleg
   D. preparturient ventral edema
   E. traumatic pericarditis

21. *Which one* of the following diseases is the *MOST LIKELY* cause of a thoracic transudate in a cat? 21. ...
   A. Cirrhosis of the liver
   B. Diaphragmatic hernia
   C. Adenocarcinoma
   D. Lymphosarcoma
   E. Cardiac hypertrophy

22. Several cows gained access to poisonous material. Though the poison contained only one ingredient, two types of symptoms were shown. Some walked in circles, appeared blind, fell, champted the jaws. Others showed severe gastro-intestinal irritation, with pain and fetid diarrhea. 22. ...
   The poisonous material was
   A. lead
   B. nitrate
   C. mercury
   D. sodium chloride
   E. copper sulfate

23. In the method of differentiating foot-and-mouth disease from vesicular stomatitis and vesicular exanthema as described by Traum, two cattle are infected with fresh vesicular fluid, one intramuscularly and the other in the mucosa of the tongue, lips, and dental pad. 23. ...
   If the vesicular fluid contained the virus of foot-and-mouth disease, the result would be:
   A. Both animals would develop the disease at the site of inoculation.
   B. Both animals would develop typical foot-and-mouth disease lesions.
   C. The animal injected intramuscularly would develop the disease while the other would remain normal.
   D. The animal injected intramuscularly would not develop the disease while the other would show typical lesions.
   E. Neither animal would develop the disease.

24. The *MOST* frequent heart disease seen in the bovine is 24. ...
   A. auriculoventricular stenosis
   B. semilunar insufficiency
   C. brisket disease
   D. traumatic pericarditis
   E. myocarditis

25. The cell-type characteristic of the leukoblastic tissues in malignant lymphoma is the: 25. ...
   A. neutrophil

B. immature lymphocyte
C. eosinophil
D. mononuclear leukocyte
E. mast cell

26. Left-sided congestive heart failure in an animal is *MOST* commonly characterized by: 26. ...
   A. Systolic murmur, liver congestion, increased heart rate, and ascites
   B. Diastolic murmur, sinus arrhythmia, cough, and fatigue
   C. Diastolic murmur, pulmonary congestion, increased heart rate, and cough
   D. Systolic murmur, sinus arrhythmia, cough, and fatigue
   E. Systolic murmur, pulmonary congestion, increased heart rate, and cough

27. Neonatal iso-erythrolysis in certain puppies occurs as a result of 27. ...
   A. gene transmission of anti-a iso-antibody from the bitch
   B. ingestion of anti-a iso-antibody from the bitch's milk during the first 24 hours of life
   C. gene transmission of anti-a iso-antibody from the sire
   D. ingestion of anti-a iso-antibody from the bitch's milk during the second week of life
   E. transplacental transfer of anti-a iso-antibody from the bitch

28. The *MOST* effective treatment of cardiac arrest is: 28. ...
   A. Intraventricular injection of 1:10,000 epinephrine chloride solution
   B. Cardiac massage and artificial pulmonary ventilation
   C. Pulmonary resuscitation and intravenous administration of fluids
   D. Cardiac stimulation and artificial pulmonary ventilation
   E. Electrical defibrillation followed by intravenous injection of ouabain

29. An acute inflammation of the lymph vessels and sometimes of the blood vessels of the legs, particularly of a rear leg, is often *mistakenly* diagnosed as lymphangitis when the *correct* diagnosis is: 29. ...
   A. Heart disease, myocarditis, or pericarditis with extensive edema
   B. Purpura hemorrhagica or dermatitis and so-called "scratches" with phlegmon
   C. Urticaria of unknown origin and sudden appearance
   D. A thrombus of the iliac arteries or veins
   E. Azoturia in the standing animal with severe myoglobinuria

30. The luteinizing hormone, in addition to causing growth of the corpus luteum, 30. ...
   A. produces alveolar growth in the mammary glands
   B. produces duct growth in the mammary glands
   C. is necessary for ovulation
   D. is responsible for the secretion of progesterone by the corpus luteum

E. is required for milk secretion

31. *MOST* recent investigations indicate that acanthosis nigricans is associated with — 31. ...
    A. hypofunction of the thyroid gland
    B. hyperfunction of the adrenal gland
    C. increase in acidophils in the pituitary gland
    D. hypofunction of the testes
    E. overproduction of thryoid-stimulating hormone

32. Puerperal tetany is generally considered to be due to — 32. ...
    A. hypopituitarism
    B. hypoparathyroidism
    C. hyperparathyroidism
    D. hyperthyroidism
    E. hyperadrenalism

33. In pregnant mares, *gonadotropin* is present in the serum in the *HIGHEST* concentration during the ______ day of pregnancy. — 33. ...
    A. 30th - 43rd
    B. 30th - 180th
    C. 43rd - 180th
    D. 80th - 180th
    E. 93rd - 180th

34. Acute gastric dilatation in the equine is *usually* the result of — 34. ...
    A. overloading with fermentable or heavy, indigestible food
    B. an enlargement of a mediastinal lymph gland
    C. working long hours in hot, humid weather
    D. a neoplasm blocking the pyloric orifice of the stomach
    E. permitting access to an unlimited amount of water before feeding

35. Replacement fluids containing dextrose, lactated sodium, and sodium and potassium chlorides are indicated for — 35. ...
    A. gastric loss
    B. protein loss
    C. duodenal loss
    D. shock
    E. water loss

36. Jaundice, a sign rather than a disease, is *usually* evidenced clinically by: — 36. ...
    A. dark and muddy discoloration of the conjunctiva
    B. pigmented areas of the skin
    C. clay-colored stools
    D. yellow discoloration of tissues and body fluids
    E. reddish discoloration of the urine

37. Salivary cysts in the dog are *MOST OFTEN* due to — 37. ...
    A. stenosis of the duct
    B. inflammatory lesions
    C. traumatic lesions
    D. obstruction of the duct
    E. congenital anomalies

38. The *CHIEF* manifestation of trichuris infestation in puppies is — 38. ...
    A. typhlitis
    B. anemia
    C. obstipation
    D. proctitis
    E. enterotoxemia

39. Hemorrhagic diarrhea in swine is *usually* indicative of 39. A...
 A. swine dysentery
 B. swine erysipelas
 C. salmonellosis
 D. hog cholera
 E. pasteurellosis

40. Nodular disease in cattle is caused by: 40. ~~A~~ C...
 A. ostertagia ostertagi
 B. chabertia bovis
 C. oesophagostomum radiatum
 D. oesophagostomum columbianum
 E. oesophagostomum venulosum

41. A stained smear of the blood of a cat with panleukopenia will *probably* show 41. E...
 A. the few remaining leukocytes to be predominantly neutrophils
 B. a marked increase in the number of young forms of neutrophils
 C. a marked decrease in the number of young forms of neutrophils
 D. lymphocyte forms
 E. microcytic hypochromic anemia to a marked degree.

42. Anaplasmosis is *MOST LIKELY* to be peracute and fatal in susceptible cattle aged 42. ~~D~~... E
 A. 1 - 6 months
 B. 4 - 18 months
 C. 18 - 24 months
 D. 1 - 2 years
 E. 3 years or more

43. The type of anemia in which a marked reduction of the hemopoietic activity of the bone marrow is typical is the 43. ~~A~~... E
 A. microcytic
 B. macrocytic
 C. hemolytic
 D. hypochromic macrocytic
 E. aplastic

44. A transient corneal opacity in one or both eyes is frequently observed in dogs following infection with 44. ~~A~~.. B
 A. canine distemper virus
 B. canine hepatitis virus
 C. canine tracheobronchitis virus
 D. neorickettsia helminthoeca
 E. leptospira canicola

45. The adult dirofilaria immitis is susceptible to medication with: 45. C...
 A. tetracyclines
 B. antimonials
 C. organic arsenicals
 D. piperazines
 E. mercurials

46. A relatively non-pathogenic nematode of dogs is 46. A..
 A. capillaria plica
 B. trichuris vulpis
 C. strongyloides sp.
 D. ancylostoma caninum
 E. dioctophyma renale

47. Feline pneumonitis in mature cats is characterized by: 47. . . .
   A. Necrotic rhinotracheitis, acidophilic intranuclear inclusions in the nasal epithelium, low morbidity, and low mortality
   B. Lobar pneumonia, serous nasal and ocular discharge, acidophilic cytoplasmic inclusions, low morbidity, and low mortality
   C. Bloody nasal discharge, pleural and peritoneal hemorrhages, swollen tonsils with petechiae, intranuclear inclusion bodies, high morbidity, and low mortality
   D. Coughing, sneezing, conjunctivitis, basophilic cytoplasmic elementary bodies, high morbidity, and low mortality
   E. Severe leukopenia, enteritis, intranuclear inclusions, high morbidity, and high mortality.

48. The *MOST* characteristic symptoms of puerperal hemoglobinemia are: 48. . . .
   A. Extreme weakness with violent nervous symptoms, the patient often lying cast for hours
   B. Chromic diarrhea with a slow pulse and general symptoms of a chronic emaciating disease
   C. Slow emaciation with a slight anemia alway before or during parturition
   D. Bloody urine with much sediment in the urine and with palpable swelling of the kidneys
   E. Pale mucosae, low hemoglobin and red cell count, tachycardia with palpitation, and increased heart impulse.

49. A chicken flock of 500 laying hens has dropped from 70 per cent to 2 per cent egg production in the course of five days. Tracheal rales and coughing were evident in the flock during this time. 49. . . .
   These symptoms are *suggestive* of
   A. avian encephalomyelitis
   B. newcastle disease
   C. chronic respiratory disease
   D. infectious laryngotracheitis
   E. fowl cholera

50. Immunity to canine distemper is related to an adequate blood level of 50. . . .
   A. receptor-destroying enzyme
   B. viral hemagglutinins
   C. virus-neutralizing antibody
   D. interferon
   E. complement-fixing antibody

# KEY (CORRECT ANSWERS)

| | | | | | | | | | |
|---|---|---|---|---|---|---|---|---|---|
| 1. | E | 11. | B | 21. | D | 31. | A | 41. | E |
| 2. | C | 12. | E | 22. | A | 32. | B | 42. | E |
| 3. | B | 13. | E | 23. | B | 33. | C | 43. | E |
| 4. | B | 14. | E | 24. | D | 34. | A | 44. | B |
| 5. | A | 15. | B | 25. | B | 35. | E | 45. | C |
| 6. | B | 16. | C | 26. | C | 36. | D | 46. | A |
| 7. | E | 17. | D | 27. | B | 37. | C | 47. | D |
| 8. | D | 18. | B | 28. | A | 38. | A | 48. | E |
| 9. | B | 19. | A | 29. | E | 39. | A | 49. | B |
| 10. | D | 20. | B | 30. | C | 40. | C | 50. | C |

# TEST 2

DIRECTIONS:
Each question or incomplete statement is followed by several suggested answers or completions. Select the one that *BEST* answers the question or completes the statement. *PRINT THE LETTER OF THE CORRECT ANSWER IN THE SPACE AT THE RIGHT.*

1. *One* of the species of coccidia *frequently* responsible for coccidiosis in cattle is: 1. ...
   A. Eimeria zurnii B. Eimeria stideae C. Eimeria necatrix
   D. Eimeria bovis E. Isospora bigemina
2. The spread of infectious canine hepatitis is difficult to control because 2. ...
   A. the infection is spread by contaminated biological products
   B. the virus is resistant to heat, drying, and disinfectants
   C. differential diagnosis is extremely difficult
   D. vaccination does not always confer immunity
   E. recovered animals may be carriers
3. A *correct* statement about immunization against canine distemper is: The 3. ...
   A. puppies of an immune dam may have levels of antibody that interfere with the production of immunity by modified live-virus vaccination during the nursing and immediate post-nursing period
   B. antiserum, as commonly employed at 10-day intervals, is incapable of producing an interference phenomenon when vaccination with modified live-virus vaccines is employed
   C. maternal protection afforded to a puppy is created both by placental transfer and by the ingestion of colostrum
   D. puppies of a distempered immune dam should be fairly well protected up to 10 weeks
   E. vaccine is most successful during the period in which the puppies are suckling
4. Anaplasma-like bodies on the red blood cells of a cat are considered pathognomonic for feline 4. ...
   A. panleukopenia B. toxoplasmosis C. infectious anemia
   D. rhinotracheitis E. pneumonitis
5. Some vaccination failures are said to be due to the fact that many dogs are exposed to canine distemper before immunity has been established. 5. ...
   In order to eliminate failures of this sort, it is necessary to
   A. use enough virus to immunize any susceptible dog
   B. inject immune serum prior to vaccination
   C. insure that puppies get their full share of colostrum
   D. use boiled syringes, insuring that they are uncontaminated by virulent virus
   E. keep puppies isolated from exposure to distemper until one week after vaccination

6. In endemic areas, a presumptive diagnosis of canine cocci-dioidomycosis can be made on the basis of 6. ...
   A. bright, shiny, hair-coat in spite of weight loss and sporadic diarrhea
   B. weight loss, deep productive cough, and loss of appetite
   C. cough, weight loss, persistent fever, and general malaise
   D. cough and lameness of long duration responsive to broad-spectrum antibiotics
   E. sporadic diarrhea without temperature elevation
7. Hypertrophic osteodystrophy, a disease most commonly seen in young dogs and characterized by subperiosteal hemorrhages, is thought to be associated with 7. ...
   A. hypovitaminosis C  B. hyperparathyroidism
   C. hypoparathyroidism  D. elevated blood phosphates
   E. deficient bone formation
8. A urine sample collected from a dog following an 18-hour water fast would indicate the *most complete* renal insufficiency if its specific gravity were 8. ...
   A. 1.005  B. 1.010  C. 1.015
   D. 1.020  E. 1.025
9. Pregnancy disease of ewes, in which there is a high mortality rate, is characterized by 9. ...
   A. marked hypocalcemia and hyperglycemia, similar to milk fever in cattle
   B. the presence of cirrhotic liver and a noticeable absence of fat throughout the body tissues
   C. its appearance in ewes which have been over-fed in the last 2 months
   D. its appearance after a sudden switch in diet from poor to luxuriant ration
   E. marked hypoglycemia, acetonemia, and acetonuria due to lack of CHO
10. Puerperal eclampsia in the bitch is characterized by: 10. ...
    A. A history of dystocia
    B. A very high temperature which is thought to cause permanent damage to the brain in many instances
    C. Sudden tetanic convulsions during which the animal usually remains conscious
    D. A gradual onset which eventually leads to semi-consciousness and collapse
    E. Sudden tetanic convulsions during which the animal usually loses consciousness
11. The cause of paraplegia in dogs whose intervertebral discs have herniated into the vertebral canal is: 11. ...
    A. Physiologic dysfunction due to myelitis
    B. The loss of the disc substance, which decreases articular movement
    C. Spinal cord compression and contusion
    D. Spinal cord and spinal nerve compression with articular ankylosis
    E. Inhibition of movement due to pain
12. In the horse, damage to the left seventh cranial nerve as it crosses the ramus of the mandible causes the 12. ...
    A. lower lip to hang slack

B. left eyelid to develop ptosis
C. right eyelid to develop ptosis
D. upper lip to be drawn to the left side
E. upper lip to be drawn to the right side

13. Symptoms resembling estrum that follow ovario-hysterectomy are usually NOT caused by 13. ...
A. vaginitis B. vulvitis C. retained ovarian tissue
D. cystitis E. nephritis

14. In cattle, chronic rhinitis accompanied by nasal granuloma is known as 14. ...
A. summer snuffles B. rhinosporidiosis
C. sarcosporidiosis D. allergic asthma
E. nasal gleet

15. Hypertrophic pulmonary osteoarthropathy is clinically characterized by 15. ...
A. chronic bronchopneumonia
B. mixed mammary tumors
C. osteoarthritis
D. coughing, dyspnea, and nasal discharge
E. bony lesions of the limbs

16. Recurrent epistaxis in dogs is NOT ordinarily associated with 16. ...
A. linguatula serrata B. thelazia californiensis
C. pulmonary neoplasms D. dirofilaria
E. pneumonyssus caninum

17. Subcutaneous emphysema in cattle is *MOST* frequently associated with 17. ...
A. verminous pneumonia B. gangrenous pneumonia
C. acute alveolar emphysema D. chronic alveolar emphysema
E. chronic bronchial pneumonia

18. Lungworm disease which occurs commonly in sheep, swine, and calves is 18. ...
A. relatively easy to prevent since no intermediate host for the parasite need be considered
B. readily overlooked on post-mortem examination when only the smaller lungworms are present, unless a low-power microscope is used
C. diminishing in frequency due to fly control by the wide use of DDT and similar products
D. confused with other types of pneumonia, except in swine where it may be easily diagnosed positively on ante-mortem examination
E. now successfully treated on a large scale, particularly in calves and sheep by the use of intratracheal injections of carbon tetrachloride

19. The treatment of choice for a cow with acute pulmonary edema due to anaphylaxis is 19. ...
A. blood transfusion
B. epinephrine, 10 cc
C. carbachol solution, 2 cc
D. norepinephrine, 1 cc
E. calcium gluconate solution, 500 cc

20. An *incorrect* statement regarding tracheobronchitis in dogs is that the 20. ...
A. cough is usually harsh and dry

B. disease responds well to broad-spectrum antibiotics
C. disease is mild and self-limiting
D. cough is easily induced by massaging the trachea
E. incubation period is 5 - 10 days

21. The *MOST* common form of pneumonia in the domestic animal is ________ pneumonia 21. ...
A. lobar B. lobular C. interstitial
D. suppurative E. verminous

22. As a preoperative rinse for the scrubbed hands of the surgeon, ethyl alcohol is *MOST* efficient in a concentration by weight of ________ per cent. 22. ...
A. 50 B. 60 C. 70 D. 80 E. 90

23. Modern chemotherapeutic agents have not permitted the abandonment of any of the principles of surgical management because the chemotherapeutic agent 23. ...
A. alleviates pain
B. stimulates healing and repair
C. is bactericidal
D. tends to control excess hemorrhage
E. is only one of a great many factors which enter into the achievement of the end result

24. The *ideal* temperature for the healing of a wound is ________ degrees C. 24. ...
A. 33 B. 36 C. 39 D. 42 E. 45

25. The *most common* indication for the removal of the spleen is 25. ...
A. splenomegaly B. the presence of hematomas
C. the presence of tumors D. nodular hyperplasia
E. traumatic rupture

26. Following systemic administration of penicillin, an adequate therapeutic level is *MOST* apt to be found in a(n) 26. ...
A. subacute circumscribed peritonitis
B. pleural empyema of the chest
C. well-localized abscess
D. subacute infection of the fetlock joint
E. acute streptococcal meningitis

27. The *MAIN* advantage of the archibald technique over other methods for the removal of the prostate is: 27. ...
A. The perineal approach causes less shock to the patient.
B. The urethra is left intact when the prostate is divided.
C. The entire gland is removed, leaving no nucleus of tissue capable of regeneration.
D. There is good visibility of all structures at all stages of the operation.
E. Electrocautery results in less hemorrhaging.

28. When a wound has been left open for a few days and the granulating surfaces have then been sutured together, the process is called healing by ________ intention. 28. ...
A. first B. second C. third D. fourth E. fifth

29. A satisfactory skin suture material should not absorb tissue fluids. 29. ...
*Which one* of the following may retain serum in a suture strand, thereby favoring invasion of the wound by microorganisms?
A. Silkworm gut B. Alloy C. Untreated silk
D. Nylon E. Fiberglas

30. Five 3-year-old litter mates in a state of normal metabolism and normal nutrition have each sustained a different kind of fracture; each fracture has been reduced promptly, aseptically, and correctly. 30. ...
The animal that will heal *MOST* rapidly is the one that has a fracture of the type:
A. Transverse epiphyseal
B. Impacted diaphyseal
C. Transverse diaphyseal
D. Oblique diaphyseal
E. Impacted epiphyseal

31. Under *optimum* conditions, first-intention healing following soft tissue surgery generally requires a *MINIMUM* of 31. ...
A. 5 - 7 days
B. 12 - 14 days
C. 41 - 44 days
D. 3 - 4 months
E. 6 - 7 months

32. The reflex stimulation of the vagus center and consequent stopping of the heart sometimes observed in chloroform anesthesia may be overcome by the 32. ...
A. preanesthetic administration of atropine
B. administration of chloroform by the choke method rather than by the drop method
C. administration of pentobarbital sodium
D. preanesthetic administration of chloral hydrate
E. use of a mixture containing alcohol, chloroform, and ether (A.C.E. mixture)

33. The *minimum* treatment with steam under pressure by which large bundles of surgical equipment can be completely sterilized is ________ degrees F for ________ minutes. 33. ...
A. 212; 15 B. 212; 30 C. 225; 30
D. 250; 15 E. 250; 30

34. When pain persists in a dog with cervical disc protrusions that have been treated with conventional drugs, the surgical procedure should consist of a 34. ...
A. ventral midline disc curettage
B. dorsal hemilaminectomy
C. dorsal laminectomy
D. dorsal disc curettage
E. lateral disc curettage

35. The *purpose* of removing the laryngeal saccules in laryngeal hemiplegia or "roaring" of horses is to 35. ...
A. produce an adhesion between the cricothyroid membrane and the vocal fold
B. give additional strength and support to the extrinsic muscles of the larynx
C. remove hypertrophied tissue in the laryngeal ventricles
D. produce a chondritis and thickening of the laryngeal cartilages
E. produce a cicatrix which holds the arytenoid cartilage and vocal fold laterally

36. *What* surgical procedure is employed for the relief of glaucoma in the dog? 36. ...
   A. Resection of the membrana nictitans
   B. Medial canthotomy
   C. Iridencleisis
   D. Cauterization of scleral vessels
   E. Conjunctival flap

37. The *MOST* common defect in the development of cheek teeth in the horse is 37. ...
   A. failure of complete cementation of the infundibuli
   B. elongation of molars
   C. growth of more than one stalk from deciduous tooth germs
   D. the occurrence of supernumerary canines
   E. the occurrence of sharp enamel points along the medial edges of the upper cheek teeth and the lateral edges of the lower cheek teeth

38. The *MOST* important feature in aural resection is 38. ...
   A. a single incision through the conchal cartilage
   B. liberal exposure of the horizontal canal at its lateral extremity
   C. the use of Kocher's forceps to control hemorrhage, and keeping the tissues well aligned
   D. liberal excision of cartilage to induce flaccidity
   E. suturing the edges of the cartilage with interrupted sutures

39. The *key* to successful capping of bovine incisor teeth is to 39. ...
   A. permit the caps to set firmly by denying the animal food and water for 12 hours
   B. half-fill the caps with cement and place them immediately on dry teeth
   C. use malleable silver alloy
   D. wait till the teeth are worn to the gum line
   E. cement the teeth of the incisor arcade together for greater support

40. A *frequently* occurring sequela to ablation of the lens for the relief of cataracts in dogs is 40. ...
   A. conjunctivitis
   B. entropion
   C. temporary corneal opacity
   D. ectropion
   E. persistent epiphora

41. The *one* of the following statements about fractures of the bones of the head in large animals that is *CORRECT* is that fractures of the 41. ...
   A. body of the mandible are repaired by ossification of endochondral bone
   B. interdental bone are usually due to abnormal fragility
   C. ramus of the mandible are most often due to extreme muscular action
   D. ramus of the mandible due to direct trauma may be simple or compound
   E. supraorbital process are often followed by loss of eyesight on the injured side

42. Anoxic anoxia results from 42. ...
   A. an insufficient delivery of oxygen to the tissues due to passive congestion
   B. decreased hemoglobin in the blood and diminished delivery of oxygen to the tissues
   C. inhibition of the utilization of oxygen by the tissues by certain chemicals
   D. an insufficient delivery of oxygen by the lungs to the blood
   E. an insufficient delivery of oxygen to the tissues due to cardiac failure

43. The heart of a dog is *BEST* exposed by an incision in intercostal space 43. ...
   A. 2 or 3 B. 4 or 5 C. 6 or 7
   D. 8 or 9 E. 9 or 10

44. In the surgery of hollow organs, the continuous Cushing suture 44. ...
   A. does not penetrate the lumen
   B. is not pulled taut
   C. requires the use of silk
   D. requires a row of reinforcing sutures
   E. everts the tissue

45. Traumatic gastritis of the bovine is *usually* the result of 45. ...
   A. increased intra-abdominal pressure incident to advanced pregnancy
   B. perforation of the anterior aspect of the reticulum by a foreign body
   C. perforation of the pericardial sac by a foreign body
   D. perforation of the wall of the rumen by a foreign body
   E. localized peritonitis between the reticulum and the diaphragm

46. Canine perineal herniae are *MOST* frequently seen in 46. ...
   A. spayed females B. normal females
   C. castrated males D. non-castrated males
   E. newborn puppies of either sex

47. The security of an intestinal suture depends upon its grasp of the 47. ...
   A. muscularis mucosae B. muscularis
   C. submucosa D. mucosa E. peritoneum

48. In the bovine, intussusception of the small intestine is *MOST* satisfactorily treated by 48. ...
   A. surgical resection of the affected portion and anastomosis of the normal ends
   B. manual manipulation of the affected bowel per rectum
   C. the administration of copious saline enemas
   D. the administration of smooth-muscle stimulants, for example, arecoline
   E. the administration of large doses of mild laxatives

49. A typhlectomy is *indicated* in 49. ...
   A. impaction B. Hirschsprung's disease
   C. ileus D. chronic whipworm infection
   E. spastic colitis

50. The Ramstedt operation is designed for the relief of — 50. ... A
A. pyloric stenosis
B. megacolon
C. duodenal ulcers
D. urinary incontinence
E. urolithiasis

---

# KEY (CORRECT ANSWERS)

| | | | | | | | | | |
|---|---|---|---|---|---|---|---|---|---|
| 1. | A | 11. | C | 21. | B | 31. | A | 41. | D |
| 2. | E | 12. | E | 22. | C | 32. | A | 42. | D |
| 3. | A | 13. | E | 23. | E | 33. | E | 43. | B |
| 4. | C | 14. | B | 24. | C | 34. | A | 44. | A |
| 5. | E | 15. | E | 25. | C | 35. | E | 45. | B |
| 6. | C | 16. | B | 26. | B | 36. | C | 46. | D |
| 7. | B | 17. | C | 27. | D | 37. | A | 47. | C |
| 8. | B | 18. | B | 28. | B | 38. | B | 48. | A |
| 9. | E | 19. | B | 29. | C | 39. | B | 49. | D |
| 10. | C | 20. | B | 30. | C | 40. | C | 50. | A |

---

# EXAMINATION SECTION
## TEST 1

DIRECTIONS: Each question or incomplete statement is followed by several suggested answers or completions. Select the one that BEST answers the question or completes the statement. *PRINT THE LETTER OF THE CORRECT ANSWER IN THE SPACE AT THE RIGHT.*

1. The lesion in an animal presented with Horner's syndrome and mild weakness in the right thoracic limb and spastic paresis in the right pelvic limb would *most likely* be located in the  1. ____
   A. $C_1$ to $C_8$ spinal cord
   B. ventral roots of $T_1$ to $T_3$ on the right side
   C. $T_1$ to $T_3$ spinal cord on the right side
   D. cranial medulla on the right side
   E. cervical sympathetic trunk

2. The postganglionic axons of the sympathetic innervation of the eye arise from the ________ ganglion.  2. ____
   A. stellate  B. nodose
   C. cranial cervical  D. ciliary
   E. trigeminal

3. It is NOT true of the pupil of Horner's syndrome that it  3. ____
   A. will NOT dilate in the dark-adapted state
   B. is NOT a pinpoint pupil
   C. is difficult to diagnose in bright light
   D. is smaller than the normal pupil
   E. will dilate approximately 3 to 4 mm in the dark-adapted state

4. Sympathetic innervation of the eye supplies ALL of the following EXCEPT the  4. ____
   A. smooth muscle of the eyelids
   B. smooth muscle of the third eyelid
   C. smooth muscle of the periorbita
   D. iris dilator muscle
   E. constrictor muscle of the iris

5. In an animal with Horner's syndrome resulting from a lesion involving the right middle ear, the associated neurologic deficits could include ALL of the following EXCEPT  5. ____
   A. a drooping lip on the right side
   B. a depressed menace reflex on the right side
   C. spastic hemiparesis on the right side
   D. inability to close eyelids properly
   E. a drooping ear on the right side

6. The MOST helpful diagnostic aid when presented with a cat with Horner's syndrome and no associated neurologic deficit or evidence of ear canal disease is *most likely*  6. ____
   A. cerebrospinal fluid tap

B. skull radiographs
C. chest radiographs
D. electroencephalogram
E. myringotomy

7. Horner's syndrome secondary to damage to the brain stem or cervical spinal cord is a result of interruption of the ________ tract. 7. ~~E~~ D
A. spinothalamic
B. spinotectal
C. propriospinal
D. lateral tectotegmentospinal
E. reticulospinal

8. The cranial cervical ganglion is located 8. ~~A~~ B
A. just inside the thoracic inlet
B. just caudomedially to the tympanic bulla
C. at the bifurcation of the common carotid arteries
D. in the middle ear
E. in the cavernous sinus

9. The lesions of paratuberculosis of cattle are found consistently in the intestinal tract and in the 9. A
A. mesenteric lymph nodes
B. kidney
C. pancreas
D. lung
E. liver

10. A gram-negative filamentous rodlike organism observed in smears from encapsulated abscesses in the wall of the rumen and the parenchymal of the liver of a cow is *most likely* 10. ~~E~~ D
A. salmonella enteritis
B. actinobacillus lignieresi
C. mycobacterium tuberculosis
D. spherophorus necrophorus
E. actinomyces bovis

11. A factor responsible for the appearence of post mortem changes resulting in pseudomelanosis of the intestinal tract is the presence of 11. B
A. excessive melanin pigments
B. hemolyzed erythrocytes
C. intestinal melanoblastoma
D. ingested carbons such as coal
E. obstructive icterus

12. Coccidia frequently produce in cattle a hemorrhagic inflamation *most commonly* located in the 12. ~~C~~ D
A. liver
B. kidney
C. small intestine
D. colon
E. mesenteric lymph nodes

13. The condition indicated by the absence of urobilinogen from the intestinal content of the icteric animal is 13. B
   A. biliary cirrhosis
   B. biliary obstruction
   C. multifocal hepatic necrosis
   D. cholesterol deficiency
   E. hemolytic anemia

14. Double operculated ova found in intestinal scrapings from a chicken indicate the presence of 14. C
   A. davainea
   B. heterakus
   C. capillaria
   D. ascaridia
   E. raillietina

15. Hepatic passive congestion without accompanying pulmonary passive congestion may be caused by 15. D
   A. cardiac sarcosporidiosis
   B. fasciola hepatica
   C. mitral insufficiency L
   D. tricuspid insufficiency R
   E. stenosis of the aortic semilunar valves

16. Vegatative endocarditis may be one of the chief lesions found in 16. B
   A. bovine traumatic gastritis
   B. swine erysipelatrix
   C. equine viral arteritis
   D. hog cholera
   E. canine toxoplasmosis

17. Partial obstruction of the esophagus can be caused by a(n) 17. C
   A. endocardial fibroblastosis
   B. patent foramen ovale
   C. persistent right aortic arch
   D. interventricular opening
   E. persistent ductus arteriosis

18. The formation of a clot in flowing blood within the vascular system is called 18. C
   A. embolism
   B. erythroblastosis
   C. thrombosis
   D. sludging
   E. infarction

19. A patent foramen ovale is NOT an unusual finding at the necropsy of newborn 19. B
   A. foals
   B. calves
   C. kids
   D. pigs
   E. lambs

20. Tricuspid stenosis results in 20. A
   A. central cirrhosis of the liver
   B. telangiectasis of the liver
   C. the lesions of sawdust liver
   D. Glissonian cirrhosis
   E. hobnail liver

21. There is a high incidence of neoplastic disease in the domestic chicken.
The type that occurs MOST frequently is the 21. C
A. osteoblastoma
B. adenoma
C. lymphocytoma
D. carcinoma
E. mysoblastoma

22. In bovine bacillary hemoglobinuria, the MOST characteristic gross lesion is 22. A
A. hemoglobinuria
B. severe renal degeneration
C. anemic infarction of the liver
D. hemosiderosis of the spleen
E. biliary obstruction due to liver flukes

23. In a dog affected with chronic intertitial nephritis, the kidneys are 23. C
A. large, pale and soft
B. large but otherwise normal
C. small, firm and pale
D. large, pale and firm
E. small but otherwise normal

24. Cystic kidneys are *most commonly* found in 24. C
A. cats
B. horses
C. swine
D. sheep
E. mules

25. The virus of infectious pustular vulvovaginitis of cattle has been identified as the same that causes 25. A
A. infectious bovine rhinotracheitis
B. foot and mouth disease
C. infectious ulcerative stomatitis
D. bovine malignant head catarrh
E. bovine pleuropneumonia

26. Hydronephrosis is a dilatation of the renal pelvis that usually results from 26. D
A. the action of toxins on the renal tubules
B. a slowly developing or intermittent obstruction of the flow of urine
C. an interference with the blood supply to the kidney
D. a complete blockage of the flow of urine
E. a deposition of amyloid in the kidney

27. Specific infectious pyelonephritis of the cow is caused by 27. E
A. actinomyces bovis
B. clostridium septicum
C. staphylococcus aureus
D. corynebacterium pyogenes
E. corynebacterium renale

28. The bacterium moraxella bovis can often be isolated from a disease of cattle characterized by inflamation of the 28. B
A. brain and spinal cord
B. cornea and conjunctiva
C. kidneys and ureters

D. trachea and bronchi
E. coronet and interdigital skin

29. Unlike the similar tumor in man, in multiple schwannomas (nerve sheath tumors) involving the peripheral nervous system in cattle, there are NO visible or palpable nodules in the skin. 29.____
But this tumor can be presumptively diagnosed upon clinical examination by
A. observing the tone of the rectal and urinary bladder sphincters
B. testing the direct and crossed pupillary reflexes
C. testing cutaneous sensation over the hindquarters
D. auscultation of the heart
E. examination of the cerebrospinal fluid

30. Granulomas in the subependymal regions of the horse brain are found in infection with 30.____
A. Japanese bovine encephalitis
B. American equine encephalomyelitis
C. equine infectious anemia
D. leptospira pomona
E. pseudorabies

31. A microscopic lesion in swine considered to be pathognomonic of the ingestion of too much salt (sodium chloride) is 31.____
A. ulcerative gastritis
B. cerebral edema
C. acute glomerulonephritis
D. eosinophilic meningo-encephalitis
E. midzonal liver necrosis

32. In listeriosis, the characteristic brain lesion is 32.____
A. the formation of microabscesses in the brain stem
B. demyelinating encephalitis
C. the occurrence of intranuclear inclusion bodies in the Purkinjie cells
D. neuronal degeneration
E. lymphocytic perivascular cuffing

33. The animal disease that CANNOT be transmitted directly from animal to man is 33.____
A. glanders
B. anthrax
C. salmonellosis
D. brucellosis
E. tetanus

34. The immediate source of energy when a muscle contracts is 34.____
A. glucose
B. ATP
C. creatinine phosphate
D. glycogen
E. adenylic acid

35. The site at which retinal detachment usually occurs is the 35.____
   A. inner nuclear layer
   B. inner plexiform layer
   C. outer plexiform layer only
   D. ganglion cell layer
   E. rod and cone layer

36. At the present time, the MOST reliable test for food allergy in the dog is 36.____
   A. test blood for reagins
   B. biopsy a skin lesion
   C. patch test with food allergins
   D. test urine for albumin
   E. eliminate single food components and observe

37. The cathartic that has irritability properties is 37.____
   A. bran
   B. methylcellulose
   C. DSS
   D. sodium sulfate
   E. cascara segrada

38. The general recommended level of salt for all swine is 38.____
   A. 0.5%
   B. 1.0%
   C. 1.5%
   D. 2.0%
   E. 2.5%

39. The MOST effective and efficient procedure for defibrillating the ventricles of the heart of a dog is the 39.____
   A. I.V. injection of calcium chloride
   B. use of intense electrical shock
   C. intracardiac injection of amphetamine sulfate
   D. intracardiac injection of 1:1000 epinephrine hydrochloride
   E. I.V. injection of 1:1000 epinephrin hydrochloride

40. The anterior drawer sign of rupture of the anterior cruciate ligament in the dog is 40.____
   A. anterior gliding of the femur
   B. anterior gliding of the tibia
   C. posteria gliding of the tibia
   D. medial luxation of the patella
   E. lateral luxation of the patella

41. In the clinical diagnosis of disease of domestic animals, it is important to remember that vomiting is 41.____
   A. rare in horses and indicative of gastric dilitation with pending rupture
   B. common in cattle and probably the main contributing factor in the low mortality rate in frothy bloat
   C. rare in swine and considered pathognomonic for hog cholera
   D. *most commonly* seen in sheep in cases of pregnancy toxemia
   E. NOT seen in cattle except in advanced vagal indigestion

42. Sudden development of fever, prostration and severe cough in nearly 100% of a herd of 190 lb. hogs is characteristic of — 42. ____
   A. hog cholera with bacterial pneumonia
   B. bordetella pneumonia
   C. mycoplasma pneumonia
   D. pasteurellosis
   E. swine influenza

43. The symptoms of limb edema, venous engorgement, ascites, hepatomegally and no respiratory signs in a dog are indicative of — 43. ____
   A. mitral insufficiency
   B. right heart failure
   C. left heart failure
   D. generalized heart failure
   E. aortic stenosis

44. The feline leukemia virus — 44. ____
   A. can be transmitted to other cats
   B. is a human health hazard
   C. can live for months outside the host
   D. stimulates production of antibodies which are detectable by the F.A. test
   E. needs rapidly dividing cells in which to replicate

45. Lungworms (Aelturostrongylus abstrusus) in the cat can be positively diagnosed by — 45. ____
   A. finding adult worms in the sputum of infected cats
   B. identification of larvae in a fecal sample
   C. tapping the chest
   D. identification of eggs by making a swab of nasal secretions
   E. identification of eggs in a fecal sample

46. The MOST effective treatment regimen for feline hemobartonellosis includes — 46. ____
   A. tetracycline
   B. chloramphenicol
   C. ampicillin
   D. tetracycline and chloramphenicol
   E. chloramphenicol and ampicillin

47. The drug that is known to have teratogenic effects if administered to the pregnant queen is — 47. ____
   A. ketamine
   B. chloramphenicol
   C. ampicillin
   D. furosemide
   E. griseofulvin

48. Undesirable drug side effects in renal failure are caused by 48. ___
A. changes in drug receptors
B. permeability changes in the blood-brain barrier
C. enzyme activity disturbances
D. metabolic load of a given drug
E. All of the above

49. The drug(s) that is (are) excreted *primarily* by the kidneys is (are) 49. ___
A. digoxin B. digitoxin C. tetracycline
D. digitoxin and tetracycline
E. All of the above

50. Which of the following are indications of beta-adrenoceptor intoxication? 50. ___
A. Depression B. Bradycardia C. Bronchospasm
D. Fever E. All of the above

---

# KEY (CORRECT ANSWERS)

| | | | | |
|---|---|---|---|---|
| 1. C | 11. B | 21. C | 31. D | 41. A |
| 2. C | 12. D | 22. C | 32. A | 42. E |
| 3. A | 13. B | 23. C | 33. E | 43. B |
| 4. E | 14. C | 24. C | 34. B | 44. A |
| 5. C | 15. D | 25. A | 35. E | 45. B |
| 6. C | 16. B | 26. D | 36. E | 46. D |
| 7. D | 17. C | 27. E | 37. E | 47. E |
| 8. B | 18. C | 28. B | 38. A | 48. E |
| 9. A | 19. B | 29. D | 39. B | 49. D |
| 10. D | 20. A | 30. C | 40. B | 50. E |

---

# TEST 2

DIRECTIONS: Each question or incomplete statement is followed by several suggested answers or completions. Select the one that BEST answers the question or completes the statement. *PRINT THE LETTER OF THE CORRECT ANSWER IN THE SPACE AT THE RIGHT.*

1. The PR interval is the time from the 1.____
   A. beginning of a P wave to the beginning of an R wave
   B. beginning of a P wave to the end of an R wave
   C. beginning of a P wave to the beginning of a QRS
   D. end of a P wave to the beginning of a R wave
   E. end of a P wave to the end of a R wave

2. Equine lampas 2.____
   A. is thickening of the hard palate in old smooth mouthed horses
   B. occurs in horses that are 8 to 10 years old
   C. is a sequelae to chronic alveolar emphysema
   D. is swelling of the soft palate
   E. is a physiologic reaction involving thickening of the hard palate

3. The MOST frequent cause of congestive heart failure in the dog is 3.____
   A. aortic insufficiency
   B. ventricular septal defect
   C. tricuspid insufficiency
   D. mitral insufficiency
   E. pulmonic stenosis

4. A physical exam of a 4-year-old intact female poodle with polyuria and polydypsia reveals bilateral cateracts which the animal's owner said appeared suddenly a few weeks ago. 4.____
   The MOST probable cause is
   A. Cushing's syndrome
   B. nephritis
   C. diabetes insipidus
   D. diabetes mellitus
   E. pyometra

5. A functional tumor of the beta cells of the pancreatic islets results in 5.____
   A. diabetes insipidus
   B. diabetic coma
   C. Cushing's syndrome
   D. hypocalcemic tetany
   E. hypoglycemic seizure

6. Pseudocyesis in the bitch and queen is due to the production of 6.____
   A. estrogens by the ovary
   B. excessive LH by the pituitary
   C. an imbalance between FSH and LH
   D. excessive FSH by the pituitary
   E. progesterone by the corpus luteum

7. The nerve block *most commonly* used as an aid in the diagnosis of navicular disease is — 7. A
   A. medial and lateral post digital
   B. common digital and deep peroneal
   C. medial and lateral volar
   D. superficial peroneal
   E. abaxial digital

8. Traumatic gastritis, a relatively common problem in cattle, is virtually non-existent in horses because they — 8. B
   A. have a shorter life span
   B. have more careful eating habits
   C. consume far less roughage
   D. are rarely exposed to foreign objects
   E. are non-ruminants, for it is next to impossible for a foreign body to penetrate the stomach wall

9. Many factors contribute to the development of cardiac arrhythmias during anesthesia.
   Among these is (are) — 9. E
   A. anxiety during induction
   B. surgical stimulation
   C. serum electrolytes, arterial pH and blood gases
   D. body temperature
   E. all of the above

10. Hepatic changes are observed following administration of — 10. D ~~B~~
   A. ether
   B. methoxyflurane
   C. ether and halothane
   D. methoxyflurane and nitrous oxide
   E. halothane and chloroform

11. In the dog, hemolytic anemia combined with basophilic stippling of reticulocytes with normoblasts on a hematologic exam suggests a tentative diagnosis of — 11. D
   A. chronic blood loss
   B. aplastic anemia
   C. chronic mercury poisoning
   D. acute lead poisoning
   E. iron deficiency anemia

12. A persistent abscess of the zygomatic salivary gland in the dog, is usually treated by — 12. A
   A. drainage of the abscess through an incision posterior to the last molar tooth
   B. administration of broad spectrum antibiotics until the fever subsides
   C. incision of the skin and underlying tissue 1cm above the zygomatic arch and 2 cm lateral to the midline
   D. incision of the ventral conjunctival sac at the junction of the bulbar and palpebral conjuctive
   E. extraction of the 4th premolar tooth

13. Congenital microspherocytosis in dogs is a manifestation of 13.____
    A. a hereditary defect in the formation of the erythron
    B. the presence of hemoparasites, such as hemobartenella or babesia
    C. a severe blood loss
    D. myelogenous leukemia
    E. iron deficient anemia

14. So called "blue eye" or hepatitis reaction is BEST treated by 14.____
    A. corticosteroids alone
    B. foreign proteins and corticosteroids
    C. foreign protein and atropine
    D. atropine and corticosteroids
    E. pilocarpine and corticosteroids

15. Which of the following is NOT a feature of dirofilaria immitis infection? 15.____
    A. Right heart enlargement
    B. An enlarged pulmonary artery segment of the cardiac silhouette
    C. Plueral effusion
    D. Areas of infarction within the lung fields
    E. Enlargement and tortuosity of the pulmonary vessels

16. Except for severity, the clinical and pathological signs of African swine fever are identical to 16.____
    A. virus pig pneumonia
    B. atrophic rhinitis
    C. hog cholera
    D. rinderpast
    E. swine influenza

17. Thickening of the colon by epithelial tissue is characteristic of 17.____
    A. BWD
    B. IPR
    C. TGE
    D. colibaccilosis
    E. Johne's disease

18. In which of the following species affected by pseudorabies is a clinical sign of pruritis absent? 18.____
    A. K-9
    B. Equine
    C. Porcine
    D. Ovine
    E. Bovine

19. In a young equine, a hard enlargement over the alveolus of the 1st, 2nd or 3rd premolar tooth is usually due to 19.____
    A. an abscess
    B. a cyst
    C. an osteoma
    D. alveolar periostitis
    E. a sarcoma

20. The B.M.R. (basal metabolic rate) is a measure of the activity of 20.____
    A. insulin
    B. cortisol
    C. aldosterone
    D. thyroxine
    E. growth hormone

21. Rumination is stimulated by 21. A
   A. the presence of coarse, fibrous material in the region of the cardia
   B. high blood sugar levels
   C. CNS stimulation
   D. abomasal distention
   E. none of the above

22. In examining a dog with suspected right leg coxofemoral luxation, a longer affected limb is revealed when it is held extended perpendicular and extended behind the body. The position of the femoral head is 22. A C
   A. anterior and dorsal
   B. posterior and dorsal
   C. posterior and ventral
   D. anterior and ventral
   E. acetabular

23. The observation MOST characteristic of a poodle with progressive retinal atrophy is 23. E
   A. abnormal protrusion of the eyes
   B. cataracts
   C. dilated pupils
   D. epiphora
   E. night blindness (nyctolopia)

24. Absorption of maternal antibody via the intestinal tract occurs for a _______ day period following birth in the dog. 24. A B
   A. 1
   B. 3
   C. 7
   D. 12
   E. 28

25. A pet cat has been found to be infected with Paragonimus kellicotti. The owner is concerned about possible infection to her children. She should be advised that 25. D
   A. her physician should initiate anthelmintic therapy to remove the adults and larvae in the children
   B. although the larval cysts have been found in human beings, they rarely occur in North America
   C. the eggs in the cat's feces can cause patent infection in children
   D. it is unlikely that the children will become infected due to life cycle requirements of the parasite
   E. visceral larva migrans is a possibility if eggs are swallowed by the children

26. A dog is presented with hypotonic eye. Which of the following would be the first to be eliminated as a possible diagnosis? 26. D
   A. Acute conjunctivitis
   B. Acute dehydration
   C. Addison's disease
   D. Anterior uveitis
   E. Episcleritis

27. A drug that can cause aplastic anemia in the dog is 27.____
   A. streptomycin
   B. penicillin
   C. estradiol
   D. atropine
   E. DNP

28. In differentiating prerenal uremia from renal uremia, the *most likely* findings in prerenal uremia would be 28.____
   A. a low specific gravity (<1.015), a large volume of urine and a trace of protein
   B. a high specific gravity (>1.030) a small volume of urine and a trace of protein
   C. a low specific gravity (<1.015), a small volume of urine and a trace of protein
   D. a specific gravity in the fixed range (1.010±.002) without proteinuria
   E. a high specific gravity (>1.030), a large volume of urine and a trace of protein

29. The BEST description of the lesions of acanthosis nigicans found in a dachshund patient is 29.____
   A. excessive coloration of the skin due to increased melanin deposition
   B. an increase in thickness of the horny (Keratin) layer of the skin
   C. an area of fibrous tissue lacking pigmentation that replaced damaged dermis or subcutaneous tissue
   D. a thick accumulation of loose fragments of the horny layer of the skin
   E. a thickening and hardening of the skin usually pigmented with exaggeration of the superficial skin markings

30. The normal $pCO_2$ of the blood is ______ mm. 30.____
   A. 760
   B. 320
   C. 40
   D. 80
   E. 10

31. Blood flow through an atrial septal defect has NO sound of its own but the murmur detected with this lesion mimics that of 31.____
   A. mitral insufficiency
   B. pulmonic stenosis
   C. aortic insufficiency
   D. ventricular septal defect
   E. mitral stenosis

32. An airbronchogram is associated *most commonly* with 32.____
   A. bronchopneumonia
   B. interstitial pneumonia
   C. pleural effusion
   D. pneumomediastinum
   E. chronic bronchitis

33. The sudden onset of marked head tilt, awkward movements, rotatory oscillation of the head and nystagmus in a cat would suggest a diagnosis of 33.____
   A. cerebellar ataxia
   B. organophosphate poisoning
   C. ear mites

D. vestibular disease
E. middle ear infection

34. The drug that would result in the highest rate of cure in treatment of uncomplicated bacterial cystitis in dogs is 34.___
A. methenamine mandelate
B. sulfasuxidine
C. D-1 methionine
D. benzathine penicillin G
E. chloramphenicol

35. A completely blind miniature poodle is presented for examination and breeding recommendation. Fundus examination reveals progressive retinal atrophy. 35.___
The *most likely* recommendation would be that this dog
A. be used for breeding since inheritance of the disease is NOT known
B. NOT be used for breeding since inheritance of the disease is NOT known
C. be used for breeding since disease is NOT inherited but is sporadic in the breed
D. be used for breeding as disease is inherited as a recessive trait
E. NOT be used for breeding as disease is inherited as a recessive trait

36. An agent which frequently produces focal, hairless and hyperkeratotic lesions of feline skin, and is transmissible to man is 36.___
A. cryptococcus neoformans
B. leptospira icterohemorrhagica
C. trichophyton verrucosum
D. microsporum canis
E. blastomyces dermatitidis

37. The MOST frequent dermatophyte isolated from ringworm lesions of cats which is also transmissible to man is 37.___
A. trichophyton mentagrophytes
B. microsporum gypseum
C. trichophyton verrrucosum
D. microsporum canis
E. trichophyton schoenleini

38. The chemical mediator at postganglionic parasympathetic nerve endings is 38.___
A. acetylcholinesterase
B. norepinephrine
C. serotonin
D. epinephrine
E. acetylcholine

39. Intravenous digoxin is indicated in acute pulmonary edema along with 39.___
A. penicillin
B. morphine
C. potassium chloride
D. 5 cc./lb. 5% dextrose
E. codeine

40. Changes in the blood count which are associated with dirofilaria in the dog include — 40.____
   A. anemia and lymphopenia
   B. eosinophilia and occasional basophilia
   C. eosinophilia and granulocytopenia
   D. leukocytosis and anisocytosis
   E. hypochromic anemia, eosinophilia and polychromasia

41. Which of the following is contraindicated in coxofemoral luxation? — 41.____
   A. Ehmer sling
   B. Toggle pin
   C. Dorsal acetabular rim prosthesis
   D. Modified Thomas splint
   E. Caudo-distal transposition of the greater trochanter

42. A wound in the equine manus or pes should be bandaged with pressure packs to prevent excessive — 42.____
   A. hoof growth
   B. contamination
   C. granulation
   D. scab formation
   E. movement

43. The *most likely* complication of repair of a ruptured cruciate ligament using the medial part of the common patellar tendon is — 43.____
   A. ankylosis of the stifle joint
   B. medial patellar luxation
   C. osteoarthritis of the patella
   D. rupture of the common patellar tendon
   E. avulsion of the tibial tuberosity

44. Given the following values: tidal volume 450 ml, expiratory reserve volume 400 ml, residual volume 210 ml, respiratory rate 22/min, and inspiratory capacity 620 ml, the minute volume is ________ L/min. — 44.____
   A. 4.6
   B. 8.8
   C. 9.9
   D. 12.4
   E. 13.6

45. Bilateral retinal detachment has been diagnosed in a 3-year-old cat.
A differential should include — 45.____
   A. feline infectious anemia, feline infectious peritonitis and toxoplasmosis
   B. feline infectious anemia, pansteatitis and toxoplasmosis
   C. lymphosarcoma, toxoplasmosis and pansteatitis
   D. lymphosarcoma, toxoplasmosis and feline infectious peritonitis
   E. rhinotracheitis, lymphosarcoma and toxoplasmosis

46. A dog with epistaxis is found to have petechial hemorrhages on mucus membranes which suggests — 46.____
   A. lack of vitamin K in the diet
   B. liver disease
   C. hemophilia A

D. thrombocytopenia
E. dicumerol toxicity

47. Electrocardiographic abnormality MOST characteristic of benign pericardial effusion is 47. D
A. ventricular premature beats
B. paroxysmal atrial tachycardia
C. atrial fibrillation
D. low amplitude recording
E. aberrant ventricular conduction

Questions 48 - 50.
Questions 48 - 50 are to be answered on the basis of the paragraphs below and the accompanying electrocardiogram.

On May 13, 1986 B. H. Brown presented his nine-year-old male poodle, Pierre, for examination. Mr. Brown complained that Pierre had been coughing off and on for the last two months. Past history revealed NO other illnesses. Pierre visited the veterinarian only for annual booster inoculations. His diet consisted of canned dog food in the morning and table food at night. He preferred table food. Questioning Mr. Brown did bring out that Pierre was NOT as active as in the past. The coughing appeared MOST severe when he was excited, particularly just after they came home from work or when company was in the house.

Examination demonstrated pink oral mucous membranes with normal capillary refill time. Precordial palpation revealed the apex cardiac beat at the left fifth intercostal space. The pulse was regular, full and moderately strong. Tonsils appeared normal and no cough would be elicited by tracheal palpation. Tracheal rings appeared to have normal contour. Lung sounds were slightly raspy in both diaphragmatic lobes. Respirations were slow and normal. A grade III/V harsh systolic murmur was heard loudest at the fifth intercostal space at the sternal border. The remaining examination found no additional abnormalities.

The problem list following the examination was:
1. Cough - particularly following excitement
2. Chronic valvular disease with mitral insufficiency
3. Decreased activity

The initial plan was:
1. Collect blood for CBC, BUN, SGPT and total protein
2. Urinalysis
3. Electrocardiogram
4. Radiograph thorax

Results:

1. PCV 36 vol%
   Hb 12 gm%
   WBC 12,500/cu mm
   Band 125/cu mm
   Neutrophil 10,000/cu mm
   Eosinophil 375/cu mm
   Lymphocyte 1,750/cu mm
   Monocyte 250/cu mm
   BUN 32 mg %
   SGPT 70 IU
   Total protein 5.8 gm%

2. Urinalysis:
   Sp. Gr. 1.020
   pH 7.0
   Glucose neg
   Ketones neg
   Protein neg
   Occult
   Blood neg
   Sediment
      Erythrocytes 1 to 2 hpf
      Leukocytes 0
      Casts - few fine granular
      Epithelial cell 1 to 3/hpf

3. Dorsoventral radiograph:
   A. Increased convexity at the left atrial area
   B. Slight decrease in distance from the left ventricle to left chest wall
   C. Pulmonary vascular congestion slight

   Lateral radiograph:
   A. Slight elevation of the left main stem bronchus
   B. Loss of the caudal waist
   C. Slight increase in left ventricular size
   D. Pulmonary vascular congestion

4. The ECG is on the following page

# 10 (#2)

I

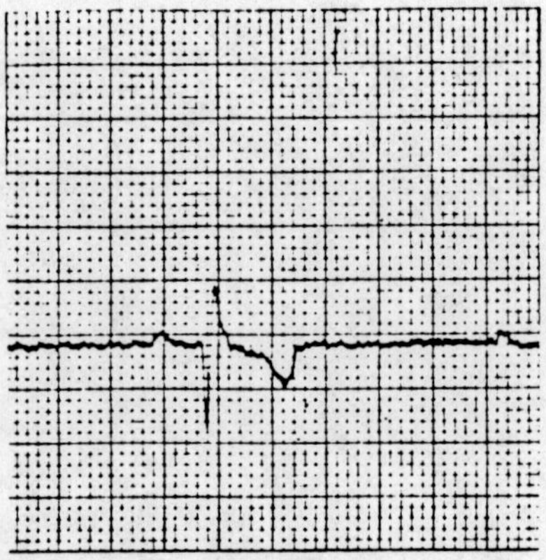

aVF

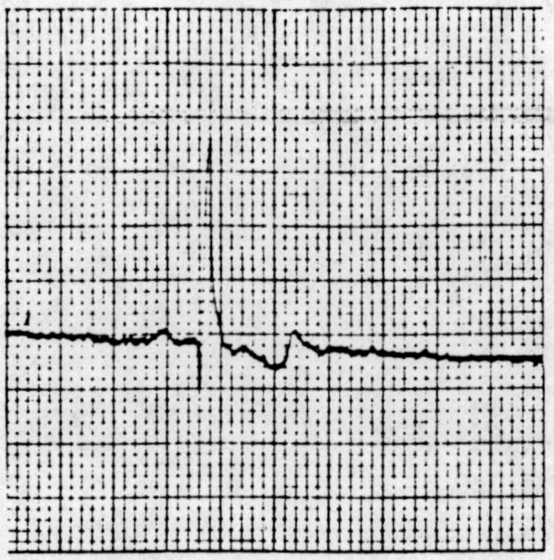

$V^{10}$

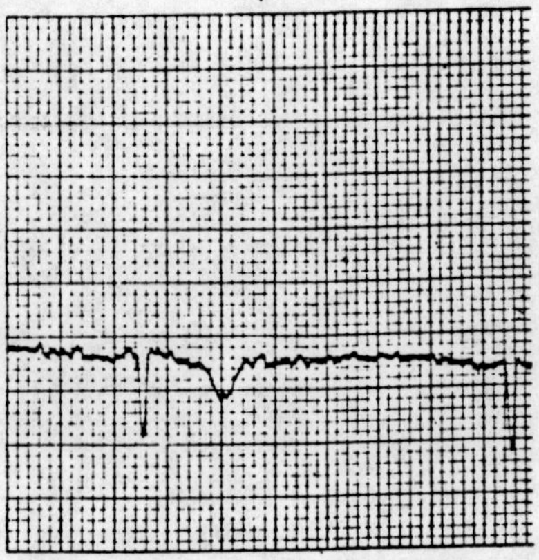

III

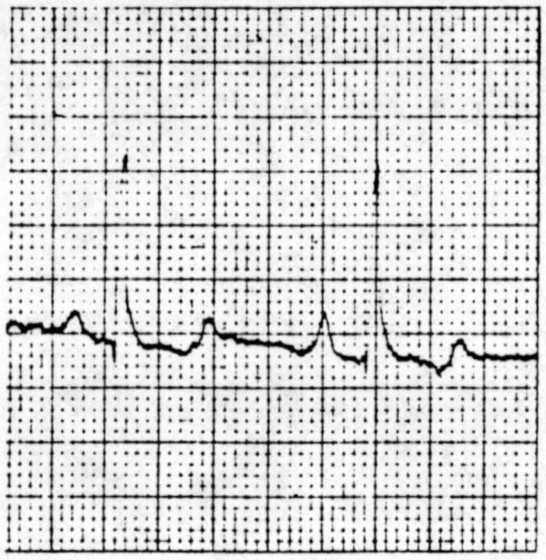

aVR

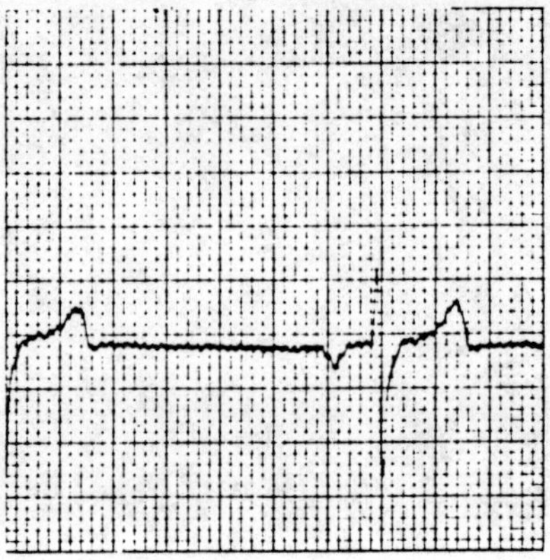

aVL

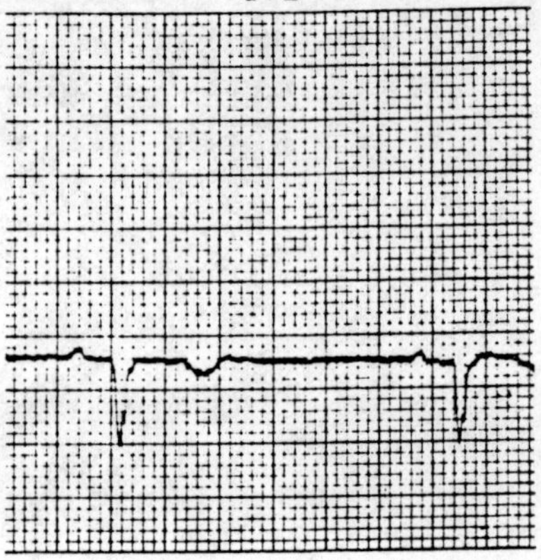

$V^{3}$

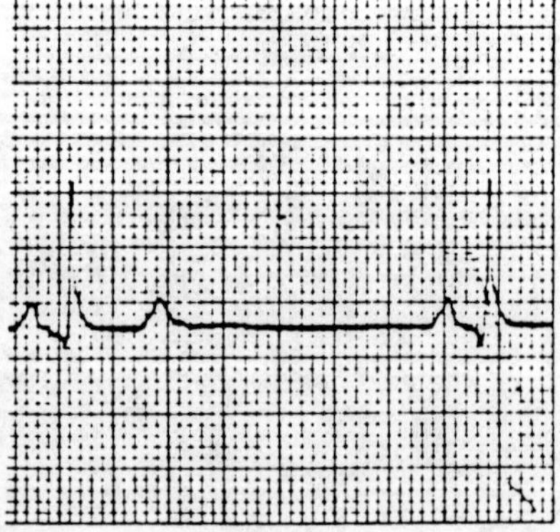

II

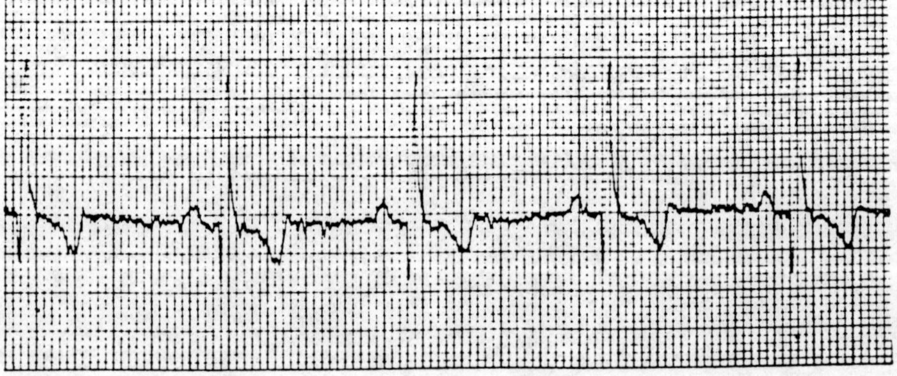

Rate ________________ b.p.m.
Rhythm ________________ o
M.E.A. ________________

P duration ________________ sec
P R interval ________________ sec
QRS duration ________________ sec
Q–T interval ________________ sec

P magnitude ________ mV
R magnitude ________ mV
T magnitude ________ mV
S–T segment ________

Interpretation:

48. Interpretation of the electrocardiogram is 48. ___
A. normal
B. left ventricular enlargment
C. right ventricular enlargement
D. left atrial enlargement
E. atrial fibrillation

49. The clinician's decision was to digitalize the patient. What additional therapeutic or management recommendation must be made to properly control the clinical signs? 49. ___
A. Sedation with phenobarbital or morphine
B. Diuresis with a carbonic anhydrase inhibitor
C. Confine to a small pen or cage
D. Restrict the sodium intake
E. Increase intake of high potassium foods such as bananas or dates

50. The blood chemistry values necessitate which of the following recommendations? 50. ___
A. High protein foods must be supplemented to elevate the total protein value
B. BUN levels are elevated so digoxin dosage must be reduced to lower than normal maintenance levels to allow for the decreased excretion rate
C. Include lipotrophic factors in the therapeutic regimen to aid in repair of hepatic necrosis
D. Add salt to the diet to increase water consumption and urine output to reduce the blood urea nitrogen
E. Run a BSP liver function test

---

# KEY (CORRECT ANSWERS)

| | | | | |
|---|---|---|---|---|
| 1. C | 11. D | 21. A | 31. B | 41. D |
| 2. E | 12. A | 22. C | 32. A | 42. C |
| 3. D | 13. A | 23. E | 33. D | 43. B |
| 4. D | 14. D | 24. B | 34. E | 44. C |
| 5. E | 15. C | 25. D | 35. E | 45. E |
| 6. E | 16. C | 26. D | 36. D | 46. D |
| 7. A | 17. E | 27. C | 37. D | 47. D |
| 8. B | 18. C | 28. B | 38. E | 48. A |
| 9. E | 19. D | 29. E | 39. B | 49. D |
| 10. D | 20. D | 30. C | 40. B | 50. B |

# TEST 3

DIRECTIONS: Each question or incomplete statement is followed by several suggested answers or completions. Select the one that BEST answers the question or completes the statement. *PRINT THE LETTER OF THE CORRECT ANSWER IN THE SPACE AT THE RIGHT.*

1. In dogs with left ventricular hypertrophy, 1.____
   A. the ratio of left ventricular plus septal weight to body weight (LV + S/BW) should be decreased
   B. the ratio of left ventricular plus septal weight to right ventricular weight (LV + S/RV) may be decreased, normal or elevated
   C. measurement of ventricular free-wall and septal thickness is the MOST reliable method of diagnosis and quantification
   D. the ratio of left ventricular plus septal weight to total cardiac weight (LV + S/TC) should be decreased
   E. the ratio of aortic circumference to pulmonic circumference (A/P) should be increased

2. In dogs with right ventricular hypertrophy, 2.____
   A. quantification requires measurement of ventricular free-wall and septal thickness
   B. the ratio of left ventricular plus septal weight to right ventricular weight (LV + S/RV) is always decreased
   C. the ratio of left ventricular plus septal weight to right ventricular weight (LV + S/RV) is usually decreased but may be normal or increased
   D. the heart is indistinguishable from normal hearts at necropsy
   E. the ratio of right ventricular weight to total cardiac weight (RV/TC) will usually be decreased

3. It has been shown that in the medical management of megaesophagus 3.____
   A. surgical management is superior
   B. the use of parasympathomimetic drugs helps greatly in reducing regurgitation
   C. dry food works BEST to reduce regurgitation in MOST affected dogs
   D. many consistencies of foods should be tried in each affected dog
   E. dogs with megaesophagus should be fed only once per day to help distend the esophagus and stimulate peristalsis

4. Which of the following is NOT true regarding the surgical treatment of megaesophagus? 4. B ?
   A. Cardiomyotomy, cardioplasty and bougienage have all been used to treat megaesophagus
   B. Surgical treatment helps restore effective peristalsis
   C. MOST experts feel that surgical treatment is associated with a higher mortality than medical management
   D. The main function of surgery is to weaken the lower esophageal sphincter
   E. Many dogs treated surgically are also managed medically

5. The description of a vaginal smear obtained from a bitch that has just been observed mating that justifies using and abortifacient is 5. ~~D~~ B
   A. a 40% intermediate epithelial cells, 10% parabasal epithelial cells, 50% superficial epithelial cells, and red blood cells, spermatozoa
   B. 95% superficial epithelial cells, and 5% superficial intermediate epithelial cells
   C. 50% superficial intermediate epithelial cells, and 50% intermediate epithelial cells
   D. neutrophils, red blood cells, 50% superficial intermediate epithelial cells, 50% superficial epithelial cells, and spermatozoa
   E. none of the above

6. Which statement is CORRECT concerning vaginal tumors in the bitch? 6. A
   A. Bitches that have them may be asymptomatic
   B. They are always benign
   C. They do NOT occur in bitches under two years of age
   D. Vaginal cytology is NOT useful in diagnosing them because tumor cells rarely exfoliate
   E. all of the above

7. Urine pooling in the cranial vagina in the bitch may occur secondary to 7. E
   A. ectopic ureters
   B. sloping cranial vagina
   C. persistent hymen
   D. vestibular tumor
   E. all of the above

8. Which of the following is NOT a property of an aeroallergen? 8. ~~A~~ E
   A. It is an antigen
   B. Stimulates formation of specific antibodies
   C. It is composed of airborne particles
   D. Produces clinical allergic reaction
   E. It is a simple protein

9. Standardization of allergens is NOT affected by 9. X E
   A. biologic complexity of materials
   B. variation of antigenicity
   C. weight of defatted allergen

D. biologic activity of allergen
E. allergen solubility in water

10. The factor that is *least* important in determining that a particle is a clinically significant aeroallergen is the 10.____
A. buoyancy of the particle
B. allergenicity of the particle
C. pollination season
D. concentration in air
E. particle size

11. Thrombosis might be anticipated in glomerulonephropathies when 11.____
A. end-stage renal failure is present
B. marked proteinuria is present in patients with near normal glomerular filtration rates
C. platelet function is reduced
D. partial thromboplastin time is prolonged
E. hypofibrinogenemia is present

12. Heparin therapy for DIC is likely to be ineffective when 12.____
A. AT III levels are markedly reduced
B. fibrinogen levels are increased
C. thrombocytopenia is present
D. partial thromboplastin time is prolonged
E. fibrin degradation products are increased

13. Which of the following statements is true concerning AT III plasma levels? 13.____
A. Mature dogs have higher AT III levels than animals of other species have.
B. Mature cats have higher AT III levels than animals of other species.
C. Neonatal foals have higher AT III levels than animals of other species have.
D. Mature horses have higher AT III levels than animals of other species have.
E. AT III levels are not significantly influenced by species or age.

14. Blood collected in which of the following would have the lowest AT III levels? 14.____
A. Citrate
B. EDTA
C. Heparin
D. Serum
E. AT III levels are not influenced by the type of anticoagulant

15. With respect to prevention of infections from indwelling urinary catheters, it is NOT true that 15.____
I. the collection system should be closed
II. the collection bag should always be at the same level as the patient
III. the catheter should be placed in a sterile manner
IV. antibiotics can help to prevent infection

The CORRECT answer is
A. I, II, III
B. II, IV
C. III, IV
D. IV *only*
E. all of the above

C

16. Secretion of an acid urine by a sheep in which gluconeogenesis occurs may be a sign of 16. D
A. excessive intake of calories
B. inadequate intake of proteins
C. inadequate intake of calories
D. excessive intake of proteins
E. inadequate intake of salt

17. The urine of a dog presented for examination has a specific gravity of 1.005. Blood urea nitrogen is 30 mg. per 100 ml. whole blood. After withholding food and water for 12 hours, a specimen of urine collected from the animal has a specific gravity of 1.008. 17. D
The animal is probably
A. dehydrated
B. a large consumer of water
C. normal
D. suffering from chronic nephritis
E. suffering from diabetes mellitus

18. The ability of the dog to digest starch 18. D
A. is absent because the gastric juice is too acid for amylolytic action to go on in the stomach
B. is so slight as to make it unsafe to add any significant amount of carbohydrate to the diet of the dog
C. varies greatly with the breed of the dog
D. is well developed in spite of the fact that dog saliva contains little or no amylase
E. is slight because dog saliva contains little or no amylase

19. In ruminant animals, the class of foodstuff which serves as substrate for volatile fatty acid production in the rumen is 19. C
A. minerals
B. vitamins
C. carbohydrates
D. proteins
E. fats

20. Canine atopy is associated with an inherited tendency to develope ________ antibodies. 20. C
A. IgA
B. IgD
C. IgE
D. IgG
E. IgM

21. The MOST consistent presenting sign of an atopic dog is 21. B
A. erythema
B. pruritis
C. alopecia
D. papules
E. wheals

22. Atopy is uncommon in the 22. _____
    A. cairn terrier B. lhasa apso
    C. dachshund D. minature schnauzer
    E. English bulldog

23. Concerning shared antigenicity of allergens, it is true that 23. _____
    A. the MOST common allergens are similar antigenically
    B. MOST grasses share at least one common antigen
    C. MOST trees share at least one common antigen
    D. MOST weeds share at least one commom antigen
    E. the house dust and kapok seldom share common antigens

24. Which of the following drugs is MOST effective in treating cryptosporidiosis in livestock? 24. _____
    A. metronidazole
    B. amprolium
    C. trimethoprim-sulfadiazine
    D. monensin
    E. there is NO satisfactory treatment

25. The disinfectant which was found to be MOST effective in destroying the infectivity of cryptosporidium oocysts is. 25. _____
    A. ammonia B. benzalkonium chloride
    C. sodium hydroxide D. sodium hypochlorite
    E. iodophor

26. Pathologic findings in sections of the intestines of animals clinically affected by cryptosporidium infection may include ALL of the following EXCEPT 26. _____
    A. varying degrees of villous atrophy
    B. fusion or bridging of adjacent villi
    C. flask-shaped ulcers
    D. cuboidal enterocytes
    E. inflammatory cells in the lamina propria of the ileum

27. Which of the following is *least likely* to lower the allergic threshold in an atopic dog? 27. _____
    A. Nutritional status B. Infection
    C. Fleas D. Environmental factors
    E. Rye grass pollen

28. Concerning treatment of the atopic dog, it is INCORRECT that 28. _____
    A. avoiding exposure to allergens is the MOST desirable therapy but the MOST difficult
    B. corticosteroids are the MOST effective drugs for medical management of atopy
    C. a therapeutic trial of antihistamine is indicated despite a normally poor therapeutic response
    D. antiseborrheic shampoos are contraindicated in the management of the atopic dog
    E. hyposensitization is the MOST effective biological method of canine atopy

29. Concerning antigens used in hyposensitization, it is CORRECT that 29. ____
   A. stability of the aqueous antigens decreases with the dilution of antigen solution
   B. sterile nodules at the site of aqueous antigen injection is a common side effect
   C. aqueous antigens generally cost more than alum-precipitated antigens
   D. more injections are required to hyposensitize an atopic dog with aqueous than with alum-precipitated antigen
   E. the MOST common side effect of hyposensitization in the atopic dog is lethargy

30. Selecting antigens for hyposensitization requires consideration of ALL of the following factors EXCEPT 30. ____
   A. history of exposure to allergen
   B. time of year tested
   C. seasonality of clinical signs
   D. strength of intradermal reaction
   E. strength of stock allergen solution

31. Bovine dermatophilosis is a serious disease in the tropics because 31. ____
   A. cattle there have a lower level of nutrition
   B. tropical climates place more stress on the animal
   C. prolonged wetting by rain weakens the natural skin barriers to the disease
   D. fewer trained people are available to treat infected cattle
   E. longer periods of sunlight cause recrudescence of the infection

32. When treatment of affected animals is indicated, the drug of choice is 32. ____
   A. penicillin
   B. polymyxin B
   C. nitrofurazone
   D. nystatin
   E. amphotericin B

33. The major end-products of carbohydrate digestion that are absorbed from the digestive tract in adult domestic animals are 33. ____
   A. volatile fatty acids (primarily acetate, propionate, and butyrate) in both simple-stomached and ruminant animals
   B. volatile fatty acids (primarily acetate, propionate, and butyrate) in simple-stomached animals and glucose in ruminant animals
   C. lactate in both simple-stomached and ruminant animals
   D. glucose in both simple-stomached and ruminant animals
   E. glucose in simple-stomached animals and volatile fatty acids (primarily acetate, propionate, and butyrate) in ruminant animals

34. In the normal ruminating animal, the reaction of the abomasal contents is 34.____
   A. acid because of hydrochloric acid
   B. acid because of volatile fatty acids
   C. neutral because of ruminal ingesta
   D. alkaline because of the backflow of duodenal contents
   E. alkaline because of the admixture of saliva

35. Circulation of the bile salts refers to 35.____
   A. secretion of these salts and their reabsorption and secretion in the urine
   B. reabsorption in the cecum and return via the blood to the liver
   C. reabsorption from the large intestine and return to the liver via the lymph and blood
   D. secretion of these salts by the liver and their reabsorption in the small intestine and resecretion by the liver
   E. secretion of these salts and their storage in the gallbladder until needed

36. The absorption of __________ through the wall of the large intestine of solipeds is of nutritional importance. 36.____
   A. maltose  B. indole
   C. lower fatty acids  D. protein
   E. fat

37. Calcium absorption from the alimentary tract is MOST efficient when the animal is on a diet that 37.____
   A. contains large amounts of phosphorus
   B. contains adequate vitamin D and phosphorus
   C. contains adequate soluble oxalates
   D. is high in cereal grains, especially oats
   E. is high in fat

38. In the digestive tract of the fowl, the proventriculus has the function of 38.____
   A. producing gastric juice
   B. producing succus entericus
   C. controlling the flow of ingesta
   D. aiding in the alkalinization of the acid chyme
   E. temporarily storing liquids and food swallowed

39. The enzyme in gastric gland secretion that changes proteins of the food into photeoses and peptones is 39.____
   A. pepsin  B. transaminase
   C. phosphoric acid  D. carboxypedtidase
   E. secretin

40. The arrest of ventricular fibrillation in dogs and larger animals can be accomplished by 40.____
   A. electrical shock
   B. artificial respiration and elevation of the posterior portion of the animal

C. massage to maintain circulation so that recovery occurs spontaneously
D. intracardial injection of acetylcholine followed in 20 to 30 seconds by norepinephrine
E. intracardiac injection of solutions of calcium chloride, followed by potassium chloride

41. In the embryo, the ductus arteriosus allows the blood to flow from the — 41. D
A. aorta to the umbilical arteries
B. aorta to the pulmonary artery
C. right to the left atrium
D. pulmonary artery to the descending aorta
E. pulmonary artery to the ductus venosus

42. An increase in blood pressure distends or stretches the baroceptors located in the wall of the carotid sinus, which in turn functions by neurogenic means to — 42. B
A. *increase* the cardiac rate WITHOUT affecting the arterioles
B. *slow* the cardiac rate and dilate the arterioles
C. *slow* the cardiac rate and constrict the arterioles
D. *increase* the cardiac rate and dilate the arterioles
E. *increase* the cardiac rate and constrict the arterioles

43. In hemorrhagic shock, the basic abnormality is — 43. ~~D~~ E
A. increased capillary permeability with the passage of large quantities of fluid into the tissues
B. histotoxic mypoxia caused by the release of histamine, serotomin and norepinephrine
C. vasomotor failure because of exhaustion of the carotid sinus and aortic arch reflex mechanisms
D. a decrease of venous return accompanied by widespread thrombosis, especially of minute vessels
E. a reduction of cardiac output, a decrease of tissue blood flow, and tissue damage

44. A bilaterally cryptorchid dog is sterile because — 44. ~~A~~ C
A. the secondary sexual organs do NOT develop completely
B. the spermatozoa produced CANNOT reach the urethra owing to kinking of the ductus deferens
C. spermatozoa are NOT produced
D. NO testosterone is produced
E. sexual desire is absent

45. Under which of the following conditions will the ratio of thyroxine:Tri-10Dothyronine secreted by the thyroid gland of a dog be highest? — 45. D
A. DNP (2,6-D11ODO-4-Nitrophenol) administration
B. high ambient temperature
C. low dietary intake of iodine (100 mg. 1/day)
D. high dietary intake of iodine (1500 mg. 1/day)
E. severe stress

46. A general statement about hormones and their functions would include the fact that hormones 46. E
   A. initiate rather than regulate reactions
   B. function primarily in a short-term, rapid response manner
   C. are excreted at a regular rate by the body
   D. become functional when the animal reaches puberty
   E. are effective in minute quantities

47. A 9 month old poodle was presented with a transverse fracture of the proximal left tibial metaphysis. The puppy had been recently obtained from a pet dealer. Therefore, the history was uncertain. The puppy had been kept in the house with NO observed trauma. On close inspection it was noted that the right tibia had an external torsional deformity of 20° and an angular deformity of 10°. All of the joints were painful. Radiographs of the pelvis and both pelvic limbs revealed the acute pathologic fracture of the left proximal tibia and malunion of an old fracture of the right tibia. The skeleton was osteoporotic as respresented by loss of density, thin cortices, and loss of trabeculation. The lab work is as follows: 47. A

| | |
|---|---|
| PVC | 41% |
| Monocytes | 2 |
| Creatinine | 1.8/mg/dl |
| RBC | 6.1m |
| Eosinophil | 1 |
| WBC | 11,500 |
| Ca | 9.3 mg/dl |
| Basophils | 0 |
| $PO_4$ | 3.8 mg/dl |
| SEG | 65 |
| Urine sp.gr. | 1.042 |
| K | 4.7 mEq/L |
| Bands | 1 |
| Na | 149 mEq/L |
| LYMPHS | 31 |
| BUN | 21mg/dl |
| Cl | 110 mEq/L |

Based on the information at hand, the MOST probable assessment of this patient's problem is
   A. primary hyperparathyroidism
   B. secondary nutritional hyperparathyroidism
   C. secondary renal hyperparathyroidism
   D. primary $PO_4$ deficiency
   E. hypocalcemia

Questions 48 - 50.
Questions 48 - 50 are to be answered on the basis of the following paragraphs.

Your patient is a miniature poodle, female six years old, in generally good physical condition. She has been in every fall since the age of 14 months for treatment of a mild pruritus. This year she comes in in July with a severe pruritus which "started on her stomach in May". Then the pruritus moved onto her sides. Now she is chewing at her feet and legs with vengeance. Last year's allergy pills seem to have provided very temporary relief. "Past episodes were nothing like this." She was bred in March, but did NOT have puppies. You see much evidence of self-trauma....she had stopped to scratch on the way into the exam room. You notice that the skin has quite a foul odor. When you ask, a child volunteers that she has been bothered by mosquito bites. The weather can be characterized as a wet spring and, so far, a dry summer.

Your diagnostic work and results:
- Fleas and flea excrement not found
- Skin scrapings negative
- Intradermals
  - control-negative
  - histamine-positive
  - molds, ragweed, feathers, housedust-intermediate
- Antibiotic and corticosteroid therapy for one week-poor progress
- Repeat exam for fleas-still no evidence
- Repeat scrapings-still negative

48. Based on the information presented, this patient's current problem can BEST be described as 48. A
    A. atopy, because of the history of previous episodes
    B. cheyletiella infestation, because of severe pruritus and poor response to corticosteroids
    C. flea bite dermatitis and atopy, even though NO evidence of fleas were found
    D. atopy overshadowed by sarcoptic scabies even though scrapings were negative
    E. sarcoptic scabies alone because of history of possible exposure (bred), bites in child, odor, and severe pruritus

49. Your plan for this patient is to 49. E
    A. continue using antibiotic and corticosteroid, waiting for a good freeze
    B. avoid corticosteroids and start hyposensitization, watching for fleas
    C. continue using antibiotic and corticosteroid, start hyposensitization
    D. continue antibiotic and corticosteroid, bath and dip series for sarcops, and hyposensitize
    E. continue antibiotic and corticosteroid, bath and dip series for sarcops, and await results before deciding on hyposensitization

50. In order to pinpoint the diagnosis while treating this patient, it will be MOST helpful to 50. A
   A. put the dog on a rice diet to check for dietary hypersensitivity
   B. check fecals for sarcoptic mites
   C. train the client to examine for fleas
   D. repeat the intradermals
   E. make scrapings from the child's lesions

---

# KEY (CORRECT ANSWERS)

| | | | | |
|---|---|---|---|---|
| 1. B | 11. B | 21. B | 31. C | 41. D |
| 2. C | 12. A | 22. C | 32. A | 42. B |
| 3. D | 13. D | 23. B | 33. E | 43. E |
| 4. B | 14. D | 24. E | 34. A | 44. C |
| 5. B | 15. B | 25. A | 35. D | 45. D |
| 6. A | 16. C | 26. C | 36. C | 46. E |
| 7. E | 17. D | 27. E | 37. B | 47. A |
| 8. E | 18. D | 28. D | 38. A | 48. E |
| 9. E | 19. C | 29. A | 39. A | 49. A |
| 10. C | 20. C | 30. E | 40. A | 50. B |

# TEST 4

DIRECTIONS: Each question or incomplete statement is followed by several suggested answers or completions. Select the one that BEST answers the question or completes the statement. *PRINT THE LETTER OF THE CORRECT ANSWER IN THE SPACE AT THE RIGHT.*

1. Enostosis (eosinophilic panosteitis), occuring in young dogs, is characterized by 1. A
   A. irregular circumscribed areas of increased density in the medullary cavity of long bone
   B. irregular areas of decreased density in the epiphysis of long bones
   C. eosinophilla accompanied by swelling and heat over the bone lesion
   D. swelling of the joints and shifting lameness
   E. fever, leukocytosis and vitamin D excess

2. A semicomatose dehydrated dog with a history of vomiting and suspected of being in shock from acute pancreatitis has a(n) 2. E
   A. elevated serum amylase which is diagnostic for pancreatitis
   B. elevated BUN which is diagnostic for renal disease
   C. high urine specific gravity (1.030), a high BUN and elevated serum amylase which rules out pancreatitis
   D. 1.011 urine specific gravity, high BUN, and elevated serum amylase which is consistent with but NOT diagnostic for pancreatitis
   E. high urine specific gravity (1.030), high BUN and elevated serum amylase which is consistent with but NOT diagnostic for pancreatitis

3. A six-week-old puppy is completely asymptomatic but has a loud, harsh, holosystolic murmur that is heard BEST on the right side of the chest near the sternum. The MOST probable diagnosis is 3. E
   A. aortic stenosis
   B. pulmonic insufficiency
   C. tricuspid insufficiency
   D. interatrial septal defect
   E. interventricular septal defect

4. The MOST satisfactory material for replacement of the cruciate ligament in the dog is 4. D
   A. dacron
   B. nylon
   C. skin
   D. fascia lata
   E. fascia pectineus

5. A five-year-old wire-haired fox terrier is examined with a direct ophthalmoscope and the fundi appear normal. However, there is a focus on the right optic disc at -2 diopters and the left optic disc at +8-10 diopters. The MOST plausible explanation is 5.____
   A. keratoconus right eye; normal left eye
   B. normal right eye; hyperopic left eye
   C. hyperopic right eye; left posterior lens luxation
   D. normal right eye; left posterior lens luxation
   E. normal right eye; left anterior lens luxation

6. Osteochondritis dissecans in the dog occurs MOST frequently in articulation of the ________ joints. 6.____
   A. scapulohumeral
   B. radiohumeral
   C. femorotibial
   D. coxofemoral
   E. anconeal

7. A low carbon dioxide tension in the blood is termed 7.____
   A. asphyxia
   B. hypercarbia
   C. hypoxia
   D. hydremia
   E. hypocapnia

8. A dog is presented by its owner for a general check up and is found to have nodules or plaques in the skin which test out as calcium salt deposits. The *most likely* diagnosis is 8.____
   A. generalized pyoderma
   B. hyperadrenocorticism
   C. hypoadrenocorticism
   D. hypothroidism
   E. naso-digital hyperkeratosis

9. The leukocyte response following steroid therapy in the dog is typified by which of the following? 9.____
   A. White blood cell count - 5,000
   B. Neutrophiles - 60, lymphocytes - 10, eosinophiles - 2, and monocytes - 28
   C. Neutrophiles - 85, lymphocytes - 0, eosinophiles - 0, and monocytes - 15
   D. Neutrophiles - 60, lymphocytes - 30, eosinophiles - 0, and monocytes - 10
   E. Neutrophiles - 70, lymphocytes - 10, eosinophiles - 12, and monocytes - 8

10. Idiopathic epilepsy usually has its onset from 6 to 18 months of age and is thought to be due to 10.____
   A. alteration of blood gas tension of the extracellular fluid
   B. hypoglycemia associated with insulin excess
   C. interference with formation of oxyhemoglobin
   D. inherited defect in the metabolism of brain neurons
   E. death of astrocytes within the central nervous system

11. In what species is spontaneous subluxation of the crystalline lens commonly seen? 11.____
   A. Airedale terrier
   B. Afghan hound
   C. Basenji
   D. Wirehair fox terrier
   E. Dachshund

12. The disease scabies incognito refers to — 12. E
   A. scabies in which many mites are recovered by skin scrapings
   B. all scabies infestations
   C. a pustular form of the disease
   D. an infestation with S. scabiei without clinical signs of the disease
   E. a condition in which clinical signs and patient history are indicative of scabies, but mites CANNOT be recovered by multiple skin scrapings

13. Pruritus refers to — 13. D
   A. erythema
   B. edema
   C. alopecia
   D. itching
   E. the same condition as pruritis

14. Pruritis implies — 14. A
   A. inflammation
   B. alopecia
   C. itching
   D. delayed sensitization
   E. dandruff

15. Scabies is diagnosed by observing — 15. E
   A. the mites
   B. mite eggs
   C. mite fecal pellets
   D. clinical signs and patient history
   E. all of the above

16. A lateral approach to the shoulder was used to repair osteochondritis dessicans in a 2-year-old golden retriever. Three weeks postoperatively, marked atrophy was present in the supraspinatous muscle. This is *most likely* a surgical complication due to — 16. C
   A. infection
   B. disuse atrophy
   C. damage to the suprascapular nerve
   D. damage to the radial nerve
   E. damage to the median nerve

17. A thrombus in the cat, in contrast to a post-mortem clot, has — 17. ~~A~~ B
   A. a smooth and uniform texture
   B. a dull and irregularly rough surface
   C. a smaller diameter than the containing vessel
   D. no attachment to the vessel wall
   E. a solid, dark-red, jelly-like appearance

18. A common radiographic manifestation of congenital renal cortical hypoplasia is — 18. A
   A. osteoporosis
   B. osteopetrosis
   C. osteogenesis imperfecta

D. osteochondritis dissecans
E. osteonecrosis

19. A heart rate of 50 beats per minute, particularly if a very faint sound at a more rapid rate can be ausculted from the heart, would lead to the diagnosis of 19. C
A. second degree (incomplete) A-V Block
B. atrial fibrillation
C. third degree (complete) A-V Block
D. sino-atrial Block
E. paroxysmal ventricular tachycardia

20. The yellow-brown color which occurs with methoxyflurane in an Ohio #8 wick vaporizer 20. D A
A. does NOT interfere with vaporization
B. inhibits vaporization
C. adds to the anesthetic action of methoxyflurane
D. results from the use of nitrous oxide with methoxyflurane
E. results from the use of halothane and methoxyflurane from different vaporizers in the same machine

21. A one-year-old female cat is presented with pruritic areas of alopecia on the chin. Close examination reveals some crusts and pus are present, along with some occluded hair follicles. 21. D
A likely diagnosis is
A. notoedric mange
B. dermatomycosis
C. scrape or bite wound
D. feline acne
E. eosinophilic ulcer

22. The MOST common cause of anemia in the cat is 22. A B
A. hemobartonella felis
B. depression anemia of infection
C. chronic parasitism
D. surgical or traumatic blood loss
E. autoimmune hemolytic anemia

23. An EKG tracing showing prolonged and notched P waves from a patient with mitral insufficiency, is *most likely* the result of 23. E B
A. right bundle branch block
B. left atrial enlargement
C. right atrial enlargement
D. left ventricular hypertrophy
E. right ventricular hypertrophy

24. Laboratory findings consistent with advanced diabetes millitus are 24. E B
A. hypoglycemia, ketonemia, ketonuria, and dehydration
B. hyperglycemia, ketonemia, ketonuria, glycosuria, and dehydration
C. hyperglycemia, hypernatremia, ketonuria, and dehydration
D. hypoglycemia, hyperkalemia, ketonuria, and dehydration
E. hypernatremia, hyperkalemia, glycosuria, hyperglycemia, and ketonuria

25. A client presents her apparently healthy cat wishing to know what can be done as the owner is pregnant and fears toxoplasmosis. 25. C
The BEST course of action is to
 A. tell the client to get rid of the cat
 B. send serum samples for titer determination
 C. do a series of fecal exams and educate the client
 D. put the cat on systemic Sulfas
 E. have the owner keep the cat indoors and feed only cooked meats and commercial cat foods

26. A client calls to report her young kitten has a swelling in the neck area with a small hole where a worm can be seen periodically. 26. D
The *most likely* diagnosis is
 A. myiasis
 B. pediculosis
 C. ticks
 D. cuterebriasis
 E. fleas

27. The agent that causes a rise in blood pressure is 27. D
 A. halothane
 B. methoxyflurane
 C. nitrous oxide
 D. ketamine
 E. acetylpromazine

28. A common sequel to long bone osteosarcoma in the dog is 28. C
 A. air bronchograms
 B. medullary sclerosis
 C. metastatic lung disease
 D. multicentric bone lesions
 E. cranial mediastinal lymphadenopathy

29. While rehydrating a patient with renal disease, the clinician should replace the 29. C
 A. rehydration fluid volumes
 B. rehydration fluid and insensible maintenance fluid volumes
 C. rehydration fluid, insensible maintenance fluid, and urine output volumes
 D. insensible maintenance fluid and urine output volumes
 E. insensible maintenance fluid volumes

30. Which of the following is a narcotic antagonist? 30. B
 A. Metrazol (pentylenetetrazol)
 B. Naloxone (narcan)
 C. Doxapram (dopram)
 D. D-propoxyphene (darvon)
 E. Mikedimide (methetharimide)

31. The results of a fat absorption test are, prefeeding - clear plasma, post feeding (2 hours) - clear plasma. 31. A
This indicates
 A. significant quantities of fatty acids are NOT absorbed from the GI tract

B. a diagnosis of pancreatic insufficiency
C. a diagnosis of malabsorption NOT related to the pancreas
D. decreased gastric acidity
E. increased intestinal motility

32. The most commonly encountered pathologic arrhythmia in dogs is — 32.____
A. atrial fibrillation
B. second degree (incomplete) A-V Block
C. paroxysmal ventricular tachycardia
D. ventricular premature beats
E. sino-atrial arrest

33. X-ray tube current is commonly measured in units called — 33.____
A. milliamperes
B. kilovolts
C. rads
D. photons
E. quanta

34. An anterior-posterior radiograph of the distal radius and ulna of an 8-month-old dog shows a premature closure of distal ulnar epiphysis. — 34.____
On physical examination, one would expect to find a
A. fracture of the anconeal process
B. lateral deviation of the forepaw
C. distraction of the radial head distally
D. medial deviation of the forepaw
E. valgus deformity of the olecranon

35. A cat is presented with a full thickness laceration of the cornea. — 35.____
You should
A. debride and suture the full thickness with 6-0 silk
B. debride and suture the full thickness with 4-0 chromic
C. debride and suture thru 1/2 the stromal thickness with 6-0 silk
D. debride and suture thru 1/2 the stromal thickness with 3-0 chromic
E. do nothing; it will heal spontaneously in 24 hours

36. A stongyle-type parasitic ova found in a fecal sample from a young dog probably is — 36.____
A. filaroides osleri
B. toxocara canis
C. dipylidium caninum
D. echinococcus granulosus
E. ancylostoma caninum

37. Animals put directly on room air after breathing a high concentraion of nitrous oxide may suffer from — 37.____
A. metabolic alkalosis
B. diffusion anoxia
C. hepatic fiebrosis
D. aortic insufficiency
E. portal shunting

38. A dog is presented with pendulous abdomen, bilateral symetrical alopecia, rough dry coat, polydipsia and polyuria. Lab findings show lymphopenia eosinopenia. Blood sugar is 200 milligrams per 100 cc.
The MOST appropriate treatment for this condition is 38. E
   A. allopurinol
   B. ACTH
   C. insulin-protamine zinc
   D. pituitary extract
   E. o', p', DDD

39. The pulmonary artery segment is BEST visualized in a(n) 39. A
   A. dorsoventral chest radiograph
   B. lateral chest radiograph
   C. angiocardiograph after injection of contrast medium into the left ventricle
   D. oblique radiograph of the right cardiac lung lobe
   E. bronchogram of the left intermediate long lobe

40. On your pharmacy shelf are a number of diuretics. A cocker spaniel is presented with acute glaucoma. You immediately drop the intraocular pressure with urea intravenously and then you wish to maintain the dog on oral medication.
The drug that is contraindicated as it is NOT an ocular diuretic is 40. ~~B~~ C
   A. acetazolamide
   B. ethozolamide
   C. furosemide
   D. mannitol
   E. glycerol

41. Antibiotic treatment of chronic bacterial cystitis in dogs should be continued 41. C
   A. for 10 to 14 days
   B. until the animal's complete blood count is normal
   C. until at least two urinalysis performed 14 to 21 days apart are normal
   D. as long as the pH of the urine is above 6.0
   E. as long as proteinuria is present

42. A cat is presented to you with NO history of trauma but the third eyelid is prolapsed, the pupil is miotic and the lid is ptotic.
Your differential diagnosis would include a number of entities but one should be considered primary 42. D
   A. traumatic uvietis
   B. foreign body
   C. superficial corneal erosion
   D. Horner's syndrome
   E. "haws"

43. An eight-week-old weimaraner is presented with grossly enlarged mandibular lymph nodes and swollen fissured lips draining a purulent material. He and one brother are the only pups affected in a litter of eight.
A likely diagnosis is 43. C
   A. impetigo (milk rash)
   B. canine acne
   C. juvenile pyoderma
   D. distemper pustules
   E. nasal pyoderma

44. A normal value for canine serum potassium is _____ mEq./l. 44. B
A. 2.2 B. 4.4 C. 6.6 D. 8.8
E. 11.0

45. In the caudal approach to the shoulder for repair of osteochondritis dissecans, exposure is obtained by incising the 45. ~~A~~ B
A. supraspinatus m. B. infraspinatus m.
C. teres minor m. D. omotransversarus m.
E. brachiocephalicus m.

46. The presence of yellow white granules in a reddish brown exudate obtained by thoracocentesis from the pleural cavity is suggestive of 46. C
A. histoplasmosis
B. heart base tumor
C. nocardiosis
D. staphylococcal infection
E. pasteurella infection

Questions 47 - 50.
Questions 47 - 50 are to be answered on the basis of the case below.

An eight-month-old male miniature schnauzer is examined by a veterinarian.

The dog is thin, a very poor eater, is small for his age, and has always appeared sickly. During the past month, the dog has had periods of intermittent diarrhea and occasional vomiting. Occasionally, he appears dazed and even blind. He becomes aggressive during these spells, appearing NOT to recognize the owner or respond to commands. The owner feels the dog's worst attacks occurred when he switched from a dry dog food to an all meat type of food. Your physical examination adds relatively little to the history. The dog appears active and alert during your exam but is very thin and appears stunted for its age.

You hospitalize the dog and although the owner had reported the dog's appetite to have been nil the past 48 hours when canned dog food was offered, he eats it readily. One hour later you return to the ward to take some preliminary blood work and note the dog appears to be demented. He is head pressing in the corner of the cage, is very ataxic, does NOT respond normally to your commands. When you reach for the dog he snaps viciously although unsuccessfully, at your hand. If the dog's head presses on the cage door, he chews constantly at the bars.

You call your kennel man to assist you in restraining the dog and draw some blood for diagnostic work and collect a catheterized urine sample, both to be run immediately.

CBC
PCV = 32%
WBC = 14.200
Neut. = 70%
Seg. = 64%
Stab. = 5%
Eos. = 10%
Baso. = 0%
Mono. = 8%
Lymph. = 12%

Urine
Specific gravity = 1.012
pH = 6.9
Color = yellow
Glucose = Neg.
Ketones = Neg.
Bilirubin = 1+Icto
Protein = Neg.
Sediment = Many biurate crystals present
WBC = Neg.
RBC = Neg.

47. You withdrew a large aliquot of blood from which serum was saved pending your CBC and urine results. From the following tests, which would you choose as likely to help establish a diagnosis? 47.____

Tests Available:
1. Blood glucose
2. Blood lead
3. SGPT
4. Alkaline phosphatase
5. BUN
6. Albumin/globulin
7. Creatinine
8. Blood ammonia
9. Uric acid
10. Amylase
11. BSP
12. Electrolytes
13. Cholesterol
14. Lipase

A. Tests 1, 2, 3, and 4
B. Tests 2, 10, and 12
C. Test 6
D. Tests 1, 2, 5, 6, 8, and 11
E. Tests 1, 5, 13, and 14

48. Based on the above data, you can conclude that 48.____

A. the dog may have a glycogen storage disease
B. some degree of impaired hepatocellular function probably exists
C. the dog may have nephrotic syndrome

D. no diagnostic information was obtained from the test results presented
E. the dog has idiopathic epilepsy

You are awaiting your lab results and observe the dog to make a slow but steady clinical improvement. By the next morning, it appears identical to when it was admitted.

You have just evaluated survey abdominal radiographs and the only remarkable finding is a greatly reduced liver size.

49. From the above information, you might likely hypothesize this dog's problem as due to 49. C
A. congenital cirrhosis of the liver
B. agenesis of one or more liver lobes
C. a congenital portal vein anomaly with liver atrophy or maldevelopment and hepatic encephalopathy
D. biliary atresia
E. neonatal hepatitis with subsequent cirrhosis

50. If you were to try to make a definitive diagnosis of a portal vein anomaly, which of the following diagnostic tests would you select? 50. ~~A~~ D
A. Cranial mesenteric angiography
B. BSP
C. Cholangiography
D. Splenoportogram
E. Hepatic veinography (retograde)

# KEY (CORRECT ANSWERS)

| | | | | |
|---|---|---|---|---|
| 1. A | 11. D | 21. D | 31. A | 41. C |
| 2. E | 12. E | 22. B | 32. D | 42. D |
| 3. E | 13. D | 23. B | 33. A | 43. C |
| 4. D | 14. A | 24. B | 34. B | 44. B |
| 5. B | 15. E | 25. C | 35. C | 45. B |
| 6. A | 16. C | 26. D | 36. E | 46. C |
| 7. E | 17. B | 27. D | 37. B | 47. D |
| 8. B | 18. A | 28. C | 38. E | 48. B |
| 9. C | 19. C | 29. C | 39. A | 49. C |
| 10. D | 20. A | 30. B | 40. C | 50. D |

# EXAMINATION SECTION

## TEST 1

DIRECTIONS: Each question or incomplete statement is followed by several suggested answers or completions. Select the one that BEST answers the question or completes the statement. *PRINT THE LETTER OF THE CORRECT ANSWER IN THE SPACE AT THE RIGHT.*

Dry eye

1. Keratoconjunctivitis sicca is easily confused with — 1. A
   A. anterior uveitis
   B. conjunctivitis
   C. episcleritis
   D. glaucoma
   E. nodular fasciitis

2. In the ventral approach to the coxofemoral joint of the dog and cat, the *only* muscle severed is the — 2. B
   A. adductor
   B. pectineus
   C. gracilis
   D. biceps femoris
   E. sartorius

3. Cats between the ages of 2 to 4 years showing signs of anemia and progressive weight loss, enlarged spleen and liver, poor appetite with blast cells in peripheral blood are likely to have — 3. D
   A. hyperthyroidism
   B. myeloproliferative disease
   C. hemabartonella
   D. infectious peritonitis
   E. aspergillosis

4. Treatment of urinary incontinence with estrogens — 4. D
   A. is usually effective regardless of etiology
   B. is often helpful in treatment of urinary incontinence associated with neurologic problems
   C. has been shown to cause neoplasia of the urinary bladder following long-term use
   D. is limited to incontinence associated with ovario-hysterectomized bitches
   E. has been shown to cause birth defects in puppies born to a treated bitch

5. The effect of circulation produced by promazine or chlor-promazine is — 5. D
   A. peripheral vasodilation
   B. positive inotropy
   C. negative inotropy
   D. peripheral vasoconstriction
   E. positive chronotropy

6. Body temperature falls fastest in an anesthetized animal that is _____ lbs. — 6. A
   A. 2
   B. 5
   C. 10
   D. 25
   E. 50

7. A dog is presented with clinical dehydration. Laboratory evaluation reveals that the serum sodium is very low. The fluid of *choice* is 7. D
   A. 5% dextrose and quarter strength saline
   B. 5% dextrose and water
   C. 2.5% dextrose and water
   D. normal saline
   E. sterile water

8. To return to normal gate [gait] earliest, ___E___ should be used to repair a dog with a transverse fractured femur. 8. E
   A. a steinmann pin plus Kirschner-Ehmer half-pinning
   B. a steinmann intramedullary pin
   C. modified Thomas splintage
   D. a plaster of Paris cast
   E. bone plating

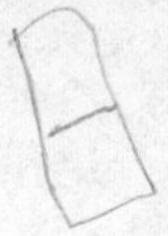

9. The outstanding clinical features of canine systemic lupus erythematosus are 9. A
   A. auto-immune hemolytic anemia and thrombocytopenia
   B. hepatomegaly
   C. erythrocyte cell membrane abnormality
   D. anemia and thrombocytosis
   E. lipid transport deficiency

10. Two 18-month-old Siamese cats (litter mates) are presented with chronic non-productive coughs. Their temperatures are normal. Radiographs reveal small radio-opaque densities throughout the lung fields. There is NO prior history of URI and NO symptoms of URI now. Both hemograms are essentially normal except for a marked eosinophilia. Both cats eat commercial canned and dry foods, although the original owner-breeder fed them raw meat combinations. Which of the following tests should be conducted next? 10. C
   A. Sputum culture
   B. Blood smear for FeLV
   C. Repeated fecal examinations
   D. Lung biopsy
   E. Lymph node biopsy

11. Renal amyloidosis is thought to be related to an immunologic disturbance and occurs *primarily* as a disease of the 11. A
   A. glomeruli and is characterized by persistent proteinemia
   B. renal tubule and is characterized by hypercalcuria
   C. interstitial tissue and is characterized by amino aciduria
   D. renal medulla and is characterized by increased catecholamines
   E. adrenals with secondary renal involvement characterized by excess sodium retention

12. Approach to the midshaft of the femur is BEST made between the 12. C
    A. vastus lateralis and biceps femoris
    B. semimembranosus and biceps femoris
    C. semitendenosus and biceps femoris
    D. vastus medialis and rectus femoris
    E. vastus intermedialis and medialis

PTH ⇒ ↑ Ca

13. Renal secondary hyperparathyroidism is characterized by 13. C
    A. hypercalcemia and hypophosphatemia
    B. hypercalcemia and hyperphosphatemia
    C. hypocalcemia and hyperphosphatemia
    D. hypocalcemia and hypophosphatemia
    E. hypercalcemia and normophosphatemia

14. One of the quickest and simplest differential diagnostic procedures to distinguish among pyometra, ascites, peritonitis, hemoperitoneum, and rupture of the bladder is 14. B
    A. x-ray examination
    B. paracentesis
    C. the white blood count
    D. determination of the pulse rate
    E. palpation

15. The drugs that should be given to a dog that collapses has pale mucous membranes, and tachycardia following intravenous promazine injection is 15. E
    A. atropine
    B. epinephrine
    C. isoproterenol HCl
    D. thiamylal Na
    E. pentobarbital Na

16. Persistence of the right instead of the left fourth aortic arch in the dog leads to ______ as an early clinical sign. 16. C
    A. coughing
    B. weakness
    C. regurgitation of solid food
    D. cachexia
    E. systolic murmur

17. The earliest that dogs with collie ectasia syndrome can be examined for the presence of the disease is 17. ___
    A. 6 weeks of age
    B. 3 months of age
    C. 6 months of age
    D. 1 year of age
    E. 2 years of age since the condition may change with age

18. A serum calcium value of 13 mg/ml in an adult dog would eliminate the need of a specific search for evidence of 18. D
    A. secondary renal hyperparathyroidism
    B. primary hyperparathyroidism
    C. hypervitaminosis D
    D. pseudohyperparathyroidism of malignancy
    E. metastatic tumor involving bone

19. A six-month-old dachshund is presented with a 2 cm in diameter red nodule on the lateral surface of the ear. The lesion is non-pruritic and has been present for two weeks. 19.___
A *likely* diagnosis is
   A. fly bite dermatitis
   B. acral pruritic nodule
   C. histiocytoma
   D. dermatomycosis
   E. mastocytoma

20. Determination of the concentration of blood urea nitrogen provides a crude index of 20.___
   A. renal tubular secretory capacity
   B. renal tubular reabsorptive capacity
   C. glomerular filtration rate
   D. renal plasma flow
   E. the nephrons' capacity to concentrate or dilute urine

21. A diagnosis of haemobartonellosis in the cat is established by the presence of 21.___
   A. a markedly reduced hemoglobin content
   B. nucleated and basophilic red blood cells in the blood film
   C. an enlarged spleen
   D. ring or rod-like bodies on the red blood cells
   E. jaundice or bile pigment in the urine

22. The Schirmer tear test as used in evaluating conjunctivitis is indicative of keratitis sicca when the amount of wetting is _____ mm. 22.___
   A. 0 to 5
   B. 6 to 10
   C. 11 to 20
   D. 21 to 30
   E. above 30

23. A 4-year-old female dachshund is presented with a purulent ocular discharge, blepharospasm and superficial corneal ulceration of the left eye (corneal wetting, left eye, 2 mm/1 min). 23.___
The initial treatment program would be to
   A. perform conjunctival flap operation
   B. treat symptomatically and begin a lacrimogenic drug
   C. shorten palpebral fissure
   D. perform parotid duct transposition
   E. treat with antibiotic and corticosteroids

24. The normal $pO_2$ of arterial blood at sea level is _____ mmHg. 24.___
   A. 760
   B. 150
   C. 120
   D. 90
   E. 60

25. A 6-year-old blood donor, DSH cat that hasn't been used in 3 months, is found in tonic seizures with downward flexion of the neck that later develops into opisthotonis. After each bleeding, the cat is given hematinics and B vitamins by injection and C/D for about a week, and then returned to a steady diet of commercial canned fish cat food. The CBC and body temperature are normal. The cat expires and NO gross or histologic lesions are found on necropsy. 25.___

The MOST probable cause of death is
- A. poisoning from Roccal-D used to disinfect cages
- B. stroke syndrome
- C. thiamine deficiency
- D. idiopathic epilepsy with grand mal seizure
- E. tetanus

26. The blood supply to the femoral head and neck in the dog is derived from 26. D
    - A. retinacular vessels alone
    - B. retinacular vessels and artery of the head of the femur
    - C. femoral medullary vessels alone
    - D. medullary and trochanteric epiphyseal vessels
    - E. external iliac arteries

27. In feline practice hypertrophy of the gland of the third eyelid is BEST treated by 27. C
    - A. cauterization of the third eyelid
    - B. flushing of the nasolacrimal duct
    - C. excision of the gland
    - D. application of antibiotic ointments
    - E. application of hot compresses

28. Which of the following agents is preferred for euthanasia? 28. E
    - A. Chloral hydrate IV
    - B. Magnesium sulfate IV
    - C. Strychnine IV
    - D. Succinylcholine dichloride IV
    - E. Pentobarbital Na IV

29. The clinical finding that differentiates tetrology of Fallot from pulmonic stenosis is 29. A
    - A. cyanosis
    - B. icterus
    - C. anemia
    - D. petechial hemorrhages
    - E. lameness

30. A simple technique for visualizing less dense urinary cystic calculi is a(n) 30. A
    - A. pneumocystogram
    - B. pneumoperitoneum
    - C. intravenous urogram
    - D. air myelogram
    - E. retropneumoperitoneum

31. Sudden death in 5-week-old English bulldog puppies with clear pleural effusion and edema in the anterior mediastinal area suggests 31. B
    - A. toxoplasmosis
    - B. toxic thymus
    - C. herpes infection
    - D. pasteurella infection
    - E. nocardiosis

32. A fracture of the distal ulna may heal because the radial splints the ulna. A fracture of the radius alone may NOT heal because 32. C
    - A. the blood supply to the radius is LESS than the ulna
    - B. the radius is thicker than the ulna

C. the ulna acts as a spring to open and close the fracture
D. the dog will NOT use the leg properly because of pain
E. excessive mobility of the carpus results

33. There is a silvery crust but NO discharges present in a circumscribed area of alopecia on the foot of a young cat being examined. The lesion is Wood's light negative. The *most likely* diagnosis is 33. ____
A. demodex felis
B. pasteurella multocida
C. microsporum felis
D. microsporum audouini
E. microsporum canis

34. Phosphate urinary calculi have just been surgically removed from a 6-year-old cocker spaniel. To avoid recurrence, the owner should be instructed to 34. ____
A. avoid all other sources of water and provide *only* distilled water
B. feed moist foods, lightly salted, and promote increased fluid intake
C. dispense calcium ethylenediamine tetraacetate orally
D. feed *only* semi-moist dog food
E. have the animal neutered

35. Which of the following is a property of x-radiation? 35. ____
A. Fluorescent effect on certain crystals
B. Visibility
C. Constant wavelength
D. Penetration of material increases with longer wavelengths
E. Non-penetration of radio-opaque objects

36. MOST likely a diagnosis of hepatocellular jaundice resulting from disease or degeneration of the hepatic cells would be made if ______ were observed. 36. ____
A. anemia and *decreased* indirect van den Bergh reaction
B. an *increase* in both conjugated and free bilirubin
C. an *increase* in conjugated bilirubin and a *decrease* in free bilirubin
D. *increased* SGOT and SGPT with *decreased* alkaline phosphatase
E. *increased* alkaline phosphatase and *decreased* indirect bilirubin

37. The use of urinary antiseptics containing methylene blue (such as Urised) are contraindicated in the feline because they may cause 37. ____
A. Heinz body production and subsequent anemia
B. frequent vomiting and subsequent staining due to the dye portion
C. an *increase* in struvite crystal formation
D. gastro-intestinal ulcers
E. severe acidosis if combined with methionine or ascorbic acid

38. A nonicteric anemic dog is evaluated with the following results: 38.___

PCV 28%
SGPT 100 F./U.
BUN 28 mg/deciliter
Total protein 8.0 gm/dl
WBC 58,600 (20 normoblasts/100 WBC)

| | |
|---|---|
| Lymphocytes | 15% |
| Total neutrophils | 78% |
| Segs. | 58% |
| Stabs. | 20% |
| Monocytes | 5% |

Coomb's test positive
The MOST probable diagnosis is

A. anemia of infection
B. anemia of chronic renal disease
C. autoimmune hemolytic anemia
D. intraperitoneal hemorrhage
E. severe blood loss through hemorrhage

39. A dog is presented with a 5 cm oval area of alopecia on the dorsal surface of the tail about 5 cm from the base of the tail. The lesion is uniformly thickened and elevated about 1 cm with a collection of sebum being present on the surface. 39.___

A *likely* diagnosis is

A. impacted anal sacs
B. inflammation of the tail shield gland
C. infected circumanal glands
D. perianal adenomas
E. stud tail

40. An 8-year-old patient is presented with a grade III holosystolic murmur over the left 4th intercostal space. Both lateral and ventro-dorsal radiographs show left atrial enlargement. 40.___

The *most likely* diagnosis is

A. aortic insufficiency
B. aortic stenosis
C. mitral insufficiency
D. mitral stenosis
E. pulmonary hypertension

41. The BEST technique for repair of olecranon fracture of the ulna is 41.___

A. crossed Kirschner wires
B. bone screw
C. a tension band and a Steinmann pin
D. neutralization plate
E. Kuentcher nail

42. The immune mechanism is thought to involve two distinct systems which are identified as 42.___

A. bursa equivalent lymphocytes and plasma cells and the thymus dependent small lymphocytes
B. the integumentary system and the bone marrow
C. the thymus gland and the spleen

D. the granulocyte series and the plasma cells
E. endothelial and plasma cells and thymus dependent lymphocytes

43. The tumors that appear to be MOST susceptible to radiation therapy are 43.___
A. chondrosarcoma and osteosarcoma
B. squamous cell carcinoma and osteosarcoma
C. perianal adenoma and astrocytoma
D. perianal adenoma and osteosarcoma
E. perianal adenoma and squamous cell carcinoma

44. The phenomenon of viral interference occurs MOST often between 44.___
A. related viruses
B. a virus and a rickettsia
C. two nonpathogenic incomplete viruses
D. two pathogenic incomplete viruses
E. a virus and a phage

45. While using a closed circuit system with an *in circle* vaporizer, the plane of anesthesia becomes too light. The MOST rapid method to attain surgical anesthesia is to 45.___
A. run high flows of carrier gas
B. run high flows of carrier gas and use controlled ventilation
C. run low flows of carrier gas
D. run low flows of carrier gas and use controlled ventilation
E. administer IV thiamalyl sodium

46. Which radiopaque contrast media is BEST suited for bronchography? 46.___
A. Dionosil B. Hypaque C. Pantopaque
D. Air E. Tantalum

47. Incision of the insertions of the superficial, middle and deep gluteal muscles is part of the _____ approach to the coxofemoral joint. 47.___
A. anterior B. posterior C. Gorman
D. dorsal E. ventral

48. The relationship of milliamperage and radiographic density is that density 48.___
A. varies *directly* and proportionally with mA increase
B. varies *indirectly* with mA increase
C. does NOT vary with mA increase
D. is *only* related to exposure time
E. is *only* related to tube-object distance

Questions 49-50.

Questions 49 and 50 are based on the following case.

A seven-year-old spayed female golden retriever is brought to your clinic for evaluation. The owner's primary complaint involves an increasingly more obvious polydipsia and polyuria over the past five months. They also complain that although their dog appears to be eating quite well, if not excessively, that she seems to be losing weight. During the past 72 hours the dog has been vomiting three to five times per day and appears very restless. Food and water are vomited back within 60 minutes of ingestion.

Your physical examination finds a moderately depressed dog that is 6% to 8% dehydrated. She has deep rapid respirations, and harsh bronchovesicular sounds are evident throughout both lung fields. Her lips and forepaws are stained with *bile colored* fluid which you presume to be vomitus. You find abdominal palpation difficult as she resents palpation, especially in the right upper quadrant. You detect what you consider to be the borders of the liver projecting approximately 2 cm caudal to the costrochondral junction.

Your initial problem list is as follows:
Problem 1 - polydipsia, polyuria, vomiting, dehydration
Problem 2 - hepatomegaly

The most likely *rule outs* for problem 1 are:
1. Acute pancreatitis
2. Diabetes mellitus (ketoacidotic)
3. Renal failure
4. Pyometra
5. Hypoadrenocorticism
6. Hepatic failure
7. Primary GI disease, ie - tumor, foreign body, intussusception, etc.

49. The *most likely* disease or diseases to rule out are 49.____
A. 1 *only*
B. 2 and 3 *only*
C. 1, 2, 3, and 4
D. 2, 3, and 6
E. 1, 2, 5, and 6

You decide to collect blood and urine for a CBC, urinalysis, BUN, amylase, SGPT and alkaline phosphatase. The results are as follows (normals in parentheses):

CBC
PCV = 56% (35-55)
WBC = 24,200 (6,000-15,000)
Neut. = 76%
Seg. = 70%
Stab. = 6%
Eos. = 0
Baso. = 0
Mono. = 10%
Lymph = 14%
BUN = 25 mg% (10-30)
Amylase = 12,500 (<3,200)
SGPT = 250 Sigma Frankel Units (10-40)
Alk. P'tase = 65 Bodansky Units (3-6)

Urine
Specific gravity = 1.036
pH = 5.0
Color = yellow
Glucose = 4+ testape
Ketones = 3+
Albumin = neg.
WBC = 3-5/High power field
RBC = Occ.
Bilirubin = 2+ Icto test

50. From the above data, your BEST assessment is that the dog has 50. A
   A. diabetic ketoacidosis, acute pancreatitis, and hepatic disease secondary to diabetes and pancreatitis
   B. primary hepatic failure and retention hyperamylasemia
   C. septic pancreatitis and stress glucosuria
   D. chronic biliary tract disease leading to acute pancreatitis
   E. primary renal diabetes (renal glucosuria) and acute pancreatitis

# KEY (CORRECT ANSWERS)

| | | | | |
|---|---|---|---|---|
| 1. B | 11. A | 21. D | 31. B | 41. C |
| 2. B | 12. A | 22. A | 32. C | 42. A |
| 3. B | 13. C | 23. B | 33. E | 43. E |
| 4. D | 14. B | 24. D | 34. B | 44. A |
| 5. A | 15. A | 25. C | 35. A | 45. D |
| 6. A | 16. C | 26. B | 36. B | 46. A |
| 7. D | 17. A | 27. C | 37. A | 47. D |
| 8. E | 18. A | 28. E | 38. C | 48. A |
| 9. A | 19. C | 29. A | 39. B | 49. E |
| 10. C | 20. C | 30. A | 40. C | 50. A |

# TEST 2

DIRECTIONS: Each question or incomplete statement is followed by several suggested answers or completions. Select the one that BEST answers the question or completes the statement. *PRINT THE LETTER OF THE CORRECT ANSWER IN THE SPACE AT THE RIGHT.*

1. Abdominal palpation reveals that the left kidney of a four-year-old dog with an unknown history seems enlarged. Subsequently, an excretory urogram (IVP) reveals that left kidney length is four times L-2 vertebrae length, and the right kidney is NOT visualized. It is *most likely* that 1.___
   - A. left kidney hypertrophy is present
   - B. left kidney hypertrophy occurred as a result of right kidney agenesis
   - C. the left kidney is actually normal in size
   - D. neoplasia of the left kidney is likely
   - E. considering the findings, the dog *probably* has an elevation of blood urea nitrogen concentration

2. With regard to triple phosphate uroliths in the dog, 2.___
   - A. NO breed predisposition exists
   - B. diet is a significant factor in stone formation
   - C. urinary acidifiers are the MOST important therapeutic tool for prevention of recurrence
   - D. inadequate treatment of infection is the MOST common cause of recurrence
   - E. frequency of occurrence is *greater* in the male than in the female dog

3. Urinary incontinence has been observed since weaning of a six-month-old intact female English bulldog. Normal urination occurs, but urine also dribbles from the vulva, particularly after the dog rises after lying for a period of time. The *most likely* cause of the incontinence is 3.___
   - A. estrogen deficiency
   - B. urinary tract infection
   - C. urachal stalk
   - D. spinal cord lesion
   - E. ectopic ureter

4. Nephrotic syndrome is caused by 4.___
   - A. abnormal liver function
   - B. azotemia and abnormal liver function
   - C. proteinuria
   - D. hyperlipidermia
   - E. hypoalbuminemia

5. Diagnostic tests on a dog with renal failure include 5.___

   Sp gr - 1.040
   Na - 124
   K - 7.5
   Serumosmolality 321 mOsm/L

Hyponatremia in this case is caused by
A. dilution of the extracellular
B. renal failure in diuresis
C. hypoaldosteronism
D. pre-renal azotemia
E. proteinuria

6. Insufficiency of exocrine function by the pancreas can be detected MOST readily by 6. C E
A. running an insulin tolerance test
B. measuring the uptake of radioactive oleic acid
C. running a glucose tolerance test
D. examining a histological section of the jejunal mucosa
E. determining the amount of trypsin in the stool

7. A correct statement referring to the appearance and composition of normal cerebrospinal fluid is that the fluid is 7. B
A. opalescent, containing myriads of chylomicrons
B. clear and colorless, containing low levels of protein
C. cloudy, containing high levels of glucose
D. clear and colorless, with the same leukocyte count as peripheral blood
E. cloudy, containing low levels of protein

8. The cerebrospinal fluid findings that is NOT usually associated with polioencephalomalacia in the bovine species is 8. D
A. elevation of pressure
B. an *increase* in the number of cells
C. a positive reaction to the pandy test
D. a predominance of neutrophils
E. the presence of globulin

9. A blood change that is associated with parturition in the cow is a(n) 9. D A
A. increase in circulating neutrophils
B. increase in circulating eosinophils
C. decrease in circulating neutrophils
D. increase in circulating lymphocytes
E. decrease in packed cell volume

10. The serum calcium level in normal adult mammals is 10. A C
A. inversely proportional to the serum phosphorus level
B. inversely proportional to the serum magnesium level
C. usually stated to be 9 to 12 mg/100 ml
D. usually stated to be 25 to 30 mg/100 ml
E. contained largely in the red blood cells

11. It is usually stated that a leukocytosis is characteristic of bacterial infections, whereas leukopenia occurs in viral disease. 11. B D
However, leukopenia *regularly* occurs in severe cases of
A. milk fever
B. acute mastitis
C. demodectic mange
D. lead poisoning
E. nervous acetonemia

12. A patient is presented to you in renal failure, with a serum creatinine concentration of 17 mg%. Concerning your course of action, which is the BEST response? 12. E

A. Tell the client it is rare that any animal will live after the creatinine goes above 6 or 7 mg%
B. Tell the client the disease process is *most likely* irreversible
C. Serum creatinines *rarely* go this high, and there MUST be a laboratory error
D. Don't waste time. Immediately perform a renal biopsy and support the patient medically
E. Tell the client you CANNOT determine reversibility or irreversibility based on serum creatinine concentration. You will support the patient and pursue a diagnosis for the renal failure and then prognosticate

13. A patient with pyometra has the following urinalysis (urine obtained by catheter) 13. ~~E~~ B

Color - pale yellow
Turbidity - clear
Specific gravity - 1.005
pH - 6.5
Glucose - neg
Ketones - neg
Bilirubin - neg
Occult blood - neg
Protein - neg
RBC - 0-1/HPF
WBC - 1-2/HPF
Casts & Epithelial cells - neg
Bacteria - neg
Crystals - none seen

Your assessment is that

A. the patient probably also has diabetes insipidus, and as soon as postsurgical recovery is complete, an ADH response test should be performed
B. patients with pyometra frequently have a urine specific gravity in the 1.005 to 1.009 range. They may retain the ability to dilute urine and for a period of time lose the ability to concentrate urine
C. patients with pyometra often have glomerulonephritis, and this urinalysis helps to prove it in this case
D. you should perform an ADH response test before surgery, because the client may be unwilling to treat diabetes insipidus
E. this urinalysis has NO particular relevance to pyometra

14. Various similar symptoms occur in traumatic gastritis and traumatic pericarditis in the bovine. However, one symptom which frequently accompanies pericarditis, but is NOT seen in traumatic gastritis alone, is 14. A

A. distention of the jugulars and edematous swellings in the region of the throat, neck, or sternum

B. complete anorexia from the onset, which persists until the death of the animal
C. *increased* pulse rate (over 100) accompanied by a substantial rise in temperature (103.5 - 105 F)
D. chronic progressive emaciation extending over a period of one to two months
E. pain on percussion or palpation in the sternal region

15. Which of the following statements concerning canine demodecosis is INCORRECT? 15.___
A. The mite causing demodecosis lives in the hair follicle and seldom in the sebaceous glands
B. Demodecosis is MORE common in pups and immature dogs than in mature dogs
C. Removal of stress factors may be of help in combatting the condition
D. Demodecosis usually presents itself as a severely pruritic condition
E. The terms red mange and demodecosis refer to the same disease entity

16. The laboratory animal MOST susceptible to dermatomycoses is the 16.___
A. rhesus monkey
B. guinea pig
C. domestic rabbit
D. Sprague-dawley rat
E. albino mouse

17. Which of the following statements about louse infestations in cattle is CORRECT? 17.___
A. Unlike animals infested with demodectic mange, lousy cattle are NOT amenable to treatment
B. Transmission to humans by contact frequently results in a malignant dermatitis
C. Cattle heavily infested with sucking lice may develop a fatal anemia
D. In some states milk from untreated animals is considered unfit for human consumption
E. Once an animal harbors the infestation, recurrences are likely for the rest of its life

18. Impetigo is a superficial pustular dermatitis that usually begins on the 18.___
A. lips
B. ears
C. back
D. udder
E. distal limbs

19. Folliculitis is usually caused by 19.___
A. C. pseudotuberculosis
B. C. pyogenes
C. beta-hemolytic streptococci
D. P. aeruginosa
E. coagulase-positive staphylococci

20. As a general rule, any abscess associated with a lymph node should be assumed to be due to 20.___
A. C. pyogenes
B. beta-hemolytic streptococci
C. C. pseudotuberculosis
D. coagulase-positive staphylococci
E. P. aeruginosa

21. The cause of caprine skin disease that has NOT been reported to cause skin disease in humans is 21.___
A. Cl. novyi
B. C. pseudotuberculosis
C. T. verrucosum
D. coagulase-positive staphylococci
E. D. congolensis

22. The disease that has been associated with the development of cutaneous horns is 22.___
A. caseous lymphadenitis
B. dermatophilosis
C. impetigo
D. dermatophytosis
E. mycetoma

23. The MOST common causal agent of dermatophytosis is 23.___
A. Ms. canis
B. T. mentagrophytes
C. E. floccosum
D. T. schoenleini
E. T. verrucosum

24. The MAJOR potential side effect of using topical captan in the treatment of dermatophytosis is 24.___
A. primary irritant contact dermatitis in treated goats
B. teratogenicity in pregnant goats
C. anorexia and depression in treated goats
D. allergic contact dermatitis in humans
E. ataxia and depression in treated goats

25. The disease that would be *lease likely* to be present as a superficial crusting dermatosis is 25.___
A. dermatophytosis
B. mycetoma
C. impetigo
D. folliculitis
E. dermatophilosis

26. Environmental contamination and contagion are apparently of NO concern in 26.___
A. dermatophytosis
B. impetigo
C. dermatophilosis
D. yeast dermatitis
E. folliculitis

27. Skin biopsy would be LEAST helpful in the diagnosis and management of 27.___
A. dermatophytosis
B. folliculitis
C. yeast dermatitis
D. dermatophilosis
E. clostridial infection

28. Urinary tract infections are a common and frequently frustrating problem in veterinary medicine. 28. D
It is the MOST accurate to say that
   A. cats with the feline urological syndrome usually have one of the enteric bacteria isolated from their urine on routine cultures
   B. a patient has NOT been on an antibiotic or chemotherapeutic agent or has been off one for at least three weeks, and a urine culture is performed, and the result is no growth. This means that there is NO urinary tract infection present
   C. A clinician can usually rule out a urinary tract infection by finding an acid urine on a fresh urine sample
   D. urinary tract infection is often superimposed on any type of renal disease; therefore, any patient with renal disease should be checked periodically for urinary tract infection
   E. the finding of abnormal numbers of leukocytes in the urine sediment is diagnostic of urinary tract infection

29. The single MOST valuable laboratory aid to follow the course of active renal disease is 29. A
   A. urinalysis
   B. PSP (phenolsulfonphtholein) excretion
   C. endogenous creatinine clearance
   D. serum creatinine concentration
   E. blood urea nitrogen

30. Given the following results obtained on urine procured by cystocentesis 30. D
color- yellow
protein - 2+
turbidity - sl. turbd
RBC - TNTC ++++
specific gravity - 1.033
WBC - TNTC
pH - 7.5
casts - 1-2/HPF
glucose - neg
epi cells - 3-5/HPF
acetone - neg
bacteria - neg
bilirubin - neg
crystals - few tri-$PO_4$
occult bl - neg
The BEST interpretation of the results obtained is that
   A. infection is ruled out since bacteria were NOT visualized
   B. cystitis is present
   C. urinary tract infection is present
   D. urinary tract inflammation is present
   E. trauma occurred as a result of cystocentesis

31. The signs of equine infectious anemia, or swamp fever, include 31. A
   A. intermittent fever and edema of the ventral abdomen and legs
   B. severe, persistent, bloody diarrhea
   C. frequent urination, the urine containing large quantities of blood
   D. bleeding from the body orifices
   E. frequent nosebleeds following exertion such as racing

32. ALL of the following are signs of acute leptospirosis in cattle EXCEPT 32. C
   A. fever, hemoglobinuria, and jaundice
   B. a fall in milk yield, the milk becoming thicker in consistency and taking on a yellow-orange color
   C. recurrent attacks of photophobia, lacrimation, conjunctivitis, keratitis, and iridocyclitis
   D. anorexia, depression, and hemolytic anemia
   E. abortion following the acute syndrome

33. The BEST method of controlling vibriosis in a dairy herd is 33. ~~D~~ C
   A. vaccination of the cows
   B. vaccination of the bulls
   C. use of artifical insemination
   D. use of a fluorescent antibody diagnostic procedure
   E. elimination from the herd of all cows that have aborted

34. A veterinarian examining an aborted 8-month fetus can make a tentative diagnosis of equine rhinopneumonitis if the lesions observed include 34. C
   A. pulmonary edema and congestion, hydrothorax, focal splenic necrosis and splenomegaly, conjunctivitis, and minimal autolysis
   B. congestion and edema of lungs, bronchi, trachea, larynx, and pharynx, hydrothorax, widespread petechia, and minimal autolysis
   C. focal hepatic necrosis, pulmonary edema, hydrothorax, generalized lymphoid necrosis, and minimal autolysis
   D. focal hepatic necrosis, pulmonary edema, hydrothorax, generalized lymphoid necrosis, and maximal autolysis
   E. congestion and edema of lungs, bronchi, trachea, larynx, and pharynx, hydrothorax, widespread petechia, and maximal autolysis

35. In a well-muscled young adult working breed, $P_2$ or $P_3$ is so badly damaged that in your opinion the respective phalanx should be amputated. 35. ~~A~~ B
The methods of amputation are
   I. $P_3$ is removed at the distal interphalangeal joint preserving the pad
   II. $P_3$ is removed along with the distal end of $P_2$ preserving the pad

III. $P_2$ is removed at the proximal interphalangeal joint preserving the pad
IV. $P_2$ is removed along with the distal portion of $P_1$ preserving the pad
V. $P_2$ is removed along with the distal portion of $P_1$ removing the pad

Which of the above is TRUE?

A. I, III  B. I, IV  C. I, V
D. II, III  E. II, IV

36. In a well-muscled young adult working breed, the entire lateral digit of the right rear foot is beyond repair and, in your opinion, should be amputated. 36.___
In amputation, the digit is disarticulated at the
I. metatarsal-phalangeal joint
II. metatarsal-phalangeal joint and sesamoids 7 and 8 are removed
III. metatarsal-phalangeal joint and the distal 4 to 5 mm of the 5th metatarsal bone is removed
IV. metatarsal-phalangeal joint and the distal 4 to 5 mm of the 5th metatarsal bone is removed together with the sesamoids
V. metatarsal-phalangeal joint and sesamoid No. 7 is removed

Which of the above is true?

A. I *only*  B. II *only*  C. III *only*
D. V *only*  E. II, IV

37. ALL of the following are threatened complications of traumatic gastritis in the bovine EXCEPT 37.___
A. traumatic pleuritis
B. metastatic pneumonia
C. hepatic abscessation
D. gangrenous pneumonia
E. pulmonary adenomatosis

38. A disease of swine MOST frequently manifested by epistaxis is 38.___
A. atrophic rhinitis  B. virus pig pneumonia
C. leptospirosis  D. lungworm infestation
E. pasteurella pneumonia

39. A mucopurulent nasal discharge in sheep is frequently a manifestation of 39.___
A. trichophytosis
B. gastrophilus larvae infestation
C. viral arteritis
D. hypoderma lineatum infestation
E. oestrus ovis larvae infestation

40. In a closed circuit anesthetic system, the function of the vaporizer is to 40.___
A. remove accumulated nitrogen from the system
B. accommodate volume fluctuations occurring during respiration
C. remove accumulations of excess water vapor

D. deliver measured concentration of anesthetic gas
E. remove accumulated carbon dioxide from the system

41. Hypertrophic pulmonary osteo-arthropathy occurs MOST frequently in association with chronic pulmonary lesions, but the important clinical characterization is — 41.___
A. hypertrophic osteodystrophy
B. vomiting, cachexia, and weight loss
C. hypertrophic lesions of the long bones
D. dyspnea, coughing, and nasal discharge
E. chronic bronchopneumonia

42. The MOST common cause of thoracic transudate in the cat is — 42.___
A. adenocarcinoma
B. diaphragmatic hernia
C. lymphosarcoma
D. viral pneumonitis
E. cardiac hypertrophy

43. Human rabies postexposure prophylaxis for an unimmunized individual may include — 43.___
A. tetanus prophylaxis
B. human diploid cell vaccine
C. human rabies immunoglobulin
D. antibiotics
E. ALL of the above

44. To determine the need for human postexposure prophylaxis, _____ should NOT be used. — 44.___
A. circumstances of the bite
B. vaccination status of the animal
C. presence of rabies in the region
D. species of biting animal
E. fluorescent antibody test of the biting animal

45. An acceptable rabies titer is $\geq$ ____ IV/ml. — 45.___
A. 0.1 B. 0.2 C. 0.3 D. 0.5 E. 5.0

Questions 46-50.

Questions 46 to 50 are based on the following case.

A 12-year-old male miniature schnauzer is presented with a history of a persistent cough, which has gotten progressively worse in the six months since it began. The cough is worse at night, and in the morning just after waking. The cough is exacerbated by exercise or excitement and even a slight amount of exercise causes him to breathe heavily. The owner reports that the dog is restless at night and has trouble sleeping.

On physical examination, he is mildly dyspneic, and has a grade V out of VI holosystolic mixed frequency murmur over the mitral area. He has a BB shot pulse, and a heart rate of 200 beats per minute. NO pulmonary rates are present. Your diagnosis is phase III congestive heart failure due to chronic left atrio-ventricular valvular insufficiency. You hospitalize the dog and record the following lead II electrocardiogram.

Lead II

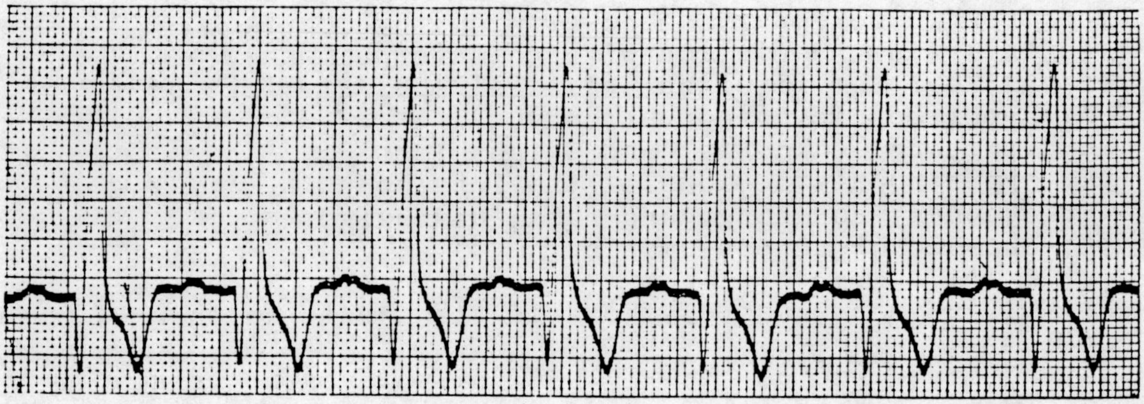

Paper Speed = 50 mm/sec, 1 cm. = 1 mv.

46. The abnormalities on this ECG include 46. E
   A. normal ECG
   B. left atrial hypertrophy
   C. biatrial hypertrophy
   D. biatrial and biventricular hypertrophy
   E. left atrial hypertrophy, biventricular hypertrophy, left bundle branch block

After two days on treatment with digoxin, you record the following electrocardiogram.

Lead II

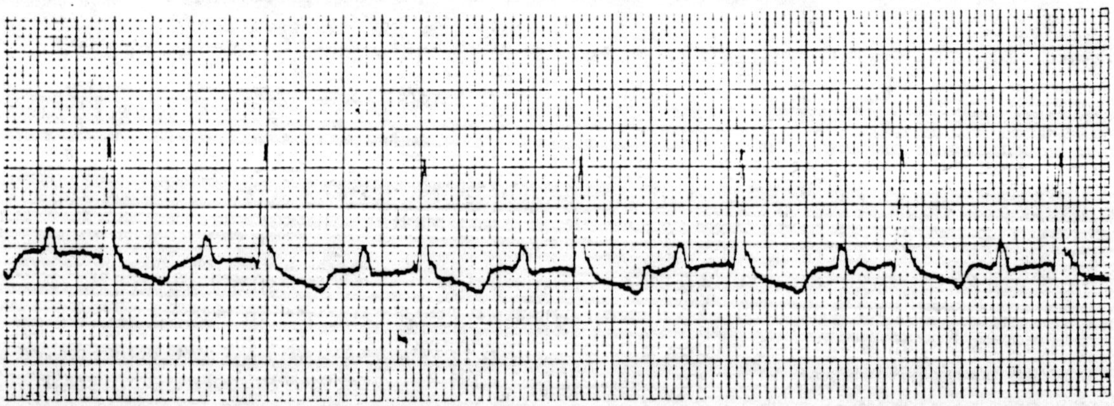

Paper Speed = 50 mm/sec, 1 cm. = 1 mv

47. The electrocardiographic diagnosis is 47. A
   A. first degree heart block
   B. second degree heart block
   C. third degree heart block
   D. complete heart block
   E. ventricular tachycardia

48. You successfully stabilize the dog on digoxin and send him home. After two weeks, the owner calls and says the dog has quit eating and is vomiting. What do you tell the owner? 48.___

A. Coax the dog to eat and keep giving the digoxin, but try to *increase* his fluid intake to promote diuresis
B. *Increase* the digoxin dosage to improve cardiac output and renal perfusion
C. *Increase* the digoxin on the next dose to avoid further toxicity
D. Stop the digoxin completely until the dog feels better and begins eating again. Then resume the digoxin at a slightly lower dosage
E. Give Kaopectate and bring in a urine and a stool sample as soon as possible

After four months of trouble-free existence, the owner calls to report that today the dog stood up, stared into space, stiffened out, and fell over on his side. He lay there unconscious for about 15 to 20 seconds, and then recovered quickly.

49. How could mitral insufficiency cause his syncopal attack? 49.___

A. His heart is fatiguing and is experiencing episodes of asystole
B. He is developing bouts of atrial tachycardia due to atrial stretching from the mitral insufficiency
C. He is beginning to have heart attacks due to coronary insufficiency, and another one may prove fatal
D. The pulmonary congestion has reached the point that the blood CANNOT be adequately oxygenated, and he experiences hypoxic syncope during exercise
E. Something else is happening now, and the dog should be hospitalized for a complete seizure workup

The owner brings the dog in at your request, and you record the following ECG:

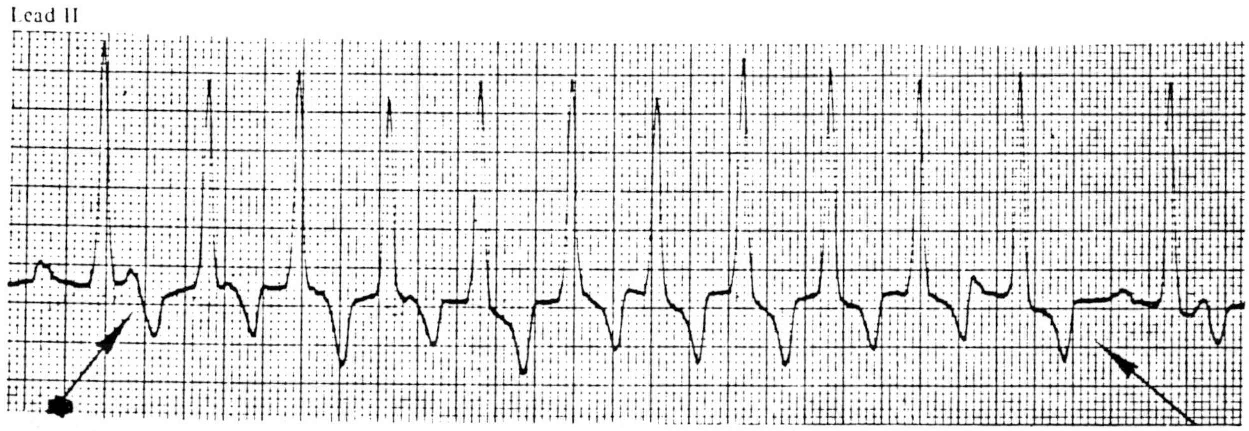


Paper Speed = 50 mm/sec. 1 cm = 1 mv.

50. Your electrocardiographic diagnosis is — 50. ____
    A. paroxysmal atrial tachycardia
    B. paroxysmal ventricular tachycardia
    C. atrioventricular dissociation
    D. first degree heart block
    E. atrial standstill

---

# KEY (CORRECT ANSWERS)

| | | | | |
|---|---|---|---|---|
| 1. A | 11. D | 21. A | 31. A | 41. C |
| 2. D | 12. E | 22. B | 32. C | 42. C |
| 3. E | 13. B | 23. E | 33. C | 43. E |
| 4. C | 14. A | 24. D | 34. C | 44. B |
| 5. C | 15. D | 25. B | 35. B | 45. D |
| 6. E | 16. C | 26. D | 36. E | 46. E |
| 7. B | 17. C | 27. E | 37. E | 47. A |
| 8. D | 18. D | 28. D | 38. A | 48. D |
| 9. A | 19. E | 29. A | 39. E | 49. B |
| 10. C | 20. C | 30. D | 40. D | 50. A |

# TEST 3

DIRECTIONS: Each question or incomplete statement is followed by several suggested answers or completions. Select the one that BEST answers the question or completes the statement. *PRINT THE LETTER OF THE CORRECT ANSWER IN THE SPACE AT THE RIGHT.*

1. Concerning fungal spores, it is INCORRECT that 1.____
   A. there is a good correlation between intensity of exposure and allergic signs
   B. dry-spore dispersal occurs during hot, windy periods
   C. slime spores become airborne during rainy periods
   D. the antigenic relationships between biologically related genera is unclear
   E. alternaria is the MOST clinically reactive airborne fungus in humans

2. ______ have NOT been associated with the house-dust allergen. 2.____
   A. Fungi
   B. Animal danders
   C. House-dust mites
   D. Plant fibers
   E. Pollens

3. The statements concerning epidermal allergens that ______ is INCORRECT. 3.____
   A. hair is a good source of allergen
   B. epidermal scale extracts are highly reactive
   C. cats are the MOST allergenic animal for humans
   D. the importance of wool as an aeroallergen is unknown
   E. aged feathers are MORE allergenic than new feathers

4. Rupture of the common digital extensor tendon can result in 4.____
   I. buckling forward at the carpus
   II. occasional stumbling when walking
   III. minimal gait abnormality
   IV. persistent lameness

   The CORRECT answer is:
   A. I, II
   B. I, II, III
   C. II, IV
   D. II, III, IV
   E. ALL of the above

5. Complete closure of the distal ulna growth plate and continued growth in the radius causes serious orthopedic problems. In time you would expect to find 5.____
   I. valgus deformity of the carpus
   II. subluxation of the carpus and elbow
   III. anterior medial bowing of the radius
   IV. osteoarthritis of the carpus and elbow
   V. *increased* joint space at the proximal radius

   The CORRECT answer is:
   A. I *only*
   B. I, II
   C. I, II, III, IV
   D. I, II, V
   E. V *only*

6. Transolecranon fractures are BEST treated by 6.A
   A. tension band wire B. single Steinmann pin
   C. Thomas splint D. double rush pin
   E. lag screw

7. An eight-month-old Yorkshire terrier with a lameness of the pelvic limb is *most likely* to have 7.A B
   A. ruptured anterior cruciate ligament
   B. Legg-Perthe's disease
   C. Osgood-Schlatter's disease
   D. avulsion of the tibial tuberosity
   E. rheumatoid arthritis

8. With a comminuted midshaft femoral fracture of the left side and a proximal femoral capital epiphyseal separation on the right side, the BEST repair for a nine-month-old Great Dane weighing 95 pounds would be 8.E
   A. IM pin and half-Kirschner on femur; femoral head/neck resection on right
   B. plate femur; femoral head/neck resection on right
   C. rush pin femur; pin cap
   D. IM pin and half-Kirschner on femur; pin cap
   E. plate femur; pin cap

9. The characteristic clinical feature of acute anterior cruciate rupture is anterior 9.A
   A. drawer motion and laxity of the lateral collateral ligament causing internal rotation of the tibia
   B. drawer motion and external rotation of the tibia
   C. drawer motion and laxity of the medial collateral ligament
   D. and posterior drawer motion
   E. drawer motion and a characteristic click caused by entrapment of the latera meniscus

10. A disease of horses which is associated with thrombosis of small branches of the mesenteric vessels, death of foals, and segmental edema of the intestine is 10.E A
   A. viral arteritis B. strongyliasis
   C. equine rhinopneumonitis D. onchocerciasis
   E. equine viral abortion

11. Medial hypertrophy, intimal fibrosis, and arteriosclerosis of the pulmonary arteries of dogs are associated with 11.A
   A. dirofilariasis
   B. canine distemper
   C. chronic failure of the left side of the heart
   D. chronic failure of the right side of the heart
   E. ehrlichosis

12. During the clinical course of African swine fever, changes occur which are similar to those of 12.A
   A. hog cholera B. pseudorabies
   C. vesicular exanthema D. foot and mouth disease
   E. brucellosis

13. The daily milk allowance for a 4-day-old, 80 pound Holstein-Friesian calf is _____ pounds. 13.___
A. 4 B. 6 C. 12 D. 14 E. 16

14. An immunity existing previous to exposure to the micro-organism is known as a(n) _______ immunity. 14.___
A. genetic
B. constitutional
C. acquired
D. acquired
E. specific

15. Canine scabies 15.___
A. resembles ringworm clinically
B. is non-pruritic
C. is not transmissible to other dogs
D. is self-limiting
E. is transmissible to man

16. Salivary cysts in the dog are MOST often due to 16.___
A. stenosis of the duct
B. inflammatory lesions
C. traumatic lesions
D. obstruction of the duct
E. congenital abnormalities

17. In the horse, failure of a *QRS* complex following a normal P wave indicates 17.___
A. normal vagal activity
B. sinus arrythmia
C. complete heart block
D. partial heart block
E. bundle branch block

18. The diagnosis of psoroptic mange in sheep requires 18.___
A. further study
B. sale of infected animals for slaughter and dipping rest
C. dipping
D. immediate reporting to a state or federal veterinarian
E. immediate slaughter

19. Traumatic gastritis in the bovine can easily be mistaken for primary indigestion because these two conditions 19.___
A. have many signs in common
B. *most commonly* affect *greedy eaters*
C. occur *only* in adults
D. are practically identical in their seasonal occurrence
E. produce the same initial rise in temperature

20. The skin lesions that may be inherited by animals via recessive genes that follow the Mendelian pattern are 20.___
A. hyperkeratosis
B. parakeratosis
C. alopecia
D. bursatti
E. skin tumors

21. Alopecia occurring in association with canine Cushing's syndrome is characterized by 21.____
   A. atrophy of the hair follicles, sebaceous glands and epidermis with loss of dermal fat
   B. connective tissue proliferation in the dermis and extensive deposition of collagen in epidermis
   C. the presence of many histeocytes laden with lipid substances in the heratinized layer
   D. dysheratesis and severe hypertrophy of the normal elastic fibers of the subcutis
   E. extensive leukocyte infiltration of the dermal adnexea

22. Anaplasmosis is MOST likely to be peracute and fatal in susceptible cattled aged 22.____
   A. 1 to 6 months
   B. 4 to 18 months
   C. 18 to 24 months
   D. 1 to 2 years
   E. 3 years or more

23. Replacement fluids containing dextrose, lactated sodium, and sodium and potassium chlorides are indicated for 23.____
   A. gastric loss
   B. protein loss
   C. duodenal loss
   D. shock
   E. water loss

24. The simplest and easiest test to differentiate between pyometra, ascites, hemoperitoneum and a ruptured bladder is the use of 24.____
   A. an x-ray
   B. paracentesis
   C. a WBC count
   D. a pulse rate
   E. palpation

25. Infectious or chick bronchitis is *usually* seen 25.____
   A. affecting ALL the birds of a young age in the same pen about the same time
   B. in ALL birds of ALL ages annually
   C. to spread *slowly* by bird to bird contact
   D. to affect *only* young when numerous ages are together
   E. to affect ALL ages with high mortality

26. A disease characterized by punched-out erosions of the esophageal mucosa is 26.____
   A. BVD
   B. MCF
   C. x-disease
   D. vitamin A deficiency
   E. winter dysentary

27. Following a gunshot injury to the rear limb, a dog does NOT have the ability to flex the ankle and extend the toes. There is loss of sensation over the dorsum of the foot. These signs may be attributed to damage of the ____ nerve. 27.____
   A. tibial
   B. saphenous
   C. fibular
   D. common digital
   E. popliteal

28. Dogs who have fractures sustained from automobile accidents frequently have injury to soft tissue. One of the MORE common injuries is 28.____
   A. ruptured urinary bladder
   B. diaphragmatic hernia
   C. damage to MAJOR nerves in the region of the fracture
   D. concussion
   E. pneumothorax

29. Fractures of the ilial body and acetabulum are BEST treated by 29.____
   A. cage rest
   B. body cast
   C. lag screws
   D. an ehmer sling
   E. a neutralization plate

30. The BEST treatment for a T-fracture of the elbow is 30.____
   A. transcondylar compression screw, IM pin in lateral condyle; oblique pin from medial condyle
   B. transcondylar compression screw, IM pin in medial condyle, oblique pin from lateral condyle
   C. transcondylar screw, bone plate along posterior lateral border of humerus
   D. transcondylar smooth pin, and IM pin into medial condyle
   E. rush pin from lateral condyle proximally, another from medial condyle proximally

31. The PRIMARY anatomic abnormality in congenital medial patellar dislocation is 31.____
   A. laxity of the lateral retinaculum
   B. tight medial retinaculum
   C. genu valgum
   D. axial distorsion of the femur
   E. plastic deformation of the tibial plateau

32. The tuberculin test is a diagnostic procedure whose usefulness depends on the allergic state in the infected animal classified as 32.____
   A. delay hypersensitivity
   B. asthma
   C. anaphylaxis
   D. atopic hypersensitivity
   E. immediate hypersensitivity

33. Tetany is common in 33.____
   A. pigs
   B. sheep
   C. cows
   D. dogs
   E. guinea pigs

34. An increase in cerebral spinal fluid in a calf and pig is due to a deficiency of 34.____
   A. vitamin A
   B. vitamin D
   C. vitamin C
   D. vitamin B
   E. thiamin

35. Persistent vomiting leads to internal changes in the fluid compartments of the body manifested by 35. E
   A. generalized edema
   B. diabetes insipidus
   C. acidosis and hyponatremia
   D. hydremia and hyperkaliemia
   E. metabolic alkalosis and hypochloremia

36. Equine encepholomyelitis is MOST prevalent during 36. D
   A. long day spells
   B. the winter
   C. the spring
   D. the summer
   E. the fall

37. Enzootic ataxia in sheep is due to a deficiency of 37. D
   A. calcium
   B. manganese
   C. iodine
   D. copper
   E. phosphorus

38. The MOST characteristic sign of guttural pouch infection is 38. B
   A. diffuse, soft tympanic swelling in the parotid area
   B. pus draining from mares when the head is lowered to eat or drink
   C. frequent coughing
   D. hard swelling on the stensens duct
   E. head tilt to the affected side

39. The MOST common cause of bronchoesophageal fistula in the dog appears to be 39. B D
   A. pulmonary infections
   B. malignancies
   C. external trauma
   D. esophageal foreign bodies
   E. esophageal diverticuli

40. Congenital bronchoesophageal fistulas 40. A C
   A. have NOT been reported in the dog
   B. are diagnosed MOST frequently in dogs under six months of age
   C. have been reported in dogs of different ages
   D. always communicate with the right caudal lung lobe bronchus
   E. have been seen MOST in dogs over 30 kg

41. Acquired bronchoesophageal fistulas MOST frequently connect the esophagus to the 41. C A
   A. right caudal and intermediate lung lobe bronchi
   B. left caudal and intermediate lung lobe bronchi
   C. left cranial lung lobe bronchus
   D. right cranial and middle lung lobe bronchi
   E. left caudal lung lobe bronchus

42. The clinical sign MOST consistently associated with bronchoesophageal fistula is 42. B
   A. regurgitation
   B. cough or cough after drinking liquids
   C. dyspnea
   D. depression
   E. lethargy

43. A previously healthy puppy begins vomiting when it is first given solid food. There is NO fever and if it is immediately returned to a liquid diet, no further vomiting occurs. 43.___ C
The congenital anomaly of the cardiovascular system that will cause such symptoms is
   A. dextrorotation of the aorta
   B. subaortic septal defect
   C. persistence of the right aortic arch
   D. patent foramen ovale
   E. patent ductus arteriosis

44. The rise in serum amylase content in acute pancreatic necrosis is of short duration if 44.___ B
   A. lipocaic limits the spread of trypsin, amylase, and lipase
   B. production of pancreatic amylase ceases and renal excretion continues
   C. vascular dilatation sequesters this substance in the splanchnic area
   D. edema shuts off venous return to the systemic circulation
   E. blood pressure falls sufficiently to interfere with renal excretion

45. In the dog, extensive tumors of the pars distalis and the pars intermedia produce 45.___ E
   A. yawning, posterior paralysis and strabismus
   B. hydrocephalus, convulsions, and terminal coma
   C. blindness, hydrocephalus, and motor irritation
   D. genital hypoplasia, oliguria, and posterior paralysis
   E. polyuria, polydypsia, obesity, bilateral alopecia and genital hypoplasia

46. In cattle, adrenal virilism connected with cystic ovaries is believed to be due to excessive secretion of androgenic hormones as a result of hyperplasia of the 46.___ B
   A. granulosa cells of the graafian follicle
   B. fetal rests of testicular tissue in the ovaries
   C. thyroid
   D. adrenal cortex
   E. pars nervosa

47. The pathologic process by which glandular epithelium of the prostate is transformed into squamous epithelium following prolonged administration of estrogens is known as 47.___ A
   A. neoplasia B. metaplasia C. hyperplasia
   D. dysplasia E. anaplasia

Questions 48-50.

Questions 48 to 50 are based on the following case.

An eight-month-old female, German short-haired pointer is referred to your hospital for evaluation of recurrent hematuria. Mr. and Mrs. Jacobsen report to you that when the dog was four months old, they had noticed gross hematuria which lasted for three days. The blood was well-mixed with the urine, occurring throughout urinations. The dog was otherwise asymptomatic, and the hematuria stopped spontaneously without treatment. When bleeding of the same character recurred at six months of age, they went to their local veterinarian for evaluation. His tests revealed the following:

| | |
|---|---|
| Specific gravity | 1.027 |
| pH | 6.5 |
| Glucose | 0 |
| Ketones | 0 |
| Albumin | 300 mg% |
| RBC | 200-300 |
| WBC | 0-1 |
| BUN | 12 |
| Abdominal x-rays | normal |
| Urine culture | negative |

The hematuria again ceased without therapy, and the dog was released for further observation. When hematuria recurred at eight months of age, the dog was referred to your hospital for reevaluation.

At that time, Mr. and Mrs. Jacobsen reported that the dog has remained in apparent excellent health despite the episodes of hematuria. Physical examination is unremarkable, and there is gross hematuria. Your laboratory tests reveal the following:

| | |
|---|---|
| BUN | 13 |
| Creatinine | 0.6 |
| Urinalysis | |
| Specific gravity | 1.032 |
| pH | 6.0 |
| Glucose | 0 |
| Ketone | 0 |
| Albumin | 300 mg% |
| Bacteria | 0 |
| RBC | 300-500 |
| WBC | 4-6 |
| Cast | 12-15 RBC |
| Abdominal x-rays | normal renal size and outline<br>bladder grossly normal |
| Cystogram | normal |

48. Further tests that should be performed include 48. A
    - A. more urine sediments, IVP
    - B. urine culture, IVP
    - C. IVP, renal biopsy
    - D. creatinine, urine culture, IVP
    - E. IVP and exploratory laparotomy

49. The prognosis with the data presented, and knowing that the IVP is normal is 49. ~~B~~ D
    - A. excellent
    - B. poor
    - C. fair
    - D. CANNOT be offered without further tests
    - E. poor with therapy

50. According to the data presented, the bleeding is originating from 50.___
A. the urethra
B. the bladder or urethra
C. the kidney
D. radiolucent bladder stones
E. any of the above

---

# KEY (CORRECT ANSWERS)

| | | | | |
|---|---|---|---|---|
| 1. A | 11. A | 21. A | 31. D | 41. A |
| 2. E | 12. A | 22. E | 32. A | 42. B |
| 3. A | 13. B | ~~23. A~~ | 33. C | 43. C |
| 4. B | 14. B | 24. B | 34. A | 44. B |
| 5. C | 15. E | 25. A | 35. E | 45. E |
| 6. A | ~~16. A~~ | 26. A | 36. D | 46. D |
| 7. B | 17. A | 27. C | 37. D | 47. B |
| 8. E | 18. D | 28. E | 38. B | 48. A |
| 9. A | 19. B | 29. E | 39. D | 49. D |
| 10. A | 20. C | 30. B | 40. C | 50. C |

---

# TEST 4

DIRECTIONS: Each question or incomplete statement is followed by several suggested answers or completions. Select the one that BEST answers the question or completes the statement. *PRINT THE LETTER OF THE CORRECT ANSWER IN THE SPACE AT THE RIGHT.*

1. A four and one-half-month-old male Great Dane with a front limb lameness is *most likely* to have 1.___
   A. rheumatoid arthritis
   B. osteochondritis dissecans
   C. panosteitis
   D. ununited anconeal process
   E. hypertrophic pulmonary osteoarthropathy

2. Complete closure of the distal radial growth plate and continued growth in the ulna *may* lead to 2.___
   I. severe shortening of the radius
   II. *decreased* joint space at the proximal radius
   III. subluxation of the elbow with osteoarthritis
   IV. *increased* joint space at the proximal radius
   V. *angular* deformity NOT being present

   The CORRECT answer is:
   A. I *only* B. I, II, V C. I, III, IV, V
   D. II, III, V E. V *only*

3. Chronic (non-acute) fractures of the palmar and plantar sesamoid bones in the dog often *only* produce lameness after exercise. 3.___
   The treatment of *choice* is
   A. phenylbutazone
   B. local injection of a corticosteroid
   C. ultrasound
   D. surgical removal
   E. mason meta splint

4. Fractures of the posterior distal border of the accessory carpal bone are BEST handled by 4.___
   A. tension band wire
   B. surgical removal of the fragment
   C. lag screw fixation
   D. mason meta splint
   E. local injection

5. The cause of paraplegia in dogs whose intervertebral discs have herniated into the vertebral canal is 5. C
   A. physiologic dysfunction due to myelitis
   B. loss of the disc substance, which *decreases* articular movement
   C. spinal cord compression and contusion
   D. spinal cord and spinal nerve compression with articular ankylosis
   E. inhibition of movement due to pain

6. Puerperal eclampsia in the bitch is characterized by 6. C
   A. a history of dystocia
   B. a very high temperature which is thought to cause permanent damage to the brain in many instances
   C. sudden tetanic convulsions during which the animal usually remains conscious
   D. a gradual onset which eventually leads to semi-consciousness and collapse
   E. sudden tetanic convulsions during which the animal usually loses consciousness

7. A cow with frontal sinusitis causes a breakdown of the bony plate between the temporal fossa and the post orbital diverticulum. Signs include 7. B
   A. bulging of the frontal sinus
   B. bulging of the eyes
   C. exudate from the nostrils
   D. exudate from the orbit
   E. exudate from the horn core

8. The presence of blood in the urine of cattle is diagnostic of 8. C
   A. anaplasmosis
   B. bacillary hemogloginuria
   C. pyelonephritis
   D. post mortem hemoglobinuria
   E. piroplasmosis

9. Chronic bloating in mature cattle is MOST suggestive of 9. B
   A. impaction of the abomasum
   B. compression stenosis of the esophagus
   C. atony of the rumen
   D. acute indigestion
   E. intussusception

10. In horses and cattle, a light red foam coming from both nostrils and harsh sounds over the trachea and bronchi indicate 10. A
   A. pulmonary hemorrhage
   B. nasal hemorrhage
   C. pharyngeal hemorrhage
   D. pulmonary congestion and edema
   E. red hepatization

11. Intracranial pressure in dogs suffering from cranial trauma is BEST treated by — 11. X E
   A. blood transfusions
   B. antibiotics and diuretics
   C. ACTH or steroids in 5% dextrose
   D. 20% saline SQ
   E. hypertonic solutions like 50% dextrose IV

12. A transient corneal opacity in one or both eyes is frequently observed in dogs following infection with — 12. A B
   A. canine distemper virus
   B. canine hepatitis virus (Blue Eye)
   C. canine tracheobronchitis virus
   D. neorickettsia helminthoeca
   E. leptospira canicola

13. Ulcers are found *most commonly* in the digestive tract of the bovine — 13. C
   A. rumen
   B. omasum
   C. abomasum
   D. reticulum
   E. esophageal groove

14. The MOST rapid depletion of body iron results from — 14. D
   A. profuse continuous vomiting
   B. a second degree burn, affecting one-fourth of the body surface
   C. low dietary iron intake
   D. slow, continuous external bleeding
   E. idiopathic diarrhea

15. Animal consumption of plants which were treated with plant hormone herbicides may result in death due to — 15. E
   A. drug allergy to the plant hormones, resulting from previous contact
   B. conversion of harmless plant starchs into toxic polysaccharide by the plants
   C. production by the plants of toxic alkoloids which cause liver cirrhosis in ruminants
   D. chemical breakdown of the plant hormones into toxoid phenols render conditions of high temperature, moisture and light
   E. accumulation of toxic quantities of niturates and nitrites in the plants

16. Partial obstruction of the esophagus can be caused by — 16. C
   A. endocardial fibroblastosis
   B. patent foramen ovale
   C. persistent right aortic arch
   D. interventricular opening
   E. persistent ductus arteriosis

17. The term *polyuria* is given to the volume of urine when there is — 17. B
   A. a *decrease* in urine
   B. an *increase* in urine volume
   C. suppression of urine
   D. LACK of variation
   E. the same volume each day

18. The clinical signs characteristic of anterior abdominal pain include — 18. E
   A. a rigid, hunched stance
   B. abduction of the elbows
   C. a grunt following pressure on the xiphoid
   D. a reluctance to move
   E. ALL of the above

19. A painful response to pressure placed on the xiphoid indicates a diagnosis of — 19. A E
   A. traumatic reticulitis
   B. traumatic pericarditis
   C. abomasal ulcer
   D. pleuritis
   E. ALL of the above

20. A positive Williams test is used for diagnosing — 20. A
   A. traumatic reticulitis
   B. a liver abscess
   C. an abomasal ulcer
   D. pyelonephritis
   E. ALL of the above

21. A cow that is NOT eating and registers a temperature of $103^{o}$ F, a neutrophil count of 5000/ul, and a fibrogen level of 1200 mg/dl is *probably* showing clinical signs of — 21. C
   A. a displaced abomasum
   B. acute indigestion
   C. traumatic reticulitis
   D. ketosis
   E. NONE of the above

22. *Increased* intensity of breath sounds heard at the trachea is — 22. A
   I. indicative of an *increase* in sound production
   II. indicative of abnormalities in transmission if there is NO concomitant *increase* in sound at the chest wall
   III. a very specific clinical indicator of disease
   IV. usually accompanied by an *increase* in intensity and change in quality of sound heard at the chest wall

   The CORRECT answer is:
   A. I, II, IV B. II, III C. III *only*
   D. III, IV E. IV *only*

23. Radiology can be used as an aid in the diagnosis of hardware disease. — 23. A C
   The MOST useful view is
   A. lateral standing
   B. dorsal ventral standing
   C. lateral in dorsal recumbency
   D. ventral dorsal in dorsal recumbency
   E. dorsal ventral standing following barium contrast

24. The cause of abomasal ulcers is 24.___
   A. an abrupt change in diet to a high concentrate and silage ration
   B. the stress of parturition
   C. the onset of lactation
   D. dry weather and heavy application of fertilizer
   E. ALL of the above

25. The onset of bacterial endocarditis is often associated with a chronic suppurative process that gives rise to sustained bacteremia and predisposes the endocardium to infection. 25.___
This chronic suppurative process can be associated with
   A. mastitis
   B. metritis
   C. foot abscessation
   D. traumatic reticulitis
   E. ALL of the above

26. Electrocardiographic findings supportive of the diagnosis of traumatic pericarditis are 26.___
   A. a depressed ST segment and *increased* P waves
   B. an *increased* P wave and negative T wave
   C. *decreased* voltages in P, QRS, and T waves
   D. *increased* voltages in P, QRS, and T waves
   E. the absence of P waves and presence of F waves

27. A culture of urine from a cow with pyelonephritis usually yields 27.___
   A. fusobacterium necrophorum
   B. corynebacterium renale
   C. salmonella typhimurium
   D. streptococcus dysuria
   E. fusobacterium renale

28. Pyelonephritis is MOST often associated with an ascending urinary tract infection involving the urethra, bladder, ureters, and kidneys. 28.___
A predisposing cause is
   A. urinary calculi
   B. obstetric procedures
   C. late pregnancy
   D. uterine prolapse
   E. any of the above

29. A common complication of arthroscopy is 29.___
   A. infection
   B. instrument breakage
   C. synovial hernia
   D. severe capsulitis
   E. none of the above

30. Traumatic plantar subluxation of the metatarsal bones is BEST handled by 30.D B
I. arthrodesis
II. rigid fixation and splinting
III. thomas splint
IV. mason meta
V. figure-eight sling
The CORRECT answer is:
A. I *only* B. I, II C. III, IV
D. IV *only* E. V *only*

31. The blood supply to a major growth plate of a long bone is comprised of the 31.A B
I. distal ramifications of the nutrient vessels
II. metaphyseal vessels
III. epiphyseal vessels
IV. cutaneous vessels
V. interosseous ligament
The CORRECT answer is:
A. I, II B. I, II, III C. I, III
D. IV, V E. V *only*

32. The usual dilution of the whole blood in a leukocyte count is 32.A B
A. 1:10 B. 1:20 C. 1:50 D. 1:100 E. 1:250

33. Inclusion bodies are found in transition epithelium of the urinary tract in 33.A B
A. canine distemper
B. infectious canine hepatitis
C. equine infectious anemia
D. equine rhinopneumonitis
E. rabies

34. The *largest* volume of blood in the body is in the 34.A D
A. large veins B. heart
C. large arteries D. capillaries
E. pulmonary vessels

35. Which of the following is LEAST toxic to cats? 35.A B
A. Toxophene B. Rotenone
C. DDT D. Malathion
E. Parathion

36. The diseases in chickens that can be egg transmitted include 36.E
A. viral arthritis
B. mycoplasma gallisepticum
C. mycoplasma synoviae
D. avian encephalomyelitis
E. ALL of the above

37. Urine specific gravity is MOST influenced by _____ in equal weight quantities. 37. A
   A. urea, $H_2O$, and electrolytes
   B. Hb, bilirubin, and sperm
   C. protein, glucose, and inflammatory cells
   D. phosphate crystals, granular casts, and urates
   E. RBC's and leukocytes

38. Inclusion body hepatitis in chickens is caused by 38. C
   A. parasites
   B. toxins
   C. a virus
   D. a fungus
   E. bacteria

39. A drug contraindicated in glaucoma is (myd. & cyclo) 39. B
   A. chloramphenicol
   B. atropine sulfate
   C. DFP
   D. estrine
   E. pilocarpine

40. A seven-year-old obese, 95 pound German shepherd has had difficulty arising from a lying down position for the last two months. A left rear leg mild lameness developed two days ago. The stifles palpate normally. The x-rays show moderate arthritis of both hips. 40. D
The best treatment at this point for the dog is
   A. bilateral femoral head and neck resection
   B. bilateral pectineotomy
   C. left femoral head and neck resection
   D. diet, rest for two weeks, and aspirin for two weeks
   E. exercise and butazolidin

41. The factor that does NOT relate to bone plates in comparison to IM pinning is that it 41. D
   A. has longer surgery time
   B. maintains length in severe comminution
   C. has *faster* return of function
   D. is less expensive in the long run
   E. is MORE stable

42. Three anatomical findings commonly seen in the *collie eye* syndrome are 42. E
   A. tortuosity of the vessels, opacity of the lens, and chorioretinal dysplasia
   B. ectasia of the optic nerve head, retinal atrophy, and chorioretinal dysplasia
   C. tortuosity of the vessels, retinal atrophy, and chorioretinal dysplasia
   D. tortuosity of the vessels, opacity of the lens, and retinal atrophy
   E. tortuosity of the vessels, ectasia of the optic nerve heads, and chorioretinal dysplasia

43. The MAJOR retinal lesions seen in the collie eye anomaly either alone or in combination are 43.___
   A. retinal hemorrhage, vascular dilation, and papilledemia
   B. microcornea, iridal heterochromia, dyscoria, cotectopia, equatorial staphylomas, retinal detachment, and cataracts
   C. microphthalmia, cortical cataracts, retinal dysplasia, and retinal detachments
   D. focal pigmentation of the area centralis, tapetal hyperreflectivity, and localized vascular constrictions
   E. chorioretinal dysplasia, colobomatous defects in the optic nerve, posterior scleral ectasia, retinal detachment and retinal hemorrhage

44. A sympathetic denervation which manifests itself clinically by unilateral miosis, ptosis, small palpebral fissure, protrusion of the nictitiating membrane, enophthalmos, and reduced intraocular pressure is called 44.___
   A. Waardenburg's syndrome
   B. unilateral microphthalmia congenita
   C. meningoencephalitis -ophthalmitis syndrome
   D. Horner's syndrome
   E. neonatal ophthalmia

45. Retinal detachments occur at the potential space between the 45.___
   A. nerve fiber layer and ganglion cell layer
   B. outer nuclear and inner nuclear layer
   C. retinal pigmented epithelium and photoreceptor layer of rods and cones
   D. retinal pigmented epithelium and tapetum lucidum
   E. tapetum lucidum and chorio-capillaries

Questions 46-50.

Questions 46 to 50 are based on the following case.

Merle Flinn presented his four and one-half-year-old male German shepherd, *Max*, for examination on September 19, 1986. The complaint at this time was lameness of the left rear leg, anorexia and lethargy of three days' duration. Polydipsia and polyuria was noted. Examination revealed a temperature of 104.4 F and pain upon palpation of the left kidney. No abnormalities of the hips or rear legs could be found. The heart rate was 160 beats per minute and heart sounds were normal.

Hemogram revealed:

| | |
|---|---|
| PCV | 43 vol% |
| Hb | 14.8 gm% |
| WBC | 22,500/cu mm |
| Band | 450/cu mm |
| Neut | 19,575/cu mm |
| Lymph | 2,250/cu mm |
| Eos | 225/cu mm |
| BUN | 22 mg% |
| SGPT | 62 IU |
| Total protein | 7.8 gm% |

| | |
|---|---|
| Urinalysis: | |
| Sp. gr. | 1.022 |
| pH | 6.8 |
| Glucose | neg |
| Ketones | neg |
| Protein | neg |
| Blood | ++ |
| Sediment: | |
| Erythrocytes | TNTC |
| Leukocytes | 8 to 10 hpf |
| Casts | none |
| Epithelial cells | few |
| Few sperm | |

A diagnosis of nephritis was made and the patient was treated with 250 mg amphycillin every six hours for seven days. Recovery seemed uneventful.

On October 4, 1986, the German shepherd was returned with a similar complaint. Anorexia and lethargy had returned and *increased* urination was noted. Temperature at this time was 103.8 F. The white blood count was 34,500 with the following distribution:

| | |
|---|---|
| Bands | 4,140/cu mm |
| Neutrophils | 25,185/cu mm |
| Lymphocytes | 4,485/cu mm |
| Eosinophils | 690/cu mm |

| | |
|---|---|
| Urinalysis: | |
| Sp. gr. | 1.028 |
| pH | 6.6 |
| Glucose | neg |
| Ketones | neg |
| Protein | neg |
| Occult Blood | neg |
| Sediment: | |
| Erythrocytes | none |
| Leukocytes | none |
| Casts | none |
| Cells | none |
| Few sperm | |

Amphycillin was repeated and much improvement was seen in three days.

On November 4, 1986, Mr. Flinn returned to the hospital with *Max* and complained that *Max* had gone downhill rapidly during the past week. Anorexia and lethargy was again a problem and swelling of the abdomen was seen. Rear limb weakness was evident.

Examination at this time revealed marked weight loss (weight 96 lb from previous 135 lb). Ascites was present. Heart rate was 230 beats per minute, and the pulse rate measured 80 per minute. There was a marked variation in intensity of heart sounds and pulse. A grade II/V systolic murmur, loudest in the left fifth intercostal space at the costo-chondral junction, was present on this entry.

46. The tests that should be run on the third hospital entry (November 6) to aid in the development of the clinical diagnosis and prognosis in this patient include a CBC, ECG, 46. A

A. radiograph thorax, and a blood culture
B. and urinalysis
C. radiograph hips, and stifles
D. and PSP renal function test
E. and BSP hepatic function test

Results of additional data November 6 are:

1. CBC

| | |
|---|---|
| PCV | 38 vol% |
| Hb | 12.2 gm% |
| WBC | 19,700/cu mm |
| Band | 197/cu mm |
| Neu | 13,396/cu mm |
| Lymph | 1,182/cu mm |
| Mono | 4,925/cu mm |
| BUN | 21.3 mg% |
| SGPT | 24 IU |
| Bilirubin | 0.25 mg% |
| Bilirubin Direct | 0.10 mg% |
| Total Protein | 5.89 gm% |
| Albumin | 1.48 gm% |
| Alkaline Phosphatase | 5.5 KKU |
| Globulin | 4.41 gm% |

2. A. Radiograph thorax - DV slight left ventricular enlargement
Lateral - loss of caudal waist
Slight pulmonary vascular congestion
B. Radiograph hips - grade I dysplasia, bilateral
C. Radiograph stifles - within normal limits
3. Blood culture - negative
4. PSP retention - 3% in 30 minutes
5. BSP retention - 5% in 30 minutes

6. The ECG is on the following page.

11. (#4)

I

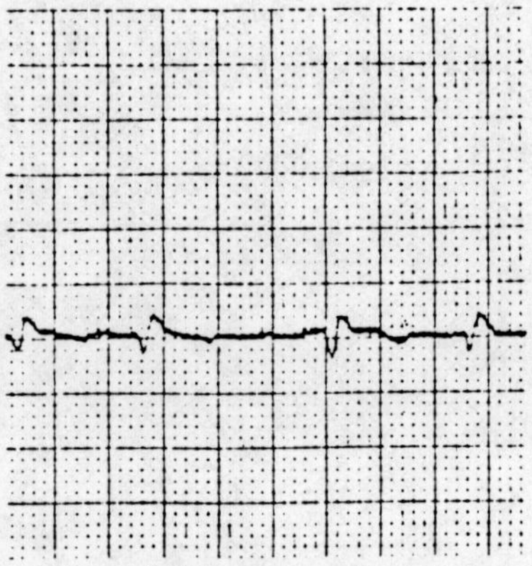

aVF

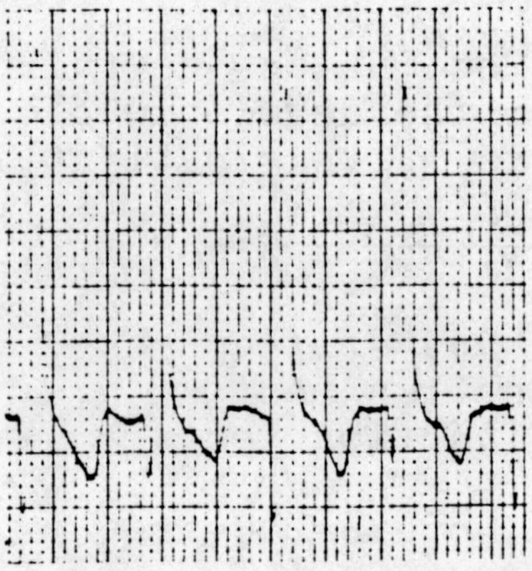

$V^{10}$

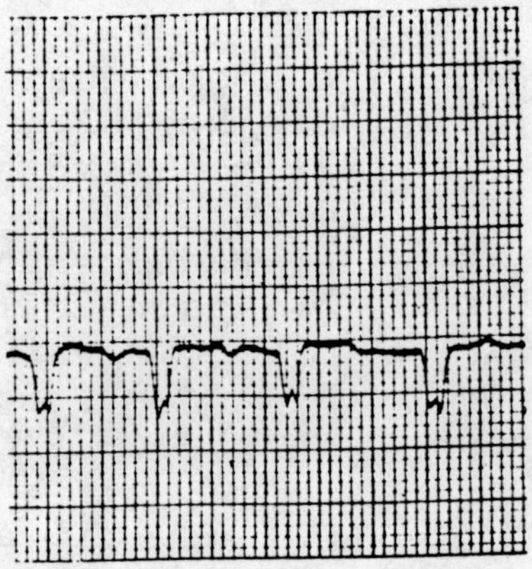

III

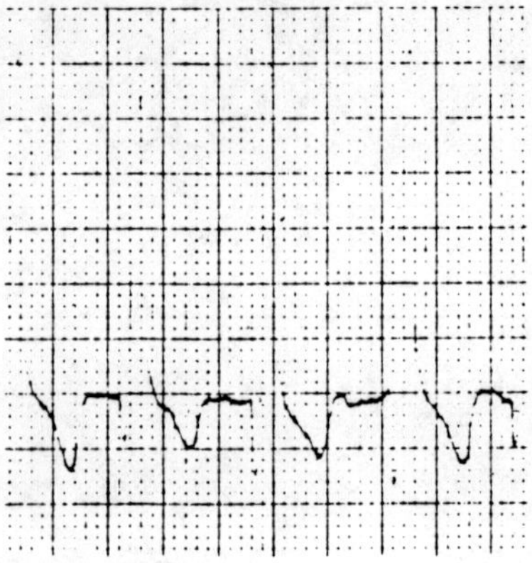

aVR

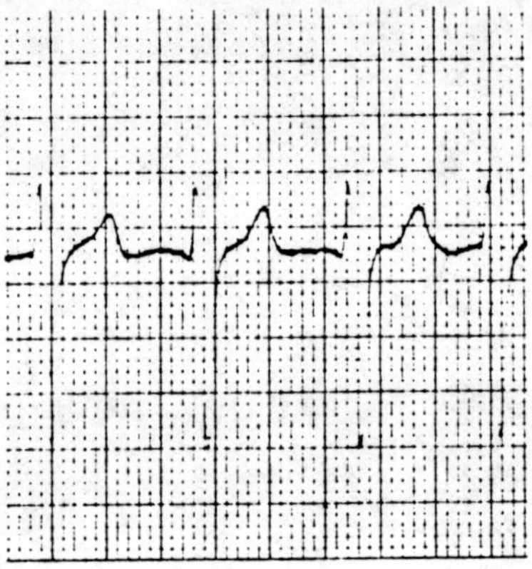

aVL

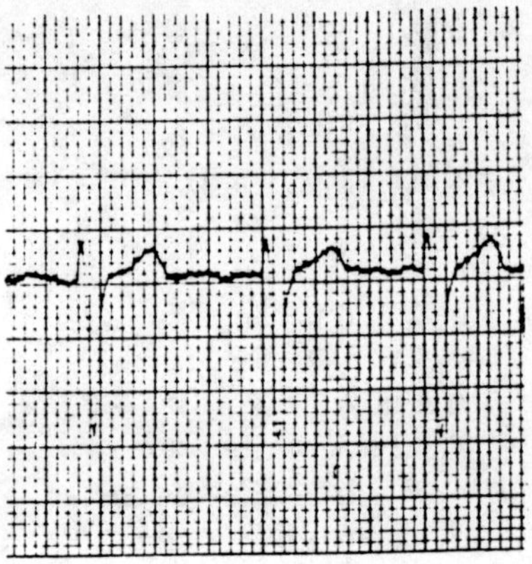

$V^3$

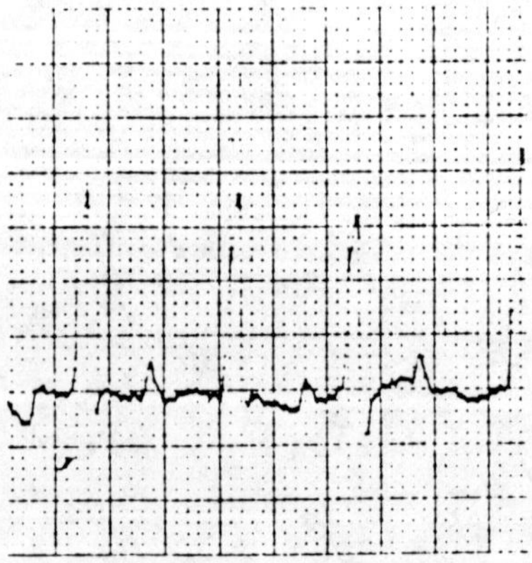

II

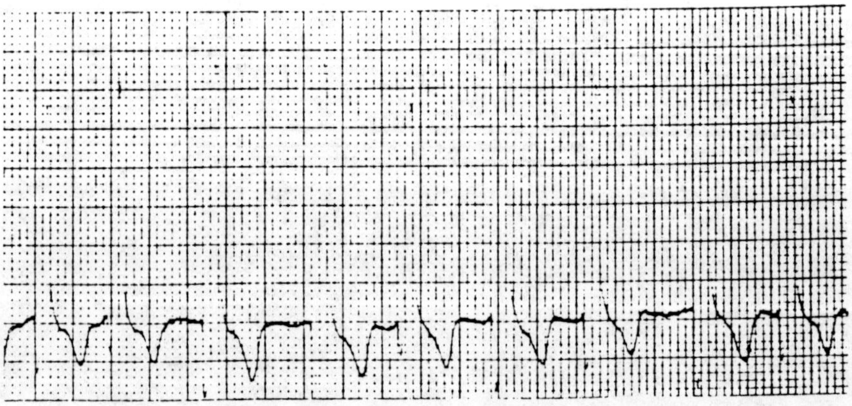

Rate ______________ b.p.m.

Rhythm ______________ o

M.E.A ______________

P duration ______________ sec

P–R interval ______________ sec

QRS duration ______________ sec

Q–T interval ______________ sec

P magnitude ______________ mV

R magnitude ______________ mV

T magnitude ______________ mV

S–T segment ______________

47. Interpretation of the electrocardiogram would be  47.___
   A. right ventricular enlargement
   B. third degree AV block
   C. sinus arrest
   D. left bundle branch block
   E. atrial fibrillation

48. *Probable* diagnosis would be  48.___
   A. idiopathic cardiomyopathy
   B. congenital third degree AV block
   C. hepatic abscess
   D. bacterial endocarditis with embolism
   E. glomerulonephritis

49. Management of the patient should include  49.___
   A. high levels of antibiotics
   B. high levels of antibiotics, digitalization, low Na+ diet
   C. *increased* salt with *increased* protein diet
   D. diuresis and corticosteroids
   E. lipotrophic factors, digitalization, and corticosteroids

50. Prognosis for this patient is  50.___
   A. poor
   B. guarded
   C. guarded with intensive therapy
   D. favorable with intensive therapy
   E. favorable

---

# KEY (CORRECT ANSWERS)

| | | | | |
|---|---|---|---|---|
| 1. B | 11. E | 21. C | 31. B | 41. D |
| 2. C | 12. B | 22. A | 32. B | 42. E |
| 3. D | 13. C | 23. C | 33. B | 43. E |
| 4. B | 14. D | 24. E | 34. D | 44. D |
| 5. C | 15. E | 25. E | 35. B | 45. C |
| 6. C | 16. C | 26. C | 36. E | 46. A |
| 7. B | 17. B | 27. B | 37. C | 47. E |
| 8. C | 18. E | 28. E | 38. C | 48. D |
| 9. B | 19. E | 29. E | 39. B | 49. B |
| 10. A | 20. A | 30. B | 40. D | 50. A |

# EXAMINATION SECTION

# TEST 1

DIRECTIONS: Each question or incomplete statement is followed by several suggested answers or completions. Select the one that BEST answers the question or completes the statement. *PRINT THE LETTER OF THE CORRECT ANSWER IN THE SPACE AT THE RIGHT.*

1. In the dog, epidural anesthesia for abdominal surgery is accomplished via puncture at the 1. ____
   A. space between the first and second coccygeal vertebrae
   B. space between the first and second sacral vertebrae
   C. space between second and third coccygeal vertebrae
   D. lumbo-sacral junction
   E. sacral-coccygeal junction

2. Satisfactory anesthesia is obtained from a paravertebral lumbar nerve block if the anesthetic is infiltrated into the 2. ____
   A. epidural space at the lumbo-sacral junction
   B. dorsal and ventral branches of the last thoracic and the first two or three lumbar nerves
   C. ventral branches of the last four thoracic nerves
   D. epidural space at the thoracolumbar junction
   E. dorsal branches of the last two thoracic and the first two lumbar nerves

3. In performing a vaginal ovariectomy in a mare, the vagina is 3. ____
   A. punctured and then partially sutured to eliminate a gaping hole
   B. minimally disturbed to facilitate locating the ovaries
   C. partially removed and then left to heal by granulation tissue
   D. punctured and then sutured to heal by primary union
   E. punctured and then left to heal by granulation tissue

4. The BEST and MOST frequently used approach for a rumenotomy is through a ____________ incision. 4. ____
   A. low right flank
   B. ventral midline
   C. high left flank
   D. high right flank
   E. low left flank

5. The strength of the suture line in an intestinal anastomosis is derived from the 5. ____
   A. serosa
   B. subserosa
   C. submucosa
   D. muscularis
   E. mucosa

6. In deciding on the amount of small bowel to be resected, an unsatisfactory criterion of gut viability is the 6.____
   A. color of the peritoneal fluid
   B. appearance of the serosa
   C. pinch reaction
   D. stab reaction
   E. peristaltic movements

7. In wound healing, vitamin C is useful as a co-factor in the formation of 7.____
   A. mucin
   B. fibroblasts
   C. collagen
   D. glycoprotein
   E. mucopolysaccharides

8. The drugs that would be indicated for use in epidural anesthesia is 8.____
   A. hexylcaine
   B. benzocaine
   C. pentobarbital sodium
   D. thiamylal sodium
   E. methoxyflurane

9. The primary disadvantage of monofilament nylon as suture material is that it 9.____
   A. does NOT hold knots well
   B. is NOT absorbed
   C. causes more sensitivity reactions than other methods
   D. is noncapillary
   E. is a synthetic material

10. Six months ago, a mammary tumor was removed from an animal which now has diffuse edematous firm swelling of the legs. X-rays show shaggy subperiosteal deposits of osteoid along ALL bones. This is probably a 10.____
   A. multiple myeloma
   B. pulmonary hypertrophic osteoarthropathy
   C. chronic osteoarthritis
   D. metastasis from the primary breast tumor
   E. giant cell sarcoma

11. In the dog, the accepted site at which to do a tap to obtain a specimen of cerebrospinal fluid for analysis is the 11.____
   A. fourth ventricle
   B. lateral ventricles
   C. subapachnoid space at the L1-2 level
   D. subapachnoid space at the L5-6 level
   E. cisterna magna

12. Surgical removal of an ununited anconeal process in a German Sheperd dog is BEST done at ________ of age. 12.____
   A. 2 months
   B. 6 months
   C. 18 months
   D. 3 years
   E. 5 years

13. The MOST common malignant tumor in the mammary gland of the dog is the 13.____
   A. fibrosarcoma
   B. multiple myeloma
   C. osteosarcoma
   D. epidermoid sarcoma
   E. adenocarcinoma

14. The MOST common complications of general anesthesia in the bovine is 14. D
   A. depression of the respiratory center
   B. increased intracranial pressure
   C. suffocation, due to extreme bloating and pressure on the diaphragm
   D. aspiration of saliva or regurgitated stomach contents
   E. ventricular fibrillation, especially when the endotracheal tube is being passed

15. The sign that is produced in a cow when the bony plate separating the temporal fossa and the postorbital diverticulum of the frontal sinus breaks down as a result of sinus infection is 15. A
   A. protrusion of the eye
   B. purulent drainage from the nostrils
   C. purulent drainage from the horn core
   D. severe bulging of the frontal bone
   E. purulent drainage from the orbital cavity

16. The stance of a horse with a fracture of the accessory carpal bone often simulates 16. E
   A. fractured navicular bone
   B. tendinitis of the superficial flexor tendon
   C. fractured proximal sesamoids
   D. bicipital bursitis
   E. radial paralysis

17. In evaluating bulls for breeding soundness potential, the electroejaculator technique for semen collection is commonly used. 17. A
A major disadvantage of this technique is that it
   A. does NOT measure ability to complete the act of copulation
   B. is relatively expensive
   C. does NOT provide a true estimate of sperm motility and percentage of abnormal cells
   D. is relatively time consuming
   E. is relatively dangerous to the operator

18. The preferred time to remove supernumerary teats in the bovine is 18. A B
   A. in the first week of life
   B. at the age of 4 to 8 months
   C. just before calving
   D. just after calving
   E. after one complete lactation

19. A statement that applies to the Caslick operation is that it 19. E
   A. has proven more effective than the Ascheim technique
   B. is indicated when damage to the left recurrent nerve has been demonstrated
   C. should be performed on horses that are bilateral cryptorchids

D. should be performed on mares that have cystic ovaries
E. is indicated when the anus of a mare is retracted and the vulva is sloped

20. The type of placenta found in the pig is correctly described as: 20.____
A. Diffuse
B. Deciduate
C. Discoidal
D. Zonary
E. Cotyledonary

21. Perineal urethrostomy is a useful surgical procedure in the treatment of recurring obstructive urolithiasis in cats. The success of this surgery is due in large part to the existence of a sufficiently large urethral opening post-surgically. 21.____
The level that the urethra must be transected and sutured to the skin in order to insure a large patent opening is just
A. posterior to the bladder sphincter
B. anterior to the bulbourethral glands
C. posterior to the insertion of the ischiocavernosus muscles
D. anterior to the reflection of the prepuce on the penis
E. posterior to the bulbourethral glands

22. Post surgical medical treatment of dogs with phosphate urolithiasis consists of 22.____
A. administration of 5,000 units of vitamin A daily and 3 hyaluronidase tablets daily for six weeks
B. a high-protein, low-carbohydrate diet and administration of 5,000 units of vitamin A daily
C. administration of 5,000 units of vitamin A daily and urinary alkalinization with sodium bicarbonate
D. urinary alkalinization and the use of an alumina carbonate gel orally
E. urinary acidification and antibacterial therapy based on in vitro sensitivity tests

23. The MOST common point of urethral obstruction in the dog is 23.____
A. at the proximal end of the os penis
B. at the ischial arch within the prostatic urethra
C. at its origin
D. in the os penis
E. in the distal part of the urethra

24. A soft, fluctuating swelling occurring in the region of the withers of the horse is usually 24.____
A. a neoplasm
B. actinobacillosis
C. a cyst
D. supraspinous bursitis
E. an abscess

25. An accurate statement concerning renal biopsy of the dog is that this procedure 25.____
   A. will detect renal lesions regardless of their distribution in the kidney
   B. is of diagnostic but NOT of prognostic value because of the type of renal diseases which affect dogs
   C. has a high percentage of complications due to development of urinary fistulas
   D. can be successfully performed through a small paralumbar incision using a Franklin Modified Vim Silverman needle
   E. is contraindicated in azoiemia because of defects in blood coagulation

26. A simple, rapid and effective method for establishing lasting hemostasis in the dehorning operation in the bovine is to 26.____
   A. apply a gauze patch
   B. apply a coagulation powder
   C. carefully ligate the vessel to the horn corium
   D. apply pressure to the cornual artery
   E. pull the cornual artery branches

27. In the dog, a uvulectomy is recommended for the correction of 27.____
   A. stenosis of the nares
   B. vegetative stomatitis
   C. chronic cough
   D. edema of the glottis
   E. prolapse of the laryngeal saccules

28. In the dog, the surgical treatment for a salivary mucocele is sialadenectomy. 28.____
The salivary glands removed in this procedure are the
   A. parotid, mandibular and posterior sublingual
   B. mandibular, posterior sublingual and zygomatic
   C. zygomatic, mandibular and parotid
   D. parotid, posterior sublingual and anterior sublingual
   E. mandibular, posterior sublingual and anterior sublingual

29. The MOST effective treatment of chronic prostatitis in older dogs is 29.____
   A. administration of broad-spectrum antibiotics
   B. administration of high levels of vitamin E
   C. injection of low levels of testosterone
   D. prolonged estrogen therapy
   E. surgical castration

30. Trichomonas foetus infection in cows frequently causes 30.____
   A. abortion after the fifth month of gestation primarily
   B. an increase in the rate of conception from first service

C. NO change in the number of abortions in the herd
D. an increase in milk production
E. abortion early in pregnancy

31. The proper location in a cow of the surgical incision to correct a small bowel intussusception palpable per rectum in the lower right quadrant is the 31.____
A. posterior right paramedian
B. mid-transverse abdominal
C. posterior midline
D. high right flank
E. low right flank

32. A 10-year-old quarterhorse mare exhibits signs of acute abdominal pain. It is determined that the animal has an obstruction at the ileocecocolic junction. 32.____
The BEST site for a laparotomy incision would be the
A. right flank or paracostal
B. left grid
C. left paramedian
D. left flank or paracostal
E. ventral midline

33. When it becomes necessary to do a standing cesarean section in a cow through a high right flank incision, the MOST important accident to avoid is 33.____
A. trauma to the duodenum
B. omental rupture resulting in peritoneal adhesions
C. aspiration of contaminated air through the incision
D. peritoneal contamination from the uterus
E. prolapse of the small bowel

34. In dogs, inguinal hernias are MOST frequently seen in 34.____
A. mature females
B. newborn males
C. spayed females
D. aged males
E. castrated males

35. A 6-year-old male dog has a sudden onset of extreme weakness. The mucous membranes are very pale and the abdomen is doughy and swollen. NO trauma has occurred. 35.____
The presumptive diagnosis would be
A. rupture of splenic tumor
B. hemobartonellosis
C. acute pancreatitis
D. rupture of the bladder
E. ingestion of a foreign body

36. A radiogram of the intestinal tract of a cat shows accordion pleating of the small intestine. 36.____
The MOST likely cause is
A. acute enteritis
B. fragments of plastic
C. paper
D. lymphoid tumor
E. string

37. A colopexy is performed to — 37. C
   A. repair a dent in the mesentery
   B. tack the fundus of the bladder to the abdominal wall
   C. secure the lower bowel to the abdominal wall
   D. secure the body of the uterus to the colon
   E. obtain internal closure of an inguinal hernia

38. The front leg of a dog is MOST frequently amputated at the — 38. D
   A. proximal third of the humerus
   B. midshaft of the humerus
   C. lower third of the humerus
   D. scapulohumeral articulation
   E. condyloid fossa

39. Bone grafts are helpful in the treatment of — 39. C
   A. femur neck fractures
   B. compound fractures
   C. non-union fractures
   D. chronic osteomyelitis
   E. acute osteomyelitis

40. The main advantage of the use of the Kuntscher nail in fracture repair is that — 40. X C
   A. insertion and removal is easy
   B. it does NOT interfere with medullary hemopoiesis
   C. rotational movement of the fracture site is limited
   D. removal following healing is NOT necessary
   E. it is inexpensive

41. The term used for a tissue graft which is of the greatest genetic disparity and, therefore, is the MOST likely to be rejected is — 41. E
   A. autograft
   B. isograft
   C. syngraft
   D. allograft
   E. xenograft

42. The surgical correction of spastic paresis in an 8-month-old dairy heifer involves the — 42. B
   A. gastrocnemius tendon
   B. gastrocnemius and superficial flexor tendons
   C. superficial and deep flexor tendons
   D. anterior tibial tendon
   E. lateral digital extensor tendon

43. A tumor is located in the fourth (caudal abdominal) mammary gland. The recommended safety procedure is to remove — 43. A
   A. glands 3, 4 and 5 on the involved side and superficial inguinal L.N.
   B. gland 4 on each side
   C. glands 3, 4 and 5 on each side
   D. ALL glands on the involved side
   E. glands 3 and 4 on each side

44. Examination of a dog that has a grossly enlarged prostrate reveals NO evidence of neoplasm or acute abscess. In treating this animal, the MOST effective procedure would be 44.____
   A. administration of stilbestrol
   B. transurethral prostatectomy
   C. androgen therapy
   D. cortisone therapy
   E. orchiectomy

45. The common tumor of young dogs that is caused by a filtrable virus, is transmissible, is self-limiting and results in immunity is the 45.____
   A. oral papilloma
   B. vaginal leiomyoma
   C. perianal adenoma
   D. salivary adenocarcinoma
   E. choroid melanoma

46. The neoplasm that is *generally* least amenable to surgical treatment is the 46.____
   A. malignant melanoma
   B. mastocytoma
   C. cholesteroloma
   D. perianal adenoma
   E. keratoacanthoma

47. The Minchev stay suture technique for correction of prolapse of the vagina in cattle consists in passing a suture from the lumen of the vagina through the lesser sciatic foramen to the outside in order to 47.____
   A. hold the vagina permanently in position through retention of the suture
   B. produce fat necrosis around the vagina and hold it in position
   C. adhere the vagina to the sacrosciatic ligament
   D. adhere the vagina to the lesser sciatic ligament
   E. produce adhesions of the vagina to the pelvic wall

Questions 48-50.
DIRECTIONS: The following passage refers to questions 48 through 50.

You are presented with a one-year-old, male, 22 lb. beagle. The complication is that of anorexia and depression of 24 hours duration. He began vomiting this morning. The history is that he was struck by a car three days ago and was treated for shock by a colleague and hospitalized for 24 hours. The following day thoracic radiographs were taken which were normal and the animal was discharged from the colleague's clinic much improved. The dog's temperature is now 100.5 F, he is moderately dehydrated (7%), has a tender abdomen and is reluctant to walk. You decide to hospitalize the animal for diagnosis and therapy.

48. In order to correct the dehydration, ______ ml of intravenous balance electrolyte solution will be required (not counting daily maintenance requirements). 48.____
   A. 300
   B. 500
   C. 700
   D. 1000
   E. 1500

49. Laboratory tests (before fluid therapy) revealed a WBC of 22,200 (seg - 51%, nonseg - 34%, L - 10%, M - 4%, - 1%), PCV = 45%, total serum protein - 7.2 gm/dl. BUN 48 mg/dl. SGPT - 70%, Sigma Frankel units and amylase - 1000 somogyi units. 49.____
From this information you can probably rule out
A. traumatic pancreatitis
B. ruptured gall bladder
C. ruptured urinary bladder
D. intestinal rupture
E. infectious peritonitis

50. Radiographs were taken and showed a fluid density in the abdomen. An abdominal paracentesis was done and the following results were obtained: 50.____
Ten milliliters of cloudy yellow, fluid
Specific gravity = 1.030, protein = 3+ blood = 2+, pH = 6.5, cells = few RBC and WBC, bilirubin - neg.
From the previous list of tentative diagnoses, which would *most likely* give the correct definitive diagnosis?
A. Barium series
B. Bacterial culture of abdominal fluid
C. Positive contrast radiograph of bladder
D. Amylase levels on peritoneal fluid
E. Cholecystogram

---

# KEY (CORRECT ANSWERS)

| | | | | |
|---|---|---|---|---|
| 1. D | 11. E | 21. B | 31. A | 41. E |
| 2. B | 12. B | 22. E | 32. E | 42. B |
| 3. D | 13. E | 23. C | 33. D | 43. A |
| 4. C | 14. D | 24. D | 34. A | 44. E |
| 5. C | 15. A | 25. D | 35. A | 45. A |
| 6. A | 16. B | 26. E | 36. E | 46. A |
| 7. C | 17. A | 27. A | 37. C | 47. E |
| 8. A | 18. B | 28. E | 38. D | 48. C |
| 9. A | 19. E | 29. E | 39. C | 49. A |
| 10. B | 20. A | 30. E | 40. C | 50. C |

# TEST 2

DIRECTIONS: Each question or incomplete statement is followed by several suggested answers or completions. Select the one that BEST answers the question or completes the statement. *PRINT THE LETTER OF THE CORRECT ANSWER IN THE SPACE AT THE RIGHT.*

1. In a suspected malignancy, the safest procedure in preventing metastasis in the absence of an accurate determination of the type of neoplasm is 1.____
   A. punch biopsy
   B. incisional biopsy
   C. aspirational biopsy
   D. complete excision
   E. smear impressions

2. In general, spastic paralysis resulting from intervertebral disc protrusion is seen in lesions involving 2.____
   A. spinal necrosis with permanent neural damage
   B. middle and lower lumbar discs
   C. acute hemorrhage into the spinal canal
   D. thoracic and anterior lumbar discs
   E. progressive spinal shock

3. The major disadvantage of ether as a selective anesthetic agent is that it 3.____
   A. is a poor analgesic
   B. is cardiotoxic
   C. is hepatotoxic
   D. causes apnea
   E. is explosive

4. When a hematoma of the penis occurs in the bovine, the BEST approximate time for surgery is within 5.____
   A. 1 hour
   B. 12 to 24 hours
   C. 48 hours
   D. 7 days
   E. 30 days

5. The currently accepted procedure for the correction of penile deviations in bulls is 6.____
   A. stabilizing the corpus cavernosum penis with fibrous tissue
   B. transecting the retractor penis muscle on the curved side
   C. injecting irritants to establish ipsilateral fibrosis
   D. amputating part of the tip of the glans penis
   E. removing wedges from the corpus cavernosum penis

6. A preputial condition in the bull, BEST treated by amputation is 7.____
   A. prolapse with fibrosis
   B. laceration with prolapse
   C. laceration with phimosis
   D. laceration with paraphimosis
   E. multiple papillomas

7. A requirement for proper correction of a urachovesical fistula in a newborn foal is  7. B
   A. amputation of the urachus and closure of the wall defect in the organ
   B. repeated cauterization of the orifice with silver nitrate sticks
   C. supportive electrolyte therapy plus antibiotic therapy until the condition corrects itself
   D. a self-retaining catheter to relieve pressure until the condition corrects itself
   E. local instillation of antibiotics and double ligation of the urachus

8. Neoplasms of the vagina occurring in older bitches are usually  8. D
   A. squamous cell carcinomas which infiltrate locally and spread to the pelvic lymph nodes
   B. pedunculated papillomas which are easily excised
   C. leiomyomas which often transform into invasive leiomyosarcomas
   D. pedunculated leiomyomas which are easily removed
   E. adenocarcinomas arising from the mucus-secreting glands of the mucosa

9. The principal advantage of a suprapubic cystotomy over a subischial urethrotomy for removal of a cystic calculus in a gelding is that  9.____
   A. healing is *more* rapid and *less* postoperative care is needed
   B. there is *less* skin scalding adjacent to the surgical wound
   C. there is NO trauma to the urethra
   D. there is *less* trauma to the bladder wall
   E. the calculus can be removed entirely

10. Torsion of the uterus is MOST commonly seen in the  10. A
    A. sow B. cow C. mare D. bitch
    E. ewe

11. Bilateral orchiectomy should ALWAYS be performed in conjunction with a(n)  11. D
    A. nephrectomy
    B. umbilical hernia repair
    C. cystotomy
    D. perineal hernia repair
    E. urethrotomy

12. Two malignancies that may show regression following orchiectomy are  12. A
    A. prostatic carcinoma and anal adenoma
    B. lymphosarcoma and anal gland carcinoma
    C. mastocytoma and metastatic sertoli cell tumors

D. basal cell carcinoma and melanosarcoma
E. prostatic cysts and thyroid carcinoma

13. The MOST common surgical treatment for urinary calculi of the bovine is 13.____
A. amputation of the distal end of the penis
B. urethrotomy performed in the area between the ischium and the sigmoid flexure
C. suprapubic urethrotomy
D. permanent fistula produced by suturing the body of the bladder to the skin of the ventral abdomen
E. urethrotomy performed in the area between the sigmoid flexure and the distal end of the penis

14. In the complete removal of the cow's udder, the MOST critical problem during surgery is 14.____
A. adequate and careful skin closure
B. isolation and ligation of the main branches of the perineal veins
C. isolation and ligation of the mammary veins
D. isolation and ligation of the external pudic artery and vein
E. availability of adequate amounts of whole blood

15. The layer that is the stongest in the small intestine and that MUST be included in the sutures in anastomosis to minimize dehiscence is the 15.____
A. peritoneum
B. tunica mucosa
C. tunica serosa
D. tunica submucosa
E. tunica muscularis

16. In the dog, MOST intestinal foreign bodies lodge in the 16.____
A. duodenum
B. ileum
C. jejunum
D. colon
E. ileocecal valve

17. At times, the castration of equine cryptorchids requires a thorough search of the abdominal cavity in order to locate the cryptic testicle. When it is necessary to search the abdominal cavity, it is recommended that the operator locate the neck of the bladder and commence from that point. 17.____
The purpose of this procedure is to locate the
A. gubernaculum of the cryptic testicle which is attached in this area
B. epididymis of the cryptic testicle and thus follow it out to the testicle
C. testicle which in about 10 percent of the cases of cryptorchidism is located in this region
D. spermatic artery which by its pulsation can be picked up and followed to the testicle
E. genital fold and the vas deferens and follow them to the testicle

18. The surgical procedure that is employed for the relief of glaucoma in the dog is 18. C
   A. resection of the membrana nictitans
   B. medial canthotomy
   C. iridencleisis
   D. cauterization of the scleral vessels
   E. conjunctival flap

19. An infra-orbital fistula usually indicates a(n) 19. B
   A. infected meibomian gland
   B. diseased root of a carnassial tooth
   C. sequester of the malar bone
   D. fracture of the zygomatic arch
   E. occlusion of the tear duct

20. Cervical salivary cysts in the dog are MOST effectively treated by 20. C
   A. removal of the persistent branchial cleft
   B. excision of the ectopic salivary tissue
   C. removal of the mandibular and sublingual salivary glands
   D. removal of the secreting cyst lining
   E. excision and anastomosis of the severed salivary duct

21. Mycotic infections of the guttural pouch can lead to 21. ~~B~~ A
   A. epistaxis
   B. facial paralysis
   C. chokes
   D. chronic catarrh
   E. emphysema

22. If the surgical approach to the hip joint of the dog is made on the cranial side, as in Brown's method, there will be 22. ~~D~~ E
   A. NO damage to the gluteal muscles
   B. a better exposure of the acetabulum
   C. less hemorrhage
   D. a greater exposure of the joint capsule
   E. less danger of injuring the sciatic nerve

23. In reducing an elbow luxation in a dog, the joint should be positioned in 23. B
   A. extreme extension
   B. extreme flexion
   C. adduction
   D. normal standing position
   E. clockwise rotation

24. In low femoral fractures, the distal segment is nearly always 24. B
   A. medially displaced
   B. posteriorly displaced
   C. rotated on its long axis
   D. laterally displaced
   E. anteriorly displaced

25. Lateral digital extensor tenotomy is commonly used in the treatment of 25.____
   A. bog spavin
   B. stringhalt
   C. bone spavin
   D. upward fixation of the patella
   E. thoroughpin

26. The MOST important consideration in corrective shoeing of a horse suffering from chronic laminitis is to 26.____
   A. apply a wide web shoe and full pads in order to decrease concussion and direct trauma
   B. trim the toe as short as possible so the horse will walk heel-toe
   C. apply weighted shoes on the front feet in order to balance them with the rear foot
   D. place large heel and toe calks on the shoe in order to keep the sole off the ground
   E. allow the horse to walk on his sole in order to prevent weight-bearing by the wall

27. A condition in horses characterized by a tenosynovitis of the tarsal sheath which encloses the deep digital flexor tendon of the hind limb is termed 27.____
   A. bog spavin
   B. omarthritis
   C. thoroughpin
   D. curb
   E. bone spavin

28. The x-ray diagnosis is osteosarcoma in a dog with a large swelling of the distal radius. The owner desires amputation. 28.____
The surgeon should feel obligated to
   A. remove the adjacent lymph glands
   B. provide a smooth, well-protected stump
   C. instruct the owner in the care of a three-legged dog
   D. x-ray the dog's chest
   E. warn the owner of surgical risk

29. Three nonmalignant neoplasms derived from epithelial tissue are 29.____
   A. lipoma, myoma and enchondroma
   B. teratoid, cystoma and pterygium
   C. melanoma, neuroma and dermoid
   D. carcinoid, neurocytoma and astroblastoma
   E. papilloma, sebaceous adenoma and adenomatous polyp

30. The ability of x-rays to penetrate the tissues is determined by the 30.____
   A. focal point
   B. time in seconds
   C. milliamperage seconds
   D. focal distance
   E. kilovolt peak

31. A caudocranial or craniocaudal radiogram of the stifle joint of an adult dog shows a radiolucent zone between the distal end of the femur and the proximal end of the tibia. Since no drawer sign is present, this zone is MOST likely 31.____
   A. abnormal and present *only* when the fibrocartilaginous menisci are injured
   B. normal and due to the fibrocartilaginous menisci
   C. abnormal and present *only* when there is achondroplasia
   D. abnormal and suggestive of arthritis
   E. normal and due to the thick articular cartilages

32. The sutural material of choice for repair of a teat laceration is 32.____
   A. any noncapillary suture
   B. a chromic catgut
   C. any capillary suture
   D. any plain catgut
   E. any chromic catgut

33. If the pleura is NOT adhered to the pericardium when a resection of the fifth rib in cattle is performed to gain access to the pericardial sac, then 33.____
   A. air will enter the thoracic cavity
   B. the cardiac lobe of the lung will prolapse through the incision
   C. the operation will NOT be successful
   D. the heart sac will NOT drain satisfactorily
   E. the heart will lose efficiency because of loss of its attachment to the body wall

34. A congenital anomaly that does NOT produce clinical disease, but often accompanies other congenital cardiac defects and may cause confusion for the thoracic surgeon is 34.____
   A. tetralogy of fallot
   B. patent ductus arteriosus
   C. persistent right aortic arch
   D. cor pulmonale
   E. persistent left cranial vena cava

35. Peri-anal adenomas are MOST commonly found near the anus, but occasionally they are located 35.____
   A. on the dorsal surface of the tail
   B. on the scrotum and in the inguinal region
   C. in the perineal region
   D. along the sacrum and along the hips
   E. on the inner surfaces of the thighs

36. A 6-year-old collie has multiple mammary tumors of the last two breasts on the right side and the rear breast on the left side. X-rays of the chest are negative and NO regional lymph node involvement is apparent. The dog has a history of recurrent pseudocyesis. 36.____
The correct recommendation is mastectomy and
   A. spaying

B. chemotherapy
C. X radiation
D. serotherapy
E. androgen administration

37. A two-hour surgical procedure with the horse in left lateral recumbency has been completed. When the horse recovers, it is noted that the left side of the lower lip is flaccid. 37.____
This is MOST likely to be a result of
A. hypoxia to the brain
B. toxicity produced by halothane
C. pressure necrosis of the masseter muscles
D. paralysis of the left recurrent laryngeal nerve
E. paralysis of the facial nerve

38. The paatsama operation stabilizes the knee joint by replacing the 38.____
A. lateral collateral ligament
B. posterior cruciate ligament
C. anterior cruciate ligament
D. patellar ligament
E. medial collateral ligament

39. An episiotomy is generally recommended to 39.____
A. remove vaginal tumors
B. treat perivulvular dermatitis
C. enlarge the external genital orifice
D. relieve the rectal sphincter
E. repair the meatus muscle

40. Coxofemoral luxation is fairly common in the 40.____
A. dog and horse
B. dog and ox
C. dog and cat
D. dog and sheep
E. sheep and ox

41. The suture material that is absorbable is 41.____
A. teflon-coated polyester fiber
B. silkworm gut
C. cotton
D. polyglycolic acid
E. non-teflon coated polyester fiber

42. Mast cell tumors are common tumors seen in small animals. 42.____
ALL of the following statements are true EXCEPT:
A. Approximately 40% to 50% of mast cell tumors may be expected to recur or metastasize
B. Mast cell tumors contain histamine
C. Mast cell tumors contain heparin
D. Mast cell tumors have NOT been reported in cats
E. Mast cell tumors may occur as multicentric proliferations involving the reticular tissues of various internal organs

43. Treatment of canine salivary mucocoeles is to — 43.____
   A. drain the mucocoele and cauterize it with iodine
   B. insert a drain tube into the mucocoele and leave it for two weeks
   C. dissect out the mucocoele surgically
   D. remove the mandibular and parotid salivary glands on the effected side and drain the mucocoele
   E. remove the mandibular and sublingual salivary glands on the effected side and drain the mucocoele

44. The surgical approach to ligate a ruptured thoracic duct in a dog is a — 44.____
   A. thoracotomy at the left fourth intercostal space
   B. thoracotomy at the right fourth intercostal space
   C. thoracotomy at the left eight intercostal space
   D. thoracotomy at the right eighth intercostal space
   E. midline sternotomy

45. You are presented with an oral tumor in a 10-year-old dog.
   The MOST common oral tumor he could have is a — 45.____
   A. melanoma
   B. squamous cell carcinoma
   C. fibrosarcoma
   D. adenocarcinoma
   E. basal cell carcinoma

46. In the postoperative treatment of urate calculi, — 46.____
   A. D-penicillamine is the drug of choice
   B. allopurinal is the drug of choice
   C. there is NO drug that will prevent recurrences
   D. long-term urinary acidification works well in the prevention of urate calculi
   E. long-term antibiotics and acidification are the treatment of choice

47. Which of the following statements about dogs with the gastric-dilation-torsion complex is NOT true? — 47.____
   A. The gastric-dilation-torsion complex is primarily a problem associated with large breed dogs
   B. As the stomach enlarges, venous return to the heart is decreased, cardiac output deceases and arterial hypotension ensues
   C. Despite surgical treatment, recurrent gastric dilations are common
   D. Pyloroplasty or pyloromyotomy are frequently used procedures to prevent recurrences
   E. Surgical decompression is NOT considered an emergency and can be delayed four to eight hours

48. The suture material that should be used to ligate bleeders in a contaminated wound is — 48.____
   A. chromic gut
   B. silk
   C. cotton
   D. dacron
   E. teflon-coated dacron

Questions 49-50.
DIRECTIONS: Questions 49 and 50 refer to the following passage.

On March 18, 1985 Mrs. Jones came into your office because her one and one-half-year-old, female, Siamese cat was acting unusual. She said the cat was crying as if she was in pain, urinating outside the litter pan, rolling all over the floor in her apartment, and walking around with her tail in the air. The cat had also not been eating well. Mrs. Jones reported that the cat went through the same type problem three weeks previously. She reported the cat was fed dry food and tuna-chicken canned food.

The only other time you had seen the cat was on July 15, 1984 to vaccinate and perform an ovariohysterectomy on it. The owner reports the cat had never had any other problems.

The physical exam was non-contributory. A CBC and differential, BUN and urinalysis were performed, as well as abdominal radiographs taken.

The radiographs were normal. The CBC

WBC $10.1 \times 10^3$
RBC $6.28 \times 10^6$
HGB 10.1 gm
Hct 40%
1 Mono
20 Lymph
77 Seg
2 band
BUN - 20 mg%

Urinalysis - expressed sample

sed - yellow clear
SG - 1.020
pH - 6.2
Prot - 0
Gluc - 0
Ket - 0
Bile - 0
Bld - None
Urob - 0
WC/h - 0
RC/h - 2

49. From the clinical data given, your MOST likely tentative diagnosis is 49._____
   A. cystitis
   B. steatitis
   C. retained ovarian tissue
   D. false pregnancy
   E. adrenal gland production of excessive endogenous estrogens

50. Your treatment of choice would be to 50. B
   A. put the cat on tranquilizers and tell the owner there is nothing to worry about with her cat
   B. perform surgery on the cat while she's acting funny to remove the retained ovarian tissue you left
   C. put the cat on antibiotics, urinary acidifiers and take her off dry foods
   D. tell the owner her cat has a rare problem that you've never heard about before and nothing can be done to stop the problem
   E. change the cat's diet, put the cat on vitamin E, antibiotics and steroids orally

---

# KEY (CORRECT ANSWERS)

| | | | | |
|---|---|---|---|---|
| 1. D | 11. D | 21. A | 31. B | 41. D |
| 2. D | 12. A | 22. E | 32. A | 42. D |
| 3. E | 13. B | 23. B | 33. A | 43. E |
| 4. D | 14. D | 24. B | 34. A | 44. C |
| 5. A | 15. D | 25. B | 35. A | 45. A |
| 6. A | 16. C | 26. A | 36. A | 46. B |
| 7. B | 17. E | 27. C | 37. E | 47. E |
| 8. D | 18. C | 28. D | 38. C | 48. A |
| 9. E | 19. B | 29. E | 39. C | 49. C |
| 10. B | 20. C | 30. E | 40. C | 50. B |

# EXAMINATION SECTION

# TEST 1

DIRECTIONS: Each question or incomplete statement is followed by several suggested answers or completions. Select the one that BEST answers the question or completes the statement. *PRINT THE LETTER OF THE CORRECT ANSWER IN THE SPACE AT THE RIGHT.*

1. A 6-year-old dog suffers an acute onset of sudden weakness, doughy abdomen, pale mucous membranes and NO history of trauma. 1.____
   The probable diagnosis is
   A. a ruptured splenic tumor
   B. a foreign body in the stomach
   C. hemabartonella
   D. pastric torsion
   E. acute pancreatitis

2. In bulls, surgical correction of a hematoma of the penis involves the repair of the 2.____
   A. retractor penis muscle
   B. corpus cavernosum urethrae
   C. prepuce as it reflects on the penis
   D. tunica vaginalis communis
   E. tunica albiginea

3. Ordinary bovine hematic mummification of the fetus is commonly said to be caused by 3.____
   A. infection of the genital organs
   B. nutritional factors or deficiencies
   C. trauma or violence
   D. hormonal factors
   E. unknown factors

4. Two malignancies that may regress after orchidectomy are 4.____
   A. prostatic carcinoma and anal gland ademona
   B. lymphosarcoma and anal gland carcinoma
   C. mastrocytoma and metastatic sertoli cell tumors
   D. basal cell carcinoma and melanosarcoma
   E. prostatic cysts and thyroid carcinoma

5. The structure(s) that would be cut in an 8-month-old holstein heifer with spastic paresis is (are) the 5.____
   A. superficial flexor and gastrocnemius tendons
   B. deep flexor tendon and gastrocnemius tendons
   C. gastrocnemium tendon
   D. deep flexor tendon
   E. superficial flexor tendon

6. According to present recommendations, an owner would be advised NOT to bring a new pup into a house where a dog had died from distemper until 6.____
   A. 1 week after the dog died

B. 2 weeks after the dog died
C. one month later
D. 9 months later
E. one year later

7. An anesthetic emergency following barbiturate anesthesia occurs. 7. C
Which of the following should be done immediately?
A. Administer corticosteroids
B. Check the weight and calculate the dosage given
C. Obtain a patent airway
D. Administer 1/150 atropine to prevent laryngospasm
E. Administer 1/1000 epinephrine to combat decreased blood pressure

8. Successful anesthesia is achieved by a paravertebral block by putting the agent: 8. ~~D~~ B
A. Epidural space at the L-S junction
B. Dorsal and ventral branches of the last thoracic and first 2-3 lumbar nerves
C. Epidural space at the thoracic lumbar junction
D. Dorsal branches of the last two thoracic and the first 2 lumbar nerves
E. Ventral branches of the first 4 lumbar nerves

9. What is released and responsible for anaphylactic reaction? 9. ~~E~~ C
A. Histamine and epinephrine
B. Epinephrine and vasoactive drugs
C. Histamine and other vasoactive amines
D. Epinephrine
E. Histamine

10. Typical human American Q fever is characterized by 10. E
A. malaise, anorexia, fever, skin rash on thighs and abdomen
B. gastrointestinal syndrome
C. a simple pneumonia condition WITHOUT systemic conditions
D. a simple pneumonia condition that is easily diagnosed
E. a pneumonia condition with malaise, fever, and pain in the muscles of the limbs and back

11. When feeding urea to cattle, it is important to supplement the diet with 11. ~~A~~ B
A. animal protein
B. carbohydrates
C. fats
D. vitamins
E. minerals

12. The post miotic phase of spermatogenesis is controlled by 12. B
A. thyroxine
B. androgen
C. luteinizing hormone
D. FSH
E. lutectrophin

13. A dog has a history of persistent vomition of solid foods. On examination NO foreign body is found. The MOST likely cause is 13. C
   A. chronic pancreatitis
   B. chronic nephritis
   C. esophageal dilatation
   D. gastric dilatation
   E. gastritis

14. Sulfonilamide used in calves for scours that is not absorbed from the gut is called 14. ~~D~~ B
   A. Sulfathiazol
   B. Phthalylsulfathiazole
   C. Sulfamerazine
   D. Sulfamethazine
   E. Sulfapyridine

15. Alveolar periostitis in dogs is MOST commonly associated with 15. C
   A. hypoplasia of enamel
   B. maloclusion
   C. tartar accumulation
   D. osteogenic sarcoma
   E. stomatitis

16. Lactogenic immunity is practical to enhance the antibody production of the dam so that more antibodies will be produced and transferred through the colostrum. This practice is used against 16. B
   A. feline rhinotracheitis
   B. transmissible gastroenteritis TGE
   C. I C H
   D. bluetongue
   E. pseudorabies

17. Plasmacytomas produce abnormal production of 17. E
   A. spinal fluid
   B. lymph
   C. albumen
   D. plasma
   E. immunoglobins

18. Dogs exposed to ragweed develop an atopic sensitivity characterized by the 18. ~~E~~ C
   A. CF reaction
   B. HI reaction
   C. Prauznitzer Haiyer reaction
   D. hemmaglutination
   E. complement - fixation reaction

19. A puppy with tenderness in the region of the stomach, a temperature of 104° enlarged tonsils, petechiae of the mucous membranes, and a clotting time of 5 minutes probably has 19. B
   A. distemper
   B. ICH
   C. a foreign body
   D. leptospirosis
   E. acute tonsillitis

20. In cattle, acute pulmonary emphysema is MOST often associated with 20. D
   A. moldy hay
   B. a high grain intake
   C. frozen forage
   D. lush pastures in the fall
   E. grazing on moutain ranges

21. In a dog, auscultation of a PDA is MOST noticeable and diagnostic of the ________ ICS. 21.____
   A. left 2-3 B. right 2-3 C. left 6-7 D. right 6-7
   E. left 7-8

22. A woods light can be used to diagnose ________ in the dog. 22.____
   A. microsporum canis
   B. trichophyton mentagrophytes
   C. North American blastomycosis
   D. madurmycosis
   E. cryptococcus

23. Systolic bruits are due to 23.____
   A. pericarditis
   B. A-V insufficiency
   C. semilunar valve insufficiency
   D. PDA
   E. A-V stenosis

24. Which of the following is NOT a primary skin lesion? 24.____
   A. Papule B. Macule
   C. Wheal D. Excoriation
   E. Pustule

25. The part of the electrocardiogram that is represented by the letter T is the 25.____
   A. isoelectric period
   B. final upward deflection
   C. upward curve corresponding to atrial contraction
   D. ventricular complex
   E. downward deflection

26. Left sided congestive heart failure is *most commonly* characterized by 26.____
   A. systolic murmur, liver congestion, increased heart rate and ascites
   B. diastolic murmur, pulmonary congestion, increased heart rate and cough
   C. diastolic murmur, sinus arrhythmia, cough and fatigue
   D. systolic murmur, sinus arrhythmia, cough and fatigue
   E. systolic murmur, pulmonary congestion, increased heart rate and cough

27. Interdigital cysts are BEST treated by 27.____
   A. cauterization B. incision and curretage
   C. surgical excision D. caustic packs
   E. icthamol packs

28. The *most common* condition resulting in congestive heart failure in the dog is 28.____
   A. aortic insufficiency
   B. ventricular septal defect
   C. mutual insufficiency
   D. tricusped insufficiency
   E. pulmonic stenosis

29. The outstanding characteristics of chronic prostatic hyperplasia in a dog are 29. E
  A. anorexia and dysuria
  B. dysuria and pain on rectal palpation
  C. urinary retention and tenesmus
  D. urinary retention and perineal
  E. constipation and tenesmus

30. Vaginal hyperplasia in the bitch occurs MOST often 30. B
  A. following copulation
  B. during estrus
  C. following estrus
  D. following whelping
  E. during vaginitis

31. A factor which will limit the future usefulness of a sow with a vaginal prolapse is 31. A
  A. recurrence during subsequent pregnancy
  B. subsequent metritis
  C. subsequent vaginitis
  D. cervical atresia
  E. subsequent vaginal structure

32. Coxo femoral lux in the dog is usually 32. A
  A. anterio dorsal
  B. anterio ventral
  C. ventral
  D. posterior dorsal
  E. posterior

33. The anterior draw sign of cranial cruciate rupture is 33. C
  A. hypermotility of the patella
  B. hyper flexion of the stifle
  C. cranial gliding of the tibia
  D. caudal gliding of the tibia
  E. prox rotation of the femur

34. The stongest layer of the small intestine that MUST be included in sutures in anastamosis to minimize dehiscence is the 34. C
  A. peritoneum
  B. tunica mucosa
  C. tunica submucosa
  D. tunica serosa
  E. tunica muscularis

35. In the dog, intestinal foreign bodies MOST frequently lodge in the 35. B
  A. duodenum
  B. ileum
  C. jejunum
  D. ilioccoal valve
  E. colon

36. Equine encephalomyelitis virus primarily attacks 36. A
  A. cerebellum causing hyperesthesis and atoxia
  B. cerebrum causing psychic changes
  C. hypo thalamus causing hypothernuia, hyperphagia and diabetes insipidus
  D. medulla causing decreased blood pressure and respiratory paralysis
  E. the respiratory system causing a decreased oxygen supply to the cerebellum

37. A dog has a dilated left pupil that is unresponsive to light in the left and right eye. This indicates damage to 37. A
   A. left optic nerve
   B. right optic nerve
   C. left oculomotor
   D. right oculomotor
   E. left corviathrocic gaglion

38. The lesions of acanthosis nigacans begin in the 38. ~~B~~ A
   A. axilla
   B. groin
   C. flank
   D. under chin
   E. ears

39. All of the following are threatened complications of traumatic gastritis EXCEPT 38. ~~B~~ E
   A. traumatic pleuritis
   B. metastatic pneumonia
   C. liver abscess
   D. gangrenous pneumonia
   E. pulmonary adenomatosis

40. The transplacental route is relatively more important than the colostral route in the transfer of maternal antibodies in the 40. B
   A. cow
   B. human
   C. horse
   D. cat
   D. dog

41. The MOST common source of microsporum gypsum is 41. B
   A. cattle
   B. soil
   D. rodents
   D. cats
   E. dogs

42. The invasion of extraintestinal abdominal organs such as the brain, lungs, and eyes of children infected with the larvae of Toricara canis, is knows as 42. E
   A. cercarind dermatitis
   B. rhabditic dermatitis
   C. hepatitis cysticercosa
   D. creeping eruption
   E. visceral larvae migrans

43. In reducing an elbow luxation of a dog, one should place the elbow in 43. A
   A. extreme flexion
   B. extreme extension
   C. adduction
   D. normal standing position
   E. rotated medially

44. The suture material of choice in teat laceration is 44. A
   A. any non capillary suture
   B. chronic gut
   C. any capillary suture
   D. #3 chronic gut
   E. #3 cat gut

45. The ideal time to castrate male swine is 45. B
   A. at birth
   B. 2 weeks after birth

C. 2 months after birth
D. during weaning
E. 6 months

46. The urine of a cat with cystitis or urolithisis is 46. B
A. usually acidic
B. usually alkaline
C. always alkaline
D. always acidic
E. bloody

47. Dexamethasone does NOT 47. ~~D~~ B
A. slow wound healing
B. lead to osteoporosis
C. dehydrate
D. increase infection
E. reduce inflammation

48. Virus disease that has a characteristically slow onset is 48. ~~E~~ C
A. rabies
B. hog cholera
C. scrapie
D. BUD
E. distemper

49. The agglutination lysis test is used in the diagnosis of 49. ~~D~~ B
A. brucella
B. lepto
C. salmonella
D. anthrox
E. HC

50. The generally recommended level of salt in any swine ration is 50. ~~C~~ A
A. 0.5%
B. 1.0%
C. 1.5%
D. 2.0%
E. 2.5%

# KEY (CORRECT ANSWERS)

| | | | | |
|---|---|---|---|---|
| 1. A | 11. B | 21. A | 31. A | 41. B |
| 2. E | 12. B | 22. A | 32. A | 42. E |
| 3. E | 13. C | 23. B | ~~33. D~~ C | 43. A |
| 4. A | 14. B | ~~24. C~~ D | 34. C | 44. A |
| 5. A | 15. C | 25. B | 35. B | 45. B |
| 6. C | 16. B | 26. E | 36. A | 46. B |
| 7. C | 17. ~~D~~ E | 27. C | 37. A | 47. B |
| 8. B | 18. C | 28. E | 38. A | 48. C |
| 9. C | 19. B | 29. E | 39. E | 49. B |
| 10. E | 20. D | 30. B | 40. B | 50. A |

# TEST 2

DIRECTIONS: Each question or incomplete statement is followed by several suggested answers or completions. Select the one that BEST answers the question or completes the statement. *PRINT THE LETTER OF THE CORRECT ANSWER IN THE SPACE AT THE RIGHT.*

1. A useful indicator regarding the state of the bovine udder is the 1.____
   A. phosphatase content of milk
   B. sediment content
   C. leukocyte count
   D. rancidity
   E. water content

2. The MOST common time for equine encephalomyelitis is during 2.____
   A. a long dry spell
   B. the summer
   C. the winter
   D. the spring
   E. the fall

3. Which is the *most commonly* found pyogenic genus in the horse? 3.____
   A. Strep
   B. Staph
   C. Pseudomenas
   D. Brucella
   E. Corynebacteria

4. The bacterial disease of cattle characterized by erythrocytes in the urine is 4.____
   A. redwater
   B. Texas fever
   C. anaplasmosis
   D. pyelonephritis
   E. leptospirosis

5. For sheep in the slaughter plant, the MOST common disease affecting the skeletal lymph nodes is 5.____
   A. actinobacillosis
   B. sarcosporidiosis
   C. TB
   D. caseous lymphadenitis
   E. lymphangitis

6. The anticoagulant which acts as an antithrombin and antithromboplastin agent is 6.____
   A. NEDTA
   B. oxalic acid
   C. KEDTA
   D. heparin
   E. citrate

7. A drug which may be used in the cow, bitch and mare to hold estrus in abeyance is 7.____
   A. estrogen
   B. oxytocin
   C. L.H.
   D. testosterone
   E. progesterone

8. Acid fast organisms associated with Johne's disease and leprosy are in the genus — 8. E
   A. erysipelothrix
   B. streptothrix
   C. actinomyces
   D. actinobacillus
   E. mycobacterium

9. The cystic ovarian follicle in a cow contains — 9. D
   A. high protein but NO estrogen
   B. glycoprotein but NO estrogen
   C. progesterone present with some estrogen
   D. estrogen, but LESS than the graffian follicle
   E. estrogen, but MORE than the graffian follicle

10. The structure that nourishes and protects the developing ovum is the — 10. ~~A~~ E
   A. corpus luteum
   B. corpus albicans
   C. graffian follicle
   D. $1^{o}$ oocyte
   E. $2^{o}$ oocyte

11. Insufficiency of endocrine function of the pancreas is BEST determined by — 11. D ~~E~~
   A. the insulin tolerence test
   B. uptake of labeled oleic acid
   C. histological examination of the jejunal mucosa
   D. the glucose tolerance test
   E. a check for trypsin in the stool

12. The normal length of time needed for an ovum to pass through the oviduct is — 12. A
   A. 10 minutes
   B. 30 to 60 minutes
   C. 4 to 6 hours
   D. 12 to 18 hours
   E. greater than 24 hours

13. The commercial hormone made from pregnant human urine is mainly — 13. ~~B~~ E
   A. mammary stimulating
   B. follicular stimulating
   C. estrogenic
   D. leutenizing
   E. ketogenic suppressing

   HCG
   FSH
   LH

14. Foal ~~heart~~ heat is ________ days after parturition in the mare. — 14. A
   A. 9
   B. 20
   C. 25
   D. 40
   E. 90

15. Which of the following is NOT a CSF characteristic, obtained from a bovine with polioencephalomalacia? — 15. ~~A~~ D
   A. Increased CSF pressure
   B. Increased number of cells
   C. Positive Pandy test
   D. Predominance of neutrophils
   E. Presence of globulin

16. Mereck's disease is classically diagnoised by extensive peripheral nerve lesions. In acute cases, visceral lesions are also present.
The etiological agent for Mereck's disease is 16. D
   A. rickettsial organism
   B. PPLO
   C. salmonella pullorum
   D. herpes virus (Group G)
   E. mycoplasma

17. The spieces that ovulates 10 to 16 hours after the start of estrus is the 17. A C
   A. sow
   B. mare
   C. cow
   D. ewe
   E. bitch

18. The ovary secretes 18. E D
   A. estrogens and corticoids
   B. LH and FSH
   C. FSH and progesterone
   D. estrogens and progestins
   E. estrogens and LH

19. Artificial light or daylight influences the ovulation rate of domestic chickens by 19. C
   A. affecting the hormonal influence of shell deposition
   B. providing more available feeding time
   C. influencing the pituitary to release hormone
   D. changing the peck order of the flock
   E. influencing the oviposition

20. A dietary deficiency of ______ is seen in parathyroid hyperplasia 20. A
   A. Ca
   B. P
   C. Mg
   D. vitamin D
   E. I

21. Big head in the horse is a disease that is morphologically characterized by 21. D
   A. osteomalacia
   B. osteoporosis
   C. ricketts
   D. osteitis (osteodystrophia) fibrosa
   E. osteitis deformans (Paget's disease)

22. Parasympathetic stimulation causes contraction of the gall bladder via release of 22. E
   A. epinephrine
   B. serotonin
   C. norepinephrine
   D. histamine
   E. acetylcholine

23. A pin in the caudal frontal sinus of the cow would gravitate directly to the 23. E
   A. pharynx
   B. lacrimal sinus
   C. maxillary sinus

D. palatine sinus
E. post-orbital diverticulum

24. In the diagnosis of rupture of the anterior cruciate ligament, a snap is heard when the 24.____
A. medial meniscus hits the flat tibial condyle
B. patella leaves its groove in the femur
C. long digital extensor tendon hits the extensor groove of the tibia
D. peroneous tendon comes in contact with the medial side of the lateral collateral ligament
E. femoral condyle comes in contact with the caudal part of medial meniscus

25. A diffuse, epitheliochorial, nondeciduate placenta is seen in the 25.____
A. horse and swine
B. cat and dog
C. rat and guinea pig
D. monkey and rabbit
E. cow and sheep

26. In the ruminant, enlargement of the spleen seen with septicemia is associated with 26.____
A. acute anthrax
B. extramedullary hematopoesis
C. massive leukocytic infiltration
D. reticuloendothelial hyperplasis of white pulp
E. lymphoid hyperplasis in the Malpighian corpuscles

27. In mercury poisoning in swine, selective coagulative necrosis occurs in the 27.____
A. renal tubules
B. urinary bladder mucosa
C. esophageal mucosa
D. splenic red pulp
E. hepatic parenchymal cells

28. In urban areas, feline infective enterities is seen in cats 28.____
A. before 2 weeks
B. before 2 years
C. prior to weaning
D. prior to sexual maturity
E. at times variable to individual circumstances

29. The method for detecting horsemeat in uncooked beef is the 29.____
A. agglutination test
B. anaphalactic test
C. allergy test
D. complement fixation test
E. precipitation test

30. When giving general anesthesia to horses and cattle, caution should be used especially in 30.____
A. cattle
B. horses
C. male horse

D. bull
E. postparturient females of both species

31. Teat surgery is MOST common in the — 31. B
A. apex of the streak canal
B. lower end of the streak canal
C. middle of the streak canal
D. upper end of the streak canal
E. entire streak canal

32. Navicular disease in the horse is associated with the — 32. D
A. insertion of the superficial digital flexor
B. insertion of the common digital extensor
C. proximal interphalangeal joint
D. insertion of the deep digital flexor
E. distal digital annular ligament

33. Which of the following has the HIGHEST concentration of protein? — 33. A
A. Plasma B. CSF C. Lymph D. Serum
E. Urine

34. Trichostrongyloidosis is *least likely* found in — 34. C
A. horses B. sheep D. C cats D. cows
E. pigs

35. The difference between the action of corticotropin and cortisone is that corticotropin — 35. B
A. is more effective
B. does NOT cause as much atrophy of the adrenal glands
C. does NOT directly cause Na retention
D. causes the release of insulin
E. causes the release of other pituitary hormones

36. Muscular dystrophy in lambs causes — 36. A D
A. markedly increased SGOT
B. elevated serum tocopherol
C. clinically detectable myoglobinuria
D. elevated plasma myoglobin
E. elevated serum selenicum

37. Antihistamines can cause problems if given — 37. C
A. orally B. I P C. I V D. I M
E. S Q

38. The disinfectant of choice for farm buildings after viral disease is — 38. B
A. NaPH B. Ca hydroxide
C. benezene hexachloride D. phenol
E. ammonia $H_2O$

39. Prevention of pseudorabics (Audjeski's disease) in cattle is prevented by — 39. E
A. disinfection of the premises

B. killing ALL infected cattle
C. decreasing ALL rodent populations of the area
D. serum immunization of cattle
E. separating cattle and swine

40. A practical method of preserving valuable breeding stock of purebred swine from brucellosis is to 40. E
A. dispose of the entire herd
B. dispose of young pigs before they are infected
C. test monthly and dispose of reactors
D. eliminate reactors to agglutination test
E. separate young at weaning, dispose of the old herd and test and eliminate

41. The clinical picture of Cushing's disease is typified by ALL of the following EXCEPT 41. E
A. alopecia
B. hyperpigmentation
C. muscle weakness
D. eosinopenia
E. hematuria

42. The MOST common vector of rabies world wide is the 42. D
A. dog
B. fox
C. skunk
D. bat
E. squirrel

43. A human infection *commonly* contracted from birds is 43. A
A. ornithosis
B. pasteurellosis
C. viriosis
D. mycoplasma
E. coccidiosis

44. Egg transmission of S. typhimurium is derived from 44. ~~C~~ D
A. air borne infection
B. contaminated feed
C. infection of the ovule
D. shell contamination
E. septicemia

45. After 60 minutes of anesthesia, the smallest difference between inspired and alveolar anesthetic concentration would exist if the agent used was 45. ~~A~~ C
A. nitrous oxide
B. ether
C. methoxyflurane
D. halothane
E. chloroform

46. The BEST single treatment for both cyanide and nitrite poisoning is 46. C
A. sodium thiosulfate
B. magnesium sulfate
C. methylene blue
D. chloral hydrate
E. amyl nitrite

47. In mammals, production of immunocompetent cells is influenced by the 47. E
A. thymus and bursa of fabricious
B. thymus and gut (associated lymphoid tissue)
C. spleen and gut (associated lymphoid tissue)
D. thymus and spleen
E. lymph nodes and spleen

48. Soon after therapy begins, resistance of all types of bacteria may soon by found with 48. B____
    A. penicillin B. streptomycin
    C. oxytetracyline D. chlortetracyline
    E. chloramphenial

49. Penicillin, streptomycin and sulfonomides are effective in treating 49. B____
    A. coccidiomycosis B. nocardiosis
    C. histoplasmosis D. aspergilliosis
    E. muccomycosis

50. The test that utilizes a specific antigen for anaplasmosis in cattle and sheep with a specificity up to 98% for carrier animals is the 50. C____
    A. ring test B. standard plate test
    C. complement fixation test D. B B A or carol test
    E. rivanol test

---

# KEY (CORRECT ANSWERS)

| | | | | |
|---|---|---|---|---|
| 1. C | 11. D | 21. D | 31. B | 41. E |
| 2. B | 12. E | 22. E | 32. D | 42. D |
| 3. A | 13. D | 23. E | 33. A | 43. A |
| 4. D | 14. A | 24. E | 34. C | 44. D |
| 5. D | 15. D | 25. A | 35. B | 45. C |
| 6. D | 16. D | 26. A | 36. D | 46. C |
| 7. E | 17. C | 27. A | 37. C | 47. E |
| 8. E | 18. D | 28. B | 38. B | 48. B |
| 9. D | 19. C | 29. E | 39. E | 49. B |
| 10. A | 20. A | 30. A | 40. E | 50. C |

---

# EXAMINATION SECTION

## TEST 1

DIRECTIONS: Each question or incomplete statement is followed by several suggested answers or completions. Select the one that BEST answers the question or completes the statement. *PRINT THE LETTER OF THE CORRECT ANSWER IN THE SPACE AT THE RIGHT.*

1. Modified Whiteside test is performed on a farm where milk is offered for sale. 1. B
   A positive reaction indicates
   A. improper cooling
   B. an abnormal leukocytes count
   C. increased lipase activity
   D. coliform contamination
   E. increased sediment

2. The increased pressure due to milk let down is due to ________ released into the blood. 2. D
   A. cortisone
   B. adrenaline
   C. glucose
   D. oxytoxin
   E. thyroxin

3. The calcium and phosphorus ratio adequate for optimal growth is 3. ~~D~~ B
   A. 2.0 : 0.05
   B. 1.7 : 1.0
   C. 2.5 : 1.0
   D. 1.2 : 1.6
   E. 1.0 : 2:0

4. A diagnosis of hepatosis dietetica and mulberry heart disease indicates a deficiency of vitamin 4. E
   A. A and Ca
   B. B and iron
   C. $B_2$
   D. D and P
   E. E and selenium

5. The BEST way to eradicate interstitial necrotic pododermatitis is to 5. D
   A. administer IV antibiotics
   B. administer IV sulfas
   C. move to wetter pastures
   D. trim feet
   E. vaccinate

6. The term "ecology" means the study of 6. A
   A. populations and their interactions with their environment
   B. host species especially concerning their roles in social structures
   C. pollution and its control
   D. symbiosis between dissimilar organism
   E. climatic factors like temperature and rainfall and their influence on seasons

7. The MOST common type of prophylactic vaccine against blackleg used today is 7.____
   A. blackleg toxoid
   B. blackleg antiserum
   C. heat killed inflammatory exudate
   D. homologous blackleg antisera
   E. bacteria composed of both Cl. chauvei and Cl. septicum

8. The BEST explanation for tuberculin reactors from a TB infected herd showing NO lesions on necropsy is that the 8.____
   A. body overcame the TB infection in the lungs
   B. body had recovered from an infection in an acid fast organism
   C. lesions were located in the bones and were NOT grossly visible
   D. tuberculin was NOT injected aseptically
   E. lesions were present but NOT developed to a size where they would be grossly visible

9. Blue tongue, an acute viral disease of sheep, is transmitted by 9.____
   A. food
   B. $H_2O$
   C. gnats
   D. 2 host ticks
   E. direct contact

10. The virus of pig pneumonia is contracted by 10.____
   A. inhalation
   B. ingestion
   C. intermediate vectors
   D. mechanical vectors
   E. fomites

11. The primary means of spreading bacillary Hb urea is 11.____
   A. ingestion
   B. inhalation
   C. coitus
   D. infection of wound
   E. insect vector

12. The biggest fault with veterinary anthelmintic is that it 12.____
   A. does NOT affect the larval stage
   B. increases susceptibility to reinfection
   C. is toxic and a prescription is needed
   D. irritates already inflamed mucosa
   E. suppresses inflammatory response

13. Vaccines and biologics are widely used as preventative measures. 13.____
   Similar techniques have been developed to prevent
   A. hookworms of dogs
   B. heart worms of dogs
   C. ural worms of chickens
   D. large roundworms of horses
   E. kidney worms of swine

14. The parasites that could prove to be a problem in cesarian produced barrier maintained dogs are 14.____
   A. sarcoptes and demodex
   B. sertoria and oncrocerca
   C. ancylostoma and ascarids (Georgi)
   D. thelazia and trichostronzylus
   E. toxoplasmosis

15. The stage of toxoplasma gondi which is MOST resistant under natural conditions is the 15.____
   A. sporocyst
   B. adult trematode
   C. fecal oocyst (Hagan)
   D. trophozoite
   E. leptotad

16. The carnivore that is *most likely* to infect man with trichinella spiralis is the 16.____
   A. black bear
   B. domestic cat
   C. dog
   D. spotted skunk
   E. red-tail fox

17. In an animal with persistent diarrheal disease, the absence of oocysts in the feces does NOT mean that the causative agent is NOT a coccidia because 17.____
   A. the oocysts are being destroyed by bacteria
   B. severe disease and death may occur prior to the production of oocysts
   C. some eimeria do NOT produce oocysts
   D. its an old infection and oocysts are no longer being produced
   E. the development of immunity is preventing the production of oocysts

18. How do you determine the number of viral particles present in a sample? 18.____
   A. Tissue culture infective $dose_{50}$ ($TCID_{50}$)
   B. $LD_{50}$
   C. Plaque assay
   D. Electron microscope
   E. Hemagglutination

19. The agglutination-lysis test is useful in the diagnosis of 19.____
   A. lepto
   B. TB
   C. brucellosis
   D. ascarosis
   E. rabies

20. The term used to describe the protein coat or shell of viral particles is the 20.____
   A. unit membrane
   B. limiting membrane
   C. cell wall
   D. envelope
   E. capsid

21. The suckling mice is used to isolate the ______ virus. 21.____
   A. arbo
   B. adeno
   C. herpes
   D. pox
   E. parvo

22. IBR is caused by a ______ virus. 22.____
   A. reo
   B. arbo
   C. herpes
   D. rhabdo
   E. myxo

23. The species of salmonella *most commonly* associated with diseases that occur in humans and animals is 23.____
   A. S. cholerasius
   B. S. derbi
   C. S. typhimerium
   D. S. typhi
   E. S. drublia

24. The chief focus of infection in bacillary Hburia of cattle is the 24.____
   A. muscle B. kidney
   C. liver D. spleen
   E. digestive system

25. The highest concentration of lead in poisoned cows is in the 25.____
   A. blood B. kidney C. liver D. brain
   E. gingivae

26. The site of choice for isolation of the pathological serotype of E. coli in a four-day-old pig with clinical colibacillosis is the 26.____
   A. duodenum B. spiral colon
   C. rectum D. spleen
   E. blood

27. A culture of salmonella is sent to the lab for sero typing. The report states that the organism is s. colesasius VI, VII, c, i, 5. 27.____
   The Roman numerals refer to
   A. H antigens, phase 2 B. H antigens, phase 1
   C. K antigens D. V antigens
   E. O antigens

28. The treatment of choice for a dog dehydrated as a result of a severe emesis is 28.____
   A. isotonic saline
   B. an isotonic solution of salt, strong acid and weak base
   C. an isotonic solution of salt, weak acid and strong base
   D. dextrose
   E. whole blood

29. Polaxalenes exert their effect for treatment of bloat by 29.____
   A. stimulating rumen motility
   B. reducing the formation of gas
   C. reducing froth
   D. stimulating rumen peristalsis
   E. increasing regurgitation

30. The steroid compound that has the least mineralocoticoid contrast effect is 30.____
   A. dexamethazone B. hydrocortisone
   C. cortisone D. prednisolone
   E. prednisone

31. Instilling lactate into an animal results in 31.____
   A. No change in the acid base metabolism
   B. NO respiratory rate due to metabolic alkalosis produced

C. alkali production due to lactate metabolism
D. acid production due to lactate metabolism
E. tachycardia due to the effect on the myocardium

32. Which of the following statements concerning neuromuscular blockade is INCORRECT? 32.____
A. Rapidly moving muscles, such as fingers, are paralyzed first.
B. Intercostals and diaphragm are last to be paralyzed.
C. Analgesia for short surgical procedures is produced.
D. Neostigmine antagonizes the blockade by curare but NOT succyntcholine.
E. Artificial respiration can be used to sustain life.

33. The species that shows the least resistance to phenothizine toxicity is the 33.____
A. goat B. cow C. horse D. sheep
E. pig

34. Phenylbutazone can be simply described as a(n) 34.____
A. anti-inflammatory analgesic
B. cataleptic agent
C. anti-inflammatory
D. local anesthetic
E. acidifying diuretic

35. It is BEST to castrate a dog 35.____
A. through the scrotum over each testis
B. anterior to the scrotum on the midline
C. along side the penis
D. lateral to the medial raphe of the scrotum
E. on the scrotal midline

36. A bacteria grown on selenite agar, has small colonies on SS agar, is urease positive, and on Krumevildes triple sugar agar, has a red slant and yellow base. 36.____
This bacteria is
A. salmonella B. aerobacter
C. paracolon D. proteus
E. e. Coli

37. In a sick, debilitated dog, the MOST rapid means of water loss is 37.____
A. through the skin B. G.I.
C. U.G. D. respiratory
E. through the breast

38. Fat steers and horses for show get epiphysitis especially at the distal radius and metacarpal epiphysis. 38.____
Signs of this are
A. protrusion of cartilage out of the epiphyseal line
B. overgrowth of bone from the metaphysis
C. crushed cartilage and disorganization

D. fragmented cartilage with some thrown into the articular area
E. hypertrophy of the area and thickening

39. Incontinence in a spayed bitch can BEST be treated with 39.____
A. drenocortisone
B. esoxycorticosterone
C. thyroxin
D. stilbesterol
E. progesterone

40. You find eosinophilia, increased BUN, increased serum K, and decreased Na+ in 40.____
A. Cushing's syndrome
B. pancreatic fibrosis
C. chronic interstitial nephritis
D. adiposogenital syndrome
E. adrenocortical insufficience

41. The flurry strain of rabies virus used to vaccinate animals is propagated in 41.____
A. rabbits
B. mice
C. horses
D. chick embryos
E. goats

42. The unique characteristic of clostridium botulinum among other pathogenic bacteria is that it 42.____
A. is found in the soil
B. survives common food processing procedures
C. does NOT invade the body
D. produces a neurotropic toxin
E. is found in sausage

43. The CORRECT statement about canine scabies is that it 43.____
A. resembles ringworm clinically
B. is non pruritic
C. is NOT transmissible to other dogs
D. is self limiting
E. is transmissible to man

44. A direct smear of a three-month-old puppy with watery diarrhea, blood tinged mucus, and a normal temperature, shows numerous fluttering organisms that are 15u long, flagellated, and concave ventrally. 44.____
The diagnosis is
A. coccidiosis
B. haemobartonella
C. girdiasis
D. babesiasis
E. anaplasmosis

45. Turkeys are susceptible to ALL of the following diseases EXCEPT 45.____
A. infectious bronchitis
B. coccidiosis
C. irysipilas
D. fowl pox
E. fowl typhoid

46. The disease that is NOT directly transmissible from animal to man is 46.____
   A. glanders B. anthrax
   C. salmonellosis D. brucellosis
   E. tetanus

47. The wildlife species that is MOST often associated with rabies in the midwest is the 47.____
   A. skunk B. raccoon C. bat D. coyote
   E. fox

48. The measure used to control swine pox, a skin disease of swine affecting all ages is 48.____
   A. the control of fleas
   B. the control of swine louse
   C. vaccination
   D. disinfection of the premises
   E. slaughter of affected animals

49. Lumpy jaw in cattle is caused by 49.____
   A. actinobacillus B. actinomyces
   C. stapn D. nocardia
   E. strepto bacillus

50. The *most commonly* reported hosts for salmonella sp in the U.S. are 50.____
   A. cattle B. swine C. poultry D. dogs
   E. sheep

# KEY (CORRECT ANSWERS)

| | | | | |
|---|---|---|---|---|
| 1. B | 11. A | 21. C | 31. C | 41. D |
| 2. D | 12. A | 22. C | 32. D | 42. C |
| 3. B | 13. A | 23. C | 33. D | 43. E |
| 4. E | 14. C | 24. C | 34. A | 44. C |
| 5. D | 15. C | 25. C | 35. B | 45. A |
| 6. A | 16. A | 26. A | 36. D | 46. E |
| 7. E | 17. B | 27. B | 37. B | 47. A |
| 8. B | 18. A | 28. B | 38. E | 48. B |
| 9. C | 19. A | 29. C | 39. D | 49. B |
| 10. A | 20. E | 30. A | 40. E | 50. C |

# TEST 2

DIRECTIONS: Each question or incomplete statement is followed by several suggested answers or completions. Select the one that BEST answers the question or completes the statement. *PRINT THE LETTER OF THE CORRECT ANSWER IN THE SPACE AT THE RIGHT.*

1. Enzootic ataxia in sheep is caused by a deficiency in 1.____
   A. Mn B. Cu C. Co D. Fe
   E. glucose

2. The National Council on Interstate Shipment of Milk has adopted an abnormal milk policy allowing for a leukocyte count of less than ________ per ml. 2.____
   A. 250,000 B. 500,000
   C. 1,000,000 D. 1,500,000
   E. 2,000,000

3. Fluid and electrolyte deficiencies created by persistent diarrhea in dogs can be corrected by the administration of 3.____
   A. 5% dextrose solution IP
   B. ammonium chloride with water per os
   C. 12% sodium bicarbonate solution IP
   D. LR solution per os or IP
   E. KCI per os with water

4. Kaolin belongs to a class of drugs knows as 4.____
   A. demulcents B. astringents
   C. absorbants D. emulsifiers
   E. emollients

5. Genetic information necessary for the reproduction of viruses is carried by the 5.____
   A. virus-related enzymes
   B. protein coat of the virus particle
   C. viruscytes
   D. lipid components
   E. nucleic acid portion of the virus particle

6. The biological vectors in which part of the life cycle of the virus is spent are usually 6.____
   A. arthropods B. mollusks
   C. mammals D. birds
   E. fish

7. A bovine hemolytic disease that is transmitted by insects without hemoglobinuria is 7.____
   A. anaplasmosis
   B. lepto
   C. piroplasmosis
   D. lympho
   E. hemolyticum septicum

8. Canine diplydium can be differentiated from other cestodes by 8.____
   A. the rostrum that has two grooves and NO hoods
   B. the shape of the gravid proglottid
   C. its human intermediate host
   D. its rabbit
   E. the motile proglottid

9. Hemoglobinuria occurs in ALL of the following diseases of animals EXCEPT 9.____
   A. piroplasmosis
   B. bracken fern
   C. anaplasmosis
   D. post-parturient hemoglobinuria
   E. bacillary hemoglobinuria

10. Leucocytozoonosis of ducks and turkeys is transmitted by 10.____
   A. ticks
   B. lice
   C. flies
   D. mosquitoes
   E. midgies

11. Abortion due to T. fetus occurs during the 11.____
   A. first trimester
   B. second trimester
   C. last trimester
   D. last week
   E. first half

12. The type of salmonella MOST common in man and animals in the U.S. is salmonella 12.____
   A. chaerasuis
   B. dublin
   C. derby
   D. typhimurium
   E. typhi

13. The MOST common source of botulism in game birds on farms is 13.____
   A. water
   B. soil
   C. feed
   D. maggot
   E. litter

14. According to MOST authorities, the one primary cause of atrophic rhinitis of swine is 14.____
   A. bordetella bronchiseptica
   B. hemophilus suis
   C. pseudomonas auerginosa
   D. pasteurella multocida
   E. corynebacterium pyogenes

15. The site of isolation of a pathogenic form of E. coli from a 4-day-old pig with clinical colibacillary is the 15.____
   A. spleen
   B. spiral colon
   C. stomach
   D. duodenum
   E. blood

16. Motility of leptospira is due to the 16.____
   A. myofibrils
   B. protoplasm
   C. elastic membrane
   D. axial filament
   E. periplast

17. Measely beef is affected with 17.____
   A. cysticercus bovis
   B. cysticercus cellulosae
   C. coenuris
   D. pentastomum denticulatum
   E. trichinella spiralis

18. In the pasteurization of raw milk, the temperature is held continuously at 161 degrees F for ______ seconds. 18.____
   A. 5
   B. 10
   C. 12
   D. 15
   E. 20

19. The MOST characteristic sign of allergic dermatitis is 19.____
   A. pruritis
   B. alopecis
   C. pain
   D. excessive exfoliation
   E. pustules

20. Suckling mice are used in the isolation of ______ viruses. 20.____
   A. arbo
   B. adeno
   C. pox
   D. parvo
   E. herpes

21. Human contact acariasis is caused by handling animals infected with 21.____
   A. caprine psoroptes
   B. canine sarcoptes
   C. canine demodex
   D. ovine psoroptes
   E. bovine chorioptes

22. A dog suffers from vitamin A deficiency. A substance that can be given as a supplement and aid in assimilation is 22.____
   A. bone meal
   B. shredded wheat
   C. vitamin E
   D. ferric citrate
   E. skimmed milk (dry)

23. Deficiency of vitamin D seldom occurs in farm animals EXCEPT when they 23.____
   A. eat pig weed
   B. over-eat on grain
   C. are confined
   D. are range fed
   E. on pasture in mid-winter

24. A characteristic of scrapie is that it 24.____
   A. has a slow onset
   B. is passed from parents to progeny
   C. is susceptible to vaccination
   D. has NO nervous signs
   E. affects lambs *only*

25. The diagnosis of leptospirosis in cattle should NOT be solely based on 25.____
   A. clinical signs and necropsy
   B. F.A.
   C. injection into G.P.
   D. H. Lysis
   E. examination for spirochetes

26. The mycotic agent that is BEST transmitted from dog to dog by direct contact is 26.____
   A. microsporum canis
   B. microsporum gypseum
   C. coccidioidin immitis
   D. blastomyces dermatidis
   E. histoplasma capsulatum

27. The semi synthetic penicillin that is broken down by the enzyme penicillinase is 27.____
   A. ampicillin
   B. cloxacillin
   C. methicillin
   D. phenethicillin
   E. polycillin

28. The virus of pig pneumonia is maintained in a herd largely through 28.____
   A. live virus vaccines
   B. ectoparasites
   C. lung worms
   D. birds and rodents
   E. carrier sows

29. A PDA in a dog is a continuous murmur heard over the 29.____
   A. right cardiac base
   B. left cardiac base
   C. left cardiac apex
   D. mid sternal border
   E. right cardiac apex

30. Classical lesions of mycotic stomotitis in cattle include 30.____
   A. necrotic inflammation of the tongue, erosions of the epidermis, and lameness
   B. ulcerative lesions of the tongue and hard palate
   C. necrotic erosions of the tongue and visicular lesions of the udder
   D. papillary lesions of the tongue, lips, nares and muzzle
   E. ulcerative erosions in and around the oral cavity, nostril and anterior turbinates

31. A dog has complete loss of the right optic nerve. The result of shining a light in the right eye *only* is 31.____
   A. normal vision but NO pupillary response in either eye
   B. loss of vision in the right eye with loss of pupillary response in the right eye *only*
   C. loss of vision in the right eye with loss of pupillary response in the left eye *only*
   D. loss of vision in the right eye with loss of pupillary response in both eyes
   E. loss of vision in the right eye with normal pupillary response in both eyes

32. A horse has an intermittent bilateral nasal discharge which is evident principally when the horse lowers its head. A unilateral pharyngeal swelling is also present. The *most likely* cause is 32.____
   A. infection of the gutteral pouch
   B. sinusitis from an infected tooth
   C. chronic pharyngitis
   D. distemper
   E. rhinosporidiosis

33. The MOST common site for neoplasm of the intestines of a dog is the 33.____
   A. duodenum B. jejunum
   C. colon D. rectum
   E. cecum

34. In an aged dog with a tumor of the distal radius, the *most likely* place to see evidence of metastasis on x-ray is the 34.____
   A. elbow B. mediastinal lymph nodes
   C. forelimb D. lung
   E. liver

35. Primary pyodermas in the dog are caused by 35.____
   A. strep B. staph
   C. corynebacterium pyogenes D. proteus vulgaris
   E. distemper virus

36. Congestive heart failure involves a complex interaction between the heart, kidney, adrenal cortex and pituitary resulting in ________ water reabsorption. 36.____
   A. *increased* Na reabsorption and *increased*
   B. *increased* Na reabsorption and *decreased*
   C. *decreased* K reabsorption and *decreased*
   D. *increased* K reabsorption and *increased*
   E. *decreased* Na reabsorption and *decreased*

37. All of the following are signs of bracken fern poison in cattle EXCEPT 37.____
   A. decreased prothrombin B. hypothiaminosis
   C. laryngeal edema D. petechial hemorrhage
   E. intestinal hemorrhage

38. Fresh froth blood from both nostrils is *most likely* due to 38.____
   A. nasal hemorrhage
   B. pulmonary hemorrhage
   C. hepatization of the lung
   D. pulmonary congestion and edema
   E. upper respiratory infection

39. Signs of polydypsia-polyuria are present in a female dog. Which of the following diseases should NOT be in the diagnosis? 39.____
   A. Diabetes mellitus B. CIN
   C. Urolithiasis D. Pyometra
   E. Cushing's

40. The cell type MOST prevalent in leukoblastic tissues in malignant lymphoma is the 40.____
   A. neutrophil B. eosinophil
   C. immature lymphocyte D. mononuclear leukocyte
   E. mast cell

41. In congestive heart failure, the production of edema is caused by 41.____
   A. hypoproteinuria
   B. renal retension of Na plus $H_2O$
   C. increased periferal vascular resistance
   D. increased periferal venous resistance
   E. increased capillary permeability

42. The MOST efficient and specific therapy for clinical gierdiasis in a young puppy is 42.____
   A. bacytrecin
   B. atabrine
   C. dihydrostreptomycin
   D. bismuth subnitrate
   E. sulfadimethoxine

43. The cause of cyanosis and brown blood in cattle and sheep is due to 43.____
   A. aldrin
   B. cyanide
   C. nitrate
   D. lead
   E. arsenic

44. Summer sores is a wound infection with excessive granulation tissue caused by 44.____
   A. eggs deposited by habronema flies
   B. larvae deposited by habronema
   C. eggs deposited by habronema in fecal material
   D. adult habronema in their normal subcutaneous migration
   E. eggs of gasterophilus intestinalis flies

45. Osteoporosis in young cats is due to 45.____
   A. hypoparathyroidism
   B. inbreeding
   C. an all organ meat diet
   D. an all commercial diet
   E. early weaning

46. A condition in budugars often characterized by dyspnea and a high pitched squeak is 46.____
   A. air sac mite infestation
   B. a ruptured air sac
   C. an impacted crop
   D. lipogranulomatosis
   E. thyroid hypertrophy

47. A six-month-old calf has a ruptured bladder. The BEST way to determine fluid level is 47.____
   A. balotment
   B. deep palpation
   C. percussion
   D. paracentesis
   E. phondoscopic auscultation

48. The BEST and MOST common way to do a ruhenotomy is at the 48.____
   A. high left flank
   B. low left flank
   C. ventral midline
   D. high right flank
   E. low right flank

49. The *most likely* cause of constant vomition following feeding is 49. ____
    A. pyloric stenosis
    B. a dilated esophagus
    C. uremia
    D. liver disease
    E. parasites

50. The breed of dog that is MOST susceptible to perianal fistulas is the 50. ____
    A. cocker spaniel
    B. German shepherd
    C. miniature poodle
    D. collie
    E. pointer

---

# KEY (CORRECT ANSWERS)

| | | | | |
|---|---|---|---|---|
| 1. B | 11. A | 21. B | 31. D | 41. B |
| 2. B | 12. D | 22. E | 32. A | 42. B |
| 3. D | 13. B | 23. C | 33. D | 43. C |
| 4. C | 14. A | 24. A | 34. D | 44. B |
| 5. E | 15. D | 25. A | 35. B | 45. C |
| 6. A | 16. D | 26. A | 36. A | 46. E |
| 7. A | 17. A | 27. A | 37. B | 47. C |
| 8. B | 18. D | 28. C | 38. B | 48. A |
| 9. C | 19. A | 29. B | 39. C | 49. A |
| 10. E | 20. E | 30. A | 40. C | 50. B |

---

# TEST 3

DIRECTIONS: Each question or incomplete statement is followed by several suggested answers or completions. Select the one that BEST answers the question or completes the statement. *PRINT THE LETTER OF THE CORRECT ANSWER IN THE SPACE AT THE RIGHT.*

1. Rabies is transmitted by the 1.____
   I. coyote
   II. squirrel
   III. rodent
   IV. racoon
   V. bat

   The CORRECT answer is
   A. I. *only*
   B. I, IV, V.
   C. II, III
   D. III *only*
   E. all of the above

2. The regulations for health certification of a bull include 2.____
   A. meeting all of the requirements of the state of destination
   B. having NO infectious diseases
   C. a physical examination
   D. a semen evaluation
   E. none of the above

3. The mite affecting dairy cows at the tail, head, and udder, with mild puritis is 3.____
   A. psoroptes
   B. ostedectes
   C. chorioptes
   D. sarcoptes
   E. any of the above

4. Fasciola hepatica is found, post mortem, in the 4.____
   A. lung
   B. liver
   C. kidney
   D. bile duct
   E. colon

5. The species target cells that indicate AIHA are 5.____
   A. IgG
   B. IgM
   C. IgA
   D. IgE
   E. none of the above

6. The food sickness that is NOT destroyed after boiling 10 minutes is 6.____
   A. botulism
   B. salmonella
   C. brucella
   D. strep
   E. staph

7. What is NOT seen in milk from mastitis 7.____
   A. *increased* CI levels
   B. *decreased* casein
   C. *increased* leukocytes
   D. *increased* lactose
   E. all of the above

8. The temperature required for short pasteurization is ________ seconds. 8.____
   A. $60^{\circ}C$ for 10
   B. $65^{\circ}C$ for 10
   C. $161^{\circ}F$ for 15
   D. $212^{\circ}F$ for 15
   E. $100^{\circ}C$ for 10

9. The minimum temperature required to destroy trichinella is ________ degrees F. 9.____
   A. 98.6
   B. 137
   C. 175
   D. 212
   E. 260

10. Toxicity occuring with rock phosphate is due to 10.____
   A. Fl
   B. Fe
   C. 2n
   D. Pb
   E. Hg

11. The analeptic that takes effect after 10-15 minutes is 11.____
   A. nikethamide
   B. doramide
   C. pikrotoxin
   D. neostigmine
   E. none of the above

12. What animal do you infect with fluids from a fetus with brucella to get a diagnosis? 12.____
   A. Rabbit
   B. Rodent
   C. Snake
   D. Guinea pig
   E. Elephant

13. Gastric rupture occurs *most commonly* in the 13.____
   A. cow
   B. dog
   C. cat
   D. horse
   E. chicken

14. Emphysema of serosa is MOST common in 14.____
   A. dogs
   B. horses
   C. cows
   D. rabbits
   E. pigs

15. The effect of aflatoxins is 15.____
   A. chronic gastritis
   B. renal failure
   C. hepatoma
   D. fibrosarcoma
   E. death

16. The electrolyte that causes electrocoupling in the heart is 16.____
   A. Na
   B. Ca
   C. Cl
   D. K
   F. Fe

17. The area that has the GREATEST ciliary action is the 17.____
   A. bronchioles
   B. alveoli
   C. intestine
   D. nostrils
   E. trachea

18. The electrolyte that causes increased electrical potential is 18.____
   A. Na
   B. Ca
   C. Cl
   D. K
   E. Fe

19. The percentage of GFR vs. blood flow through the kidney is ________ percent. 19.____
   A. 10 B. 25 C. 50 D. 75
   E. 90

20. The fibers that make neurosecretory fibers different from other neurons are increased numbers of 20.____
   A. golgi bodies B. secretory granules
   C. endoplasmic reticula D. all of the above
   E. none of the above

21. Hemoglobinuria is caused by 21.____
   A. Pb B. Hg
   C. SLE D. pyruvate kinase
   E. babesia

22. The cause of meningitis is 22.____
   A. scrapie B. glassers
   C. hog cholera D. rabies
   E. mononucleosis

23. EIA is found in 23.____
   I. blood
   II. saliva
   III. manure
   IV. any secretions
   The CORRECT answer is
   A. I *only* B. I, II
   C. III *only* D. IV *only*
   E. all of the above

24. The main source of histoplasmosis infections is 24.____
   A. aireborne B. feces
   C. soil D. feed
   E. water

25. The test used to determine lepto is the 25.____
   A. agglutination test B. CF
   C. IF D. CBC
   E. serum neutralization test

26. Glucagon acts in the 26.____
   A. muscle B. fat
   C. stomach D. brain
   E. liver

27. The stroke volume of the heart is equal to the 27.____
   A. $\frac{\text{cardiac output per minute}}{\text{minute volume}}$
   B. $\frac{\text{minute volume}}{\text{pulse rate per minute}} \times 100$
   C. $\frac{\text{cardiac output per minute}}{60}$

D. $\dfrac{\text{stroke volume}}{\text{pulse rate per minute}} \times 60$

E. $\dfrac{\text{total blood volume}}{\text{minute blood volume}}$

30. A decrease in the mortality of cattle due to broncho-pneumonia in the last 15 years is the result of the — 30.____
   - A. use of blood transfusions
   - B. development of bacterin
   - C. development of serological test enabling early diagnosis
   - D. use of sulfonamides and antibiotics
   - E. better sanitation methods

31. A dog is presented to you with an eye injury two days old, there is myosis, blepharospasm, photophobia, and a clear normal cornea. The diagnosis is — 31.____
   - A. acute iritis
   - B. glaucoma
   - C. peripheral synechia
   - D. traumatic conjunctivitis
   - E. iris bombe

32. The site of edema in causes of pulmonary edema is in the — 32.____
   - A. alveoli
   - B. bronchi
   - C. bronchioles
   - D. interlobular
   - E. connective tissue

33. The nerve to the extensors of the forearm is — 33.____
   - A. radial
   - B. musculo cutaneous
   - C. axillary
   - D. median
   - E. ulnar

34. With urinary calculis in a tom cat, the urine is — 34.____
   - A. *always* alkaline
   - B. *always* acid
   - C. *usually* alkaline
   - D. *always* bloody
   - E. *usually* acid

35. The MOST common long bone fracture in fatigue of the horse is — 35.____
   - A. phalange #1
   - B. phalange #2
   - C. phalange #3
   - D. radius
   - E. metacarpal #3

36. The C.L. does NOT persist in the ________ through pregnancy. — 36.____
   - A. horse
   - B. cow
   - C. goat
   - D. pig
   - E. sheep

37. The treatment of a well circumscribed cellulitis from a local wound should consist of — 37.____
   - A. massage
   - B. thermal packs
   - C. forced excerise
   - D. excision
   - E. incision

38. Which of the following glands is neurohumoral? 38.__B__
    A. Thyroid
    B. Adrenal medulla
    C. Parathyroid
    D. Ovary
    E. Adrenal cortex

39. A mammary gland is classified as 39.__C__
    A. apocrine
    B. holocrine
    C. merocrine
    D. mesenchymal
    E. epithelial

40. The MOST suitable anesthetic for C-section in the bitch is 40.__E__ A
    A. ether
    B. chloroform
    C. nubercaine
    D. pentobarbitol
    E. thiopental

41. A sign that may be seen during the sternal recumbency stage of hypocalcemia in the cow is 41.__A__
    A. subnormal temperature
    B. increased passage of urine and feces
    C. moist muzzle and skin warm to the touch
    D. constriction of the pupils
    E. NO changes related to the circulatory system

42. A horse has bilateral pneumothorax after being gored by a steer. The horse will die if it is unable to meet the requirements of 42.__A__
    A. tidal volume
    B. inspiratory capacity
    C. supplemental air
    D. vital capacity
    E. complemental air

43. If semen is placed at the cervix, it will take ________ to reach the oviduct. 43.__A__
    A. less than 10 minutes
    B. 10 minutes to 1 hour
    C. 1 hour to 4 hours
    D. 4 hours to 12 hours
    E. more than 12 hours

44. The type of placentation due to chorionic villi distribution is termed zonary in the 44.__E__ A
    A. dog
    B. pig
    C. horse
    D. cow
    E. sheep

45. Which of the following is MOST radiolucent? 45.__B__
    A. Metal
    B. Gas
    C. Muscle
    D. Fat
    E. Bone

46. When a cow is being fed urea, ________ must be supplied in adequate levels in the diet. 46.__B__
    A. fat
    B. carbohydrates
    C. proteins
    D. minerals
    E. vitamins

47. The parasite that does NOT have an intermediate host is 47.X C
A. paragonamous
B. setaria
C. habronema
D. bunostomum
E. megacanthornicus

48. Cystine calculi are seen *most commonly* in the 48.A
A. male dalmation
B. female dalmation
C. male and female cocker spaniel
D. male dachshund
E. female dachshund

49. To destroy sensation to a part, the nerve can be transcected physiologically with 80% ethyl alcohol 49.D
A. by IV at the rate of 1cc/100#
B. in the stomach at 8cc/100#
C. in the nerve
D. around the nerve
E. in a compress over the part

50. The slowest acting cardiac glycoside when used in the heart is 50.C
A. ouobaine
B. digoxin
C. digitoxin
D. lanacide C
E. deslanacide

# KEY (CORRECT ANSWERS)

| | | | | |
|---|---|---|---|---|
| 1. B | 11. C | 21. E | 31. A | 41. A |
| 2. A | 12. D | 22. B | 32. A | 42. A |
| 3. C | 13. D | 23. B | 33. A | 43. A |
| 4. D | 14. E | 24. C | 34. C | 44. A |
| 5. A | 15. C | 25. A | 35. E | 45. B |
| 6. E | 16. B | 26. E | 36. A | 46. B |
| 7. D | 17. E | 27. D | 37. D | 47. C |
| 8. C | 18. A | 28. D | 38. B | 48. A |
| 9. B | 19. B | 29. E | 39. C | 49. D |
| 10. A | 20. D | 30. D | 40. A | 50. C |

# EXAMINATION SECTION

# TEST 1

DIRECTIONS: Each question or incomplete statement is followed by several suggested answers or completions. Select the one that BEST answers the question or completes the statement. *PRINT THE LETTER OF THE CORRECT ANSWER IN THE SPACE AT THE RIGHT.*

1. An episiotomy is performed to  1. B
   A. remove vulvar tumors
   B. enlarge external genital orifice
   C. amputate the clitoris
   D. treat cheilitis

2. The proper procedure to a C-section in the dog is the  2. B
   A. flank approach
   B. midline with ventral incision into the body of the uterus
   C. midline with dorsal incision into the body of the uterus
   D. midline with the incision into both uterine horms

3. The action of muscle relaxant drugs such as d-tubocurarine and gallamine triethiodicte is the  3. A
   A. motor end plate
   B. cerebral cortex
   C. autonomic ganglia
   D. motor end ganglia

4. A 7-year-old fox terrier injured the right stifle 12 days ago. The dog still has pain and swelling, and occasionally places weight on it.
   The BEST diagnostic procedure to perform is to  4. D C
   A. inject procaine into the joint then evaluate
   B. inject the joint with corticosteroid
   C. use short acting anesthesia and try the Paatsama anterior drawer sign
   D. use tranquilizer and take radiographs in A-P and lateral views

5. To perform a posterior digital neurectomy, it is important to know the arrangement of the artery, vein and nerve at this region of the pastern.
   The arrangement from anterior to posterior is  5. C
   A. artery, vein, and nerve
   B. nerve, artery, and vein
   C. vein, artery, and nerve
   D. vein, nerve, and artery

6. For the diagnosis of navicular disease in a horse, you would block the  6. A
   A. posterior digital
   B. volar
   C. anterior digital
   D. plantar

7. Although the clinical signs indicate a cat has pansteatitis, you CANNOT be sure until you — 7.____
   A. have examined cut surfaces of body fat
   B. do a complete hemogram
   C. do a fecal exam
   D. do a gross micro exam of sub. Q fat

8. In the treatment of cows for milk fever with Ca salts, heart block can occur but can be corrected with the administration of — 8.____
   A. atropine sulfate
   B. sodium bicarbonate
   C. epinephrine
   D. norepinephrine

9. The treatment that would be the BEST for a valuable 4-year-old heifer with a hygroma of the knee is — 9.____
   A. extripation
   B. incision and drainage
   C. antiphylligistine pack
   D. to allow the animal to rest

10. A satisfactory pre-anesthetic agent for cats is — 10.____
   A. chlorpromazine
   B. morphine
   C. thiapental sodium
   D. none of the above

11. Atropine sulfate given in acute pancreatitis — 11.____
   A. *decreases* secretions of the pancreas
   B. *increases* secretions of the pancreas
   C. *increases* gut motility
   D. *decreases* intestinal motility

12. The MOST important criteria for assessing the viability of gut is — 12.____
   A. comparative diameter
   B. color
   C. contractility with pinched
   D. warmth

13. Acute pulmonary edema in cattle is characterized by — 13.____
   A. open-mouth breathing and frothed fluid at the lips and nostrils
   B. mild dyspnea with reduced pulse and respiratory rates
   C. cyanosis and hemoglobinuria due to hemolyzed RBC's
   D. none of the above

14. When the horse's head is lowered, purulent discharge from the nose is caused by — 14.____
   A. sinusitis
   B. gutteral pouch
   C. rhinosporidiosis
   D. laryngeal paralysis

15. A horse shows stupor, incoordination, and spells of aimless walking. He drags his hind hoof, and has an icterus index greater than 5. — 15.____
The *most likely* diagnosis is
   A. cirrhosis of the liver
   B. encephalomalacia
   C. congestion
   D. severc gastritis

16. A clinical case of trichophyton equinum in the horse would appear as 16.____
    A. raw ulcerated disc shaped lesions that leave a permanent scar
    B. skin blisters filled with a watery fluid
    C. disc shaped skin-lesions devoid of hair, covered with gray to white scales
    D. wart-like lesions covered with hair

17. The reduction in mortality in bronchopneumonia in cattle in the past five years is due to 17.____
    A. improved sanitation today by livestock growers
    B. development of specific and satisfactory bacterin and serum
    C. laboratory tests to detect early cases
    D. sulfonamide and antibiotic therapy

18. A suture material that absorbs fluid is 18.____
    A. untreated silk
    B. silk worm gut
    C. nylon
    D. alloy

19. Abdominocentesis provides a definitive diagnosis in case of 19.____
    A. torsion of the colon
    B. diffuse adhesive peritonitis
    C. malignant carcinomas
    D. ruptured bladder

20. In an abdominal equine cryptorchoid castration, the surgeon locates the testicle by 20.____
    A. grasping the testicle directly
    B. pushing it into the inguinal canal
    C. drawing an imaginary line from the kidney to the inguinal ring
    D. following the vas deferns or gubernaculum

21. The MOST common heart disease in the equine is 21.____
    A. left A-V insufficiency
    B. pericarditis
    C. myocarditis
    D. cardiac hypertrophy and enlargement

22. With congestive heart failure in the dog, the most important initial consideration is 22.____
    A. relieve fluid accumulation caused by retention of Na+ and $H_2O$ by the kidney
    B. decide how serious the disease is
    C. ascertain whether problem is right or left sided
    D. relieve the paroxysomal coughing

23. Infectious bovine rhinotracheitis has been associated with ALL of the following EXCEPT 23.____
    A. conjunctivitis
    B. malillitis
    C. encephalitis
    D. vaginitis

24. Hyperkeratosis of the foot pad, in dogs, is sometimes associated with 24. A
A. distemper
B. lepto
C. histo
D. I C H

25. Traumatic gastritis is MOST common in 25. X A
A. yearling dairy heifer
B. range beef cattle
C. range beef heifers
D. grain fed dairy cows

26. The MOST urgent need of a cat blocked with urinary sand is 26. D
A. a low ash diet
B. a urinary antiseptic
C. a culture and sensitivity of the urine
D. relief from the obstruction

27. Anthrax and blackleg in a cow is present with swelling. The swelling in anthraxis is 27. B D
A. in the dorsal tail
B. edematous
C. emphysematous
D. crepitant

28. A(n) ___________ is used to increase the antigenicity of a substance. 28. B
A. complement
B. adjuvant
C. immunoceptor
D. amboceptor

29. The diagnosis of hemorrhagic colitis and idiopathic thrombocytopenia are BEST differenciated by the fact that in 29. C
A. hemorrhagic colitis there is projectile vomiting
B. hemorrhagic colitis there is palor of the mucus membranes
C. thrombocytopenia purpura there is subcutaneous and subscleral edema
D. thrombocytopenia purpura there are deep ulcers in the gums

30. Pyloric stenosis is BEST treated by 30. B
A. giving a paragoric
B. incising the serosa and muscularis of the pylorus
C. passing the stomach tube
D. incising the mucosa and submucosa

31. A swagged on taper point needle is BEST for intestinal surgery because 31. B
A. it is easily adapted to needle holder
B. it causes less tissue trauma
C. easily passes through the intestine
D. it can be reautoclaued easily

32. Chronicity, lack of pruritis, bilateral alopecie, and bilateral hyper pigmentation are all important characteristics of 32. D
A. parasitic dermiatitis

B. bacterial infection
C. an allergic skin condition
D. an endocrine imbalance

33. Muco purulent nasal discharge of sheep is a manifestation of  33.____
A. hypoderma infestation
B. gasterophilus
C. uiral arteritis
D. oestrus ovis

34. HPO is frequently associated with chronic lung lesion but its MOST characteristic signs are  34.____
A. cachexia, vomiting, and weight loss
B. broncho pneumonia and weight loss
C. hypertrophic lesions of long bones
D. nasal discharge, and coughing

35. Neoplasms involving the eye and its appendages in cattle are *most likely* related to a(n)  35.____
A. adeno carcinoma
B. carcinoma
C. adenoma
D. papilloma

36. The MOST common ringworm in cats is  36.____
A. microsporum canis
B. microsporum gypsum
C. tricophyton floculosum
D. none of the above

37. To reduce routine plate on pasteurized milk at the plant, action would be directed at  37.____
A. cooling and refrigeration
B. cleaning and sanitizing utensils
C. clip and clean udder
D. all of the above

38. The type of neoplasm *most likely* to be found diseminated throughout the bovine body is  38.____
A. carcinoma
B. lympho
C. sarcoma
D. adenoma

39. A leukopenia is observed in  39.____
A. mastitis
B. milkfever
C. lead poisoning
D. gutteral pouch

40. Melanin is produced in the skin of a dog with  40.____
A. a tumor of the acidophils of adenohypophysis
B. hyperadrenal corticism
C. a sertoli cell tumor producing estrogen
D. hypoadrenal corticism

41. Selective ventilation, in reference to gas flow through the lungs means that  41.____
A. $CO_2$, $O_2$ and $N_2$ pass across alveoli
B. $CO_2$ is passed from alveoli to blood but NOT from blood to alveoli
C. the passage of gases in and out depends on their partial pressures in both blood and alveolar air
D. components of air pass into the blood via osmosis

42. Newborn puppies that are NOT able to recognize their mother or handlers one week to ten days after their eyelids open are suffering from 42.____
   A. congenital coleboma
   B. incomplete development of neural pathways
   C. a persistent puppilary membrane
   D. no abnormality, this is a common condition

43. Injection of an adult bull with chorionic gonadotropin would be expected to 43.____
   A. stimulate spermiogenesis
   B. stimulate division of interstitial cells
   C. stimulate production of testosterone via Zeydig cells
   D. cause testicular atrophy

44. A fluid loss of ________ is non-compatible with life in animals. 44.____
   A. 10%   B. 20%   C. 30%   D. 40%

45. Thiobarbiturates are ultra-short acting because of their 45.____
   A. rapid elimination by active transport out of brain tissue
   B. poor penetration through the blood-brain barrier
   C. rapid excretion by the kidney
   D. rapid redistribution from the brain to parenchymetous tissue, and ultimately to fat depots

46. Mold that is extremely dangerous to handle as it bursts into spores is 46.____
   A. coccidiodimites
   B. histo
   C. blasto
   D. cryptococcus neoformas

47. The Humane Slaughter Act of 1958 states that ALL 47.____
   A. animals processed in Federal establishments MUST be humanely slaughtered
   B. poultry additives going into red meat products MUST come from humanely slaughtered fowl
   C. red meat products for interstate shipments MUST have come from humanely slaughtered animals
   D. red meat on government consignment must have come from humanely slaughtered animals

48. Squamouscell carcinoma has spread from the eye to the parotid lymph node.
The proper course of action would be to condemn 48.____
   A. the animal
   B. the head and tongue
   C. the head, tongue, and liver
   D. the lungs, spleen, and liver

49. A food borne disease caused by intoxication is 49.____
   A. botulism
   B. salmonella
   C. trichinella
   D. shigella

50. The use of pit-type milking parlors may result in the spread of 50. D
A. rhino
B. anthrax
C. rabies
D. lepto

# KEY (CORRECT ANSWERS)

| | | | | |
|---|---|---|---|---|
| 1. B | 11. A | 21. C | 31. B | 41. C |
| 2. C | 12. B | 22. A | 32. D | 42. B |
| 3. A | 13. A | 23. B | 33. D | 43. A |
| 4. D | 14. A | 24. A | 34. C | 44. D |
| 5. C | 15. A | 25. A | 35. B | 45. D |
| 6. A | 16. C | 26. D | 36. A | 46. D |
| 7. D | 17. D | 27. B | 37. B | 47. A |
| 8. A | 18. A | 28. B | 38. B | 48. B |
| 9. B | 19. D | 29. C | 39. C | 49. A |
| 10. A | 20. D | 30. B | 40. C | 50. D |

# TEST 2

DIRECTIONS: Each question or incomplete statement is followed by several suggested answers or completions. Select the one that BEST answers the question or completes the statement. *PRINT THE LETTER OF THE CORRECT ANSWER IN THE SPACE AT THE RIGHT.*

1. The factors that influence the frequency of infection at different seasons of the year is 1.____
   A. dosage B. the vector
   C. the vehicle D. water

2. VE causes disease in 2.____
   A. dogs B. cattle C. swine D. goats

3. Genetic information of virus is contained in the 3.____
   A. nucleic acid B. protein coat
   C. viral enzymes-neurinimidas D. lipid coat

4. Bluetongue is transmitted by 4.____
   A. ticks B. gnats C. lice D. fleas

5. The MOST significant chemical sign of infectious feline enteritis is 5.____
   A. depression B. increased temperature
   C. inappetance D. leukopenia

6. A chemical substance that is legal to add to meat products is 6.____
   A. formaldehyde B. sulfuric acid
   C. salicylic acid D. salt peter

7. Congenital microspherocytosis in the dog is due to 7.____
   A. a hereditary defect in erythron
   B. fedef anemia
   C. trauma anemia
   D. hemoparasites

8. The obvious difference between the semen of a boar and a bull is in 8.____
   A. chemical composition B. volume
   C. color D. appearance

9. The MOST common cause of parathyroid hyperplasia in the dog is 9.____
   A. chronic interstitial nephritis
   B. chronic interstitial nepititis
   C. diet
   D. chronic gastritis

10. In diabetes mellitus there is a hyperglycemia and polyphagia, yet weight is lost. 10.____
This is because
A. glucose is metabolized MORE slowly
B. enzymes for glucose metabolism are inhibited
C. glucose transport across cells is inadequate
D. of the lower renal threshold for glucose

11. Persistent dribbling of urine in a one-week-old female calf is *most likely* due to 11.____
A. Meckel's diverticulum
B. hypospodius
C. persistent patent urachus
D. allantois

12. MOST of the blood passing from the caudal vena cava to the left atrium in the fetus goes through the 12.____
A. ductus arteriosum
B. ductus venosus
C. foramen orale
D. lung

13. A change in the composition of milk during mastitis is due to a 13.____
A. casein increase
B. lactose increase
C. chloride increase
D. decrease in neutralized fats

14. To test trichinosis free swine at a U.S. slaughter plant, ________ is needed. 14.____
A. squash preparations
B. a direct microscopic exam
C. heat preparation
D. a gross exam

15. The temperature and time for pasteurization is ________ seconds. 15.____
A. 143$^{o}$ for 30
B. 161$^{o}$ for 15
C. 212$^{o}$ for 15
D. 161$^{o}$ for 30

16. When biopsying a subcutaneous hemangioma ______ should be used. 16.____
A. a punch biopsy
B. an excision biopsy
C. an incision biopsy
D. paracentesis

17. Equine influenza is caused by ________ virus. 17.____
A. myxo
B. adena
C. papovo
D. herpes

18. At which stage of development of chlamydial organisms does binary fission occur? 18.____
A. Initial body
B. Elementary body
C. Binary body
D. none of the above

19. The ______ virus is characterized by basophilic intracellular inclusion bodies. 19.____
A. myxo
B. papovo
C. herpes
D. adeno

20. The typical signs of primary hyperparathyroidism in the dog are 20.____
    A. hypocalcemia, hypercalcuria, hypophosphatemia, and hypophosphoturia
    B. hypercalcemia, hypocalcuria, hypophosphotemia, and hyperphosphoturia
    C. hypercalcemia, hypercalcuria, hyperphosphotemis, and hyperphosphaturia
    D. hypocalcemia, hypercalcuria, hyperphosphtemia, and hyperphosphaturia

21. Pyloric stenosis is BEST differentiated from pyloric spasm by 21.____
    A. a clinical exam
    B. radiology
    C. a CBC
    D. anticholinergic drugs

22. Vomition in the equine is associated with 22.____
    A. severe gastritis
    B. laryngeal paralysis
    C. severe gastric dilitation
    D. sinusitis

23. Non-absorbable sutures should be left in the cornia before removal for _______ days. 23.____
    A. 7
    B. 14 to 21
    C. 30
    D. 60

24. Teat canal obstruction are MOSTLY 24.____
    A. upper
    B. lower
    C. entire
    D. medial

25. During blood transfusions in the cat, crossmatching is 25.____
    A. ALWAYS important
    B. NOT important as it rarely affects the recipient
    C. important if it comes from more that one donor
    D. NEVER important

26. The main contraindication for barbiturate use in C-sections is 26.____
    A. agalactia
    B. vomition
    C. depression of the fetus
    D. temporary paralysis of the hind legs

27. A number of mature toms are dying in a large flock. Signs exhibited are listlessness, weakness, and diarrhea, with a number showing purple-red caruncles. The diagnosis is *most likely* 27.____
    A. eripipilathrix insidiosa
    B. vibrio
    C. mycoplomagallinarum
    D. none of the above

28. In the Kingdom Protista, the Eucarions have 28.____
    A. nuclei that are free in the cytoplasm
    B. discrete nuclei within the cytoplasm
    C. chromatin that isn't contained in the nuclei
    D. no endoplasmic reticulum

29. Use of bulk tanks in storing milk (repeat) - cause for higher incidence of 29.____
A. contamination
B. mesoyshike bact.
C. spore forming
D. strep ag.

30. Death from anthrax is caused by 30.____
A. mechanical blockage of the capillaries
B. thrombi of the capillaries
C. toxin destroying kidneys and blood vessels
D. endotoxin causing mass hemorrhage

31. Rancid milk is caused by 31.____
A. lipase activity
B. improper cooling
C. coliform container
D. increased leukocytes

32. A cow presented for slaughter with cancer is cachectic and has open abscesses. 32.____
The cow should be
A. slaughtered for cooking
B. condemned, slaughtered and tanked
C. passed, and the head condemned
D. sold for treatment

33. The parasite that causes cardiovascular problems in the dog is 33.____
A. T. canis
B. strongyloides
C. dirofilaria immitus
D. diplydium caninuin

34. Bluetongue is transmitted by 34.____
A. the tabanid
B. the gnat
C. the tick
D. contact

35. The virus type that is known for its latency is
A. corona
B. reo
C. herpes
D. pacorna ona

36. Vibriosis is self-limiting in the 36.____
A. boar, nanny, and billy goat
B. mare, ewe, and billy goat
C. ram, ewe, and billy goat
D. ewe, cow, and stallion

37. Potassium may exert a synergistic effect with other drugs used on the heart by 37.____
A. reversing sinus tachycardia due to overdoses of quinidine
B. decreasing atrial fibrillation
C. increasing the effect of procaine
D. increasing the effect of fluid elimination of carbonic anhydrase inhibitors

38. The MOST successful means of treating an ununited anconeal process is 38.____
A. surgical removal
B. steroids
C. to cast it in extension
D. cage rest

39. With fluid depletion and shock due to severe burns, whole blood infusion is contraindicated primarily because 39.____
    A. Na levels are too high
    B. it causes decreased colloid osomotic pressure
    C. the erythrocyte count is already too high
    D. increased potassium ions produce a toxic effect

40. Stenotic nares in a dog are due to 40.____
    A. collapsed alar cartilages
    B. a malformed septum
    C. cleft palate
    D. an elongated soft palate

41. Cauterization is BEST used for treating the equine cannon bone with 41.____
    A. suppurative arthritis
    B. aseptic periostitis
    C. fractured splints
    D. osteomyelitis

42. The time-temperature relationship of pasteurization is MOST concerned with 42.____
    A. killing milk borne pathogens
    B. delaying spoilage
    C. killing all pathogens
    D. removing reductase

43. The complement fixation test exhibits the presence of 43.____
    A. specific complement
    B. specific antigen
    C. specific antibody
    D. amboceptors

44. A cow at a slaughterhouse with antemortem signs of milk fever should be 44.____
    A. condemned and tanked
    B. treated with calcium and returned in 10 days
    C. treated as a suspect and slaughtered at the end of the day
    D. slaughtered normally

45. The principal vector of canine babesiasis is 45.____
    A. dermocentor
    B. rhipicephalus
    C. demodex
    D. linognathus

46. The chief sign of fibrotic or ossifying myositis in the horse is ______ phase of stride. 46.____
    A. a shortened anterior
    B. a shortened posterior
    C. abduction in the anterior
    D. abduction in the posterior

47. The BEST diagnosis sign of pyelonephritis in the cow is 47.____
    A. temperature, pulse, and respiration
    B. the size of the ureters
    C. small amounts of urination of hb urine
    D. pain on deep palpation of the right paralumbar fossa

48. Leucopenia is *most commonly* seen with 48.____
A. hog cholera
B. anthrax
C. IBR
D. circumscribed peritonitis

49. A case is presented of several dead cows in a dairy herd. 49.____
Post mortem examination showed Septicerma, enlarged spleen, hemolyzed blood, and petechial hemorrhages.
The diagnosis is
A. anthrax
B. hemorrhagic Septicemia
C. malignant edema
D. bracken fern

50. A cow suffers from bilaterally distended jugulars and submandibular edema. 50.____
The *most likely* cause is
A. actinobacillosis
B. snake bite
C. traumatic pericarditis
D. intestinal parasitism

# KEY (CORRECT ANSWERS)

| | | | | |
|---|---|---|---|---|
| 1. B | 11. C | 21. B | 31. A | 41. B |
| 2. C | 12. C | 22. C | 32. B | 42. A |
| 3. A | 13. A | 23. B | 33. C | 43. B |
| 4. B | 14. B | 24. B | 34. B | 44. B |
| 5. D | 15. B | 25. B | 35. C | 45. A |
| 6. D | 16. C | 26. C | 36. D | 46. A |
| 7. A | 17. A | 27. A | 37. C | 47. B |
| 8. B | 18. A | 28. B | 38. A | 48. A |
| 9. A | 19. A | 29. A | 39. C | 49. A |
| 10. C | 20. B | 30. C | 40. A | 50. C |

# EXAMINATION SECTION

## TEST 1

DIRECTIONS: Each question or incomplete statement is followed by several suggested answers or completions. Select the one that BEST answers the question or completes the statement. *PRINT THE LETTER OF THE CORRECT ANSWER IN THE SPACE AT THE RIGHT.*

1. Intussusception in a dog is BEST treated by 1.____
   A. gastroenterastomy  B. entero-enterastomy
   C. enterotomy  D. choleceptotomy

2. Vaginal hyperplasia in a bitch is seen in 2.____
   A. proestrus  B. estrus
   C. metestrum  D. pseudocycosis

3. The TB strain(s) that affect swine is (are) 3.____
   A. human  B. avian and human
   C. avian, human, and bovine  D. bovine and avian

4. K+ is added to electrolytes when cellular hydration is desired because it 4.____
   A. is the chief intracellular cation
   B. balances the electrolyte solution
   C. aids in the excretion of Na+
   D. is beneficial to the heart

5. Blackleg infection in sheep is MOST common 5.____
   A. at 6 months to 2 years of age
   B. after ingestion of contaminated feed
   C. following wound infection from docking, shearing, or lambing
   D. after inhalation of contaminant

6. The MOST common leptospira in cattle and swine is 6.____
   A. icterohemorrhagicum  B. pomona
   C. canicola  D. hadjuri

7. The latent period is a particularly important consideration for 7.____
   A. picorna  B. myxo
   C. herpes  D. parvo

8. Feline infectious peritonitis shows 8.____
   A. enteritis  B. anorexia
   C. depression  D. leucopenia

9. Relief of a visoid mucus is provided with 9.____
   A. atropine  B. pilocarpine
   C. oxygen  D. a steam chamber

10. The MOST irritating anesthetic to the respiratory tract is 10.____
    A. halothane  B. ether
    C. chloroform  D. thiopental

11. Atropine sulfate, a drug used in the treatment of periodic opthalmia of horses is used to 11.____
    A. decrease tear production and reduce facial scald
    B. decrease pain because of relaxation of smooth muscle spasm
    C. decrease damage to internal ocular structures due to light by constricting the pupil
    D. prevent adhesions of the iris to the lens

12. Immune tolerance is due to 12.____
    A. exposure to an antigen before the development of immune competence
    B. repeated injection of an antigen
    C. exposure to large doses of toxic substance
    D. exposure to an antigen after the development of immune competence

13. Cl. perfringens in sheep causes 13.____
    A. malignant edema
    B. blackleg
    C. enterotoxemia
    D. agalactia

14. When using sodium pentobarbitol for euthanasia, death is caused by 14.____
    A. respiratory failure
    B. cardiac failure
    C. cerebral anoxia
    D. heart block

15. The tissue of choice for examination in suspected mycotic abortion in the bovine is the 15.____
    A. placenta
    B. fetal skin
    C. fetal liver
    D. fetal heart

16. Leptospirosis in swine can be prevented by 16.____
    A. vaccination with MOST prevalent bacterin in the herd
    B. elimination of ALL positive blood tested animals
    C. the introduction of non-injected males into the herd
    D. any of the above

17. Hepatized lung from pneumonia would show in exudate of alveoli 17.____
    A. lymphocytes
    B. leucocytes
    C. fibroblasts
    D. neutrophils

18. Adenomatous hyperplasia of the parathyroid results in 18.____
    A. gignatsin and skeletal gravity
    B. osteomaleria and kidney cysts
    C. loss of hair and abeneria
    D. paralysis

19. In hepatogenous photosensitization, the sensitizing agent is 19.____
    A. indole
    B. phylcerythrin
    C. chlorophyl
    D. none of the above

20. The action of heparin is promptly terminated by. 20.____
A. menedion
B. methylene blue
C. vitamin $K_1$
D. protamine sulfate

21. Quinidine sulfate is used in heart disease because it 21.____
A. depresses cardiac muscle
B. stimulates cardiac muscle
C. abolishes sympathetic response
D. abolishes parasympathetic response

22. To make a diagnosis of anthrax in swine, a ________ sample should be taken. 22.____
A. blood
B. bronchial lymph node
C. pharyngeal lymph node
D. kidney

23. Botulism is UNLIKE other food poisonings in that 23.____
A. its signs may NOT be only gastrointestinal
B. it has a shorter incubation period
C. it has a longer incubation period
D. its toxin is NOT killed by cooking

24. A moderately affected hog carcass with cysticercus cellulosa should be 24.____
A. condemned
B. passed
C. passed after heating to 143° F
D. passed after removing affected parts

25. Avain Arizona infections affect ________ *only*. 25.____
A. ducks
B. fowls
C. turkeys
D. geese

26. The intermediate host for dipylidium canis is the 26.____
A. culex
B. ctenocephalide
C. tick
D. louse

27. Following the removal of interdigital fibroma, immobilization of the claws is BEST affected by 27.____
A. a paster cast
B. electricians tape
C. clip shoes
D. wiring the toes

28. Skin penetration of the cercaid form of fluke is MOST often found in the 28.____
A. lungs
B. small intestine
C. liver
D. blood

29. Dermatophyte isolated from ring worm of the cat that is transmissible to man is 29.____
A. microspyrum gypseum
B. tricophytom verticosun
C. microsporum canis
D. tricophyton mentagraphytes

30. Non-inherited cerebellar hypoplasia in the bovine calf is caused by 30.____
A. IBR
B. BVD

C. lepto
D. bovine enzootic pheuropneumonia

31. Extrinsic pancreatic function can BEST be determined by Jasper's test for 31.____
A. lipase
B. amylase
C. pepsin
D. trypsin

32. Bone grafts are BEST indicated with 32.____
A. a femoral head fracture
B. a compound fracture
C. non-union healing
D. osteomylitis

33. The use of a Kurshner nail is advantageous because it 33.____
A. allows for improved rotational stability
B. is easy to insert and remove
C. need NOT be removed
D. does NOT interfere with medullary hematopoesis

34. Contrast radiography of the esophagus in the cat reveals a rough separated mucosal surface in the caudal third of the organ. 34.____
This indicates
A. a normal pattern
B. esophagitis
C. dilatation
D. neoplasm

35. The two fungi that cause bovine abortion *most commonly* are 35.____
A. mucomycosis of asprigellus
B. asprigillus histoplasmoses
C. histoplasmosis and blastomycoses
D. coccidiodomycosis and histoplasmosis

36. The adults of S. vulgaris are found in the 36.____
A. stomach
B. cecum of the colon
C. anterior mesenteric artery
D. heart

37. The common testicular tumors listed in decreasing order of frequency are the ________ tumors. 37.____
A. seminoma, interstitial, and sertoli
B. tubular carcinoma, seminoma, and sertoli
C. interstitial cell, seminoma, and sertoli
D. other variations of above

38. On auscultation of the chest of an animal, one side is devoid of tubular and vessicular sounds. 38.____
The MOST helpful diagnostic procedure would be
A. to hold the animal off feed for 95 hours
B. to attempt to aspirate fluid from the pleural cavity
C. the application of a counter-irritant to the other side of the chest
D. to cast the animal and see if the lung sounds change

39. The treatment of choice for an ununited anconeal process in a cat is to 39.____
   A. use a stainless steel screw
   B. wire it
   C. fire it
   D. remove it

40. In a fracture of a long bone, the FIRST consideration by the veterinarian should be o+ 40.____
   A. shock and its complication
   B. proper fixation
   C. muscle action on fixation
   D. the extent of the fracture

41. The MOST frequent cause of purulent pericarditis in the cow is 41.____
   A. foreign body traumatism
   B. congenital heart disease
   C. allergic reaction due to strep infection
   D. cancer of the pericardium

42. An intracapsular femoral fracture is MORE severe than an extracapsular fracture because 42.____
   A. it destroys the blood supply
   B. it destroys the nerve supply
   C. fracture pieces cause arthritis
   D. all of the above

43. An immunity existing as a result of previous exposure to a micro-organism is called a(n) ________ immunity. 43.____
   A. genetic
   B. constitutional
   C. acquired
   D. artificial passive

44. For a laboratory diagnosis of anthrax in swine, the ________ is necessary. 44.____
   A. spleen
   B. liver
   C. lymph node
   D. kidney

45. A stag-like hog is presented at slaughter. At P-M it has one retained testicle.
The hog should 45.____
   A. be condemned at P-M
   B. have been condemned at A-M
   C. pass for slaugher
   D. be tested with heat and the olfactory test before making any decisions

46. The urinary antiseptic action of methenamine is due to 46.____
   A. formic acid
   B. phenol
   C. cresol
   D. formaldehyde

47. Suturing the dorsal commissure of the vulva in a barren mare with a genital infection 47.____
   A. elongates the perimum and strengthens the vaginal walls
   B. prevents atrophy of the vagina in old mares
   C. prevents the dorsal commissure of the vagina from tipping anterially
   D. prevents aspiration of debris and air into the anterior vagina

48. A valuable young bitch suffers from dystocia due to two live pups in a hysterocele. 48.____
It is BEST to follow through with
   A. a herniagraphy C-Section
   B. 1 cc of POP every 30 to 60 minutes
   C. forceps retraction
   D. a C-section of hysteropexy

49. The proper technique for dog castration is to make 49.____
   A. 2 incisions on each side of median raphae
   B. 1 incision paralleling the median raphae
   C. 1 incision in the middle of the scrotum
   D. 1 incision on the midline anterior to the scrotum

50. A dog is presented with bilateral dilated pupils, episcleral congestion, corneal edema, an insensitive cornea, epiphora, and pain. 50.____
The *most likely* diagnosis is
   A. acute glaucoma
   B. neoplasia
   C. acute iridocyclitis
   D. acute conjunctivitis

# KEY (CORRECT ANSWERS)

| | | | | |
|---|---|---|---|---|
| 1. C | 11. D | 21. A | 31. D | 41. A |
| 2. B | 12. A | 22. C | 32. C | 42. A |
| 3. C | 13. C | 23. A | 33. A | 43. C |
| 4. B | 14. A | 24. A | 34. A | 44. C |
| 5. C | 15. A | 25. C | 35. A | 45. D |
| 6. B | 16. B | 26. B | 36. B | 46. D |
| 7. C | 17. C | 27. D | 37. C | 47. D |
| 8. C | 18. B | 28. C | 38. B | 48. A |
| 9. A | 19. B | 29. C | 39. D | 49. D |
| 10. B | 20. D | 30. B | 40. A | 50. A |

# TEST 2

DIRECTIONS: Each question or incomplete statement is followed by several suggested answers or completions. Select the one that BEST answers the question or completes the statement. *PRINT THE LETTER OF THE CORRECT ANSWER IN THE SPACE AT THE RIGHT.*

1. Hemoglobinuria is NOT seen in 1.____
   A. anaplasmosis
   B. toxemias
   C. bacillary hemoglobinuria
   D. parturient hemoglobinuria

2. Aldosterone is responsible for the absorption of 2.____
   A. K B. Na C. Ca D. H

3. The cerebro-spinal fluid from the ventricles communicates with that of the sub-arachnoid space by the 3.____
   A. foramen of monro
   B. central canal of the spinal cord
   C. foramen of magendse
   D. foramen magnum

4. An equine sarcoid is 4.____
   A. a keratinized neoplasm of the skin
   B. found in old horses
   C. found in young horses
   D. found in more than one animal on a farm

5. The muscle that causes extension of the hock when the stifle is extended in the horse is the 5.____
   A. long digital extensor
   B. superficial digital extensor
   C. deep digital extensor
   D. anterior tibialis

6. The nerve to the flexor carpi radialis is the 6.____
   A. laterial femoropatellar
   B. laterial collateral
   C. medial collateral
   D. medial patellar

7. Hematuria at the end of micturition is indicative of a lesion in the 7.____
   A. bladder B. kidney C. ureters D. urethra

8. The MOST resistant non-parasitic larva in the external environment is 8.____
   A. oxyuris equi B. parascaris equorum
   C. megastomum D. none of the above

9. A horse with encephalitis with a febrile response has 9.____
   A. rabies B. sleeping sickness
   C. ETA D. rinderpest

10. The type of leptosporosis *most commonly* seen in cattle and swine in the U.S. is 10.____
   A. ictero hemorrhagica B. grippo
   C. pommona D. serjo

11. The MOST common cause of alveolar periostitis in the first upper cheek tooth in the horse is 11.____
   A. patent infundibulum
   B. permanent teeth eruption
   C. enamel points
   D. sinusitis

12. In the fetus blood flow follows post cava to the umbilical vein via the 12.____
   A. ductus arteriosus
   B. foramen ovale
   C. interventricular defect
   D. pulmonary artery

13. The medial pulmonary artery is usually hypertrophied in the 13.____
   A. cow B. dog C. equine D. swine

14. Puerperal hemoglobinemia of cattle is caused by 14.____
   A. metabolic disorder B. anaplasmosis
   C. piroplasmosis D. overeating

15. Mycotic stomatitis is an important clinical disease because it is difficult to differentiate from ________ stomatitis. 15.____
   A. vesicular B. necrotic
   C. allergic D. any

16. Scrotal hernias in the dog occur 16.____
   A. never B. rarely
   C. commonly D. in young dogs

17. A pre-natal infestation of puppies with hookworms occurs 17.____
   A. by maternal passage
   B. by skin penetration of the pups
   C. by ingestion of the eggs by the pups
   D. during delivery

18. In a barbiturate overdose, what should be done first? 18.____
   A. Metrazol
   B. Artificial respiration
   C. Epinephrine (1 cc) in the heart
   D. Shock treatment

19. In addition to stimulating intestinal motility, carbachol will 19.____
   A. increase bile secretion
   B. cause polyuria
   C. dilate the pupils
   D. increase salivation

20. Transmission of viral pneumonia in a swine herd is perpetuated by 20.____
   A. lungworms
   B. infected brood sow carriers
   C. birds and other vermin
   D. vaccinations

21. Post mortem examination of a beef carcass shows one live cysticercoid. The disposition should be to 21.____
   A. condemn entirely
   B. condemn the cyst and pass the carcass
   C. condemn the head and pass the carcass
   D. pass unrestricted

22. To contrast a radioluscent cystic calculi, _________ should be used 22.____
   A. air
   B. water
   C. didrast
   D. 15% NaI

23. The BEST approach to ooporhorectomy in the horse with respect to the safest surgical technique is 23.____
   A. vaginal
   B. flank
   C. midline
   D. paramedian

24. The term describing the abnormal decrease of the angle between the femoral shaft and the femoral neck is 24.____
   A. coxa plana
   B. coxa valga
   C. coxa vara
   D. coxitis senilas

25. The incision site in a colt to correct an intussusception is at the 26.____
   A. right flank
   B. left flank
   C. midline
   D. paralumbar fossa

26. Ornithosis *commonly* invades the _________ system. 26.____
   A. reticulo-endothelial
   B. hepatic
   C. respiratory epithelium
   D. marrow

27. The MOST unusual crystals found in the urine of female dogs and castrated male cats are 27.____
   A. citrates
   B. oxalates
   C. phosphates
   D. uric acid

28. The parasympathetic nerve supply to the rectum is via the _________ nerve. 28.____
   A. lumbar-splanchnic
   B. pelvic
   C. vagus
   D. pudendal

29. The tissue that is MOST susceptible to radiation is in the 29.____
A. brain
B. skin
C. gonads
D. striated muscles

30. If you see swelling above the maxillary bone in cattle, you should suspect 30.____
A. cysts
B. actinomycosis
C. alveolar periostitis
D. abscess

31. Less oxygen is taken up by the systemic tissues when 31.____
A. $CO_2$% within the circulation *increases* from .3% to 3%
B. body temperature *increases* 2 to 4 degrees
C. activity level *increases*
D. hemoglobin levels within the circulation is *decreased*

32. A virus that affects mucous membranes primarily is 32.____
A. rinderpest
B. ICH
C. distemper
D. panleukopenia

33. On auscultation, harsh vesicular sounds are diagnostic of 33.____
A. pneumothorax
B. hydrothorax
C. emphysema
D. consolidation

34. In a 30 cm. thick well muscled limb, the BEST way to eliminate secondary radiation is by 34.____
A. using a long cone
B. a sheet of aluminum over the plate
C. a reciprocating potter grid
D. increasing the film-target distance

35. The breed(s) of dog that *most commonly* have mastocytoma is (are) the 35.____
A. boxer and bull terrier
B. manchester and chihuahua
C. collie
D. poodle

36. You can palpate a non-radioopaque calculi in a dog's bladder. 36.____
The contrast media that you would use is
A. air
B. 15% iodine
C. barium sulfate
D. diodrast

37. The *most likely* site of tumors in the long bones is the 37.____
A. metaphysis
B. diaphysis
C. epiphysis
D. periosteum

38. What is the name of the inverting suture used on the rumen? 38.____
A. Gobbler
B. Mattress
C. Continuous
D. Quill

39. To be fertile semen, _______ percent must be normal, active structures. 39.____
   A. 20 B. 40 C. 60 D. 80

40. The ureters of the chicken empty into the 40.____
   A. urodeum
   B. proctodeum
   C. coprodeum
   D. rectum

41. Chickens are presented for necropsy. Some are dead, and some are shaking their tails, heads, and bodies. They have 41.____
   A. encephalomalacia
   B. Newcastle's disease
   C. avian encephalitis
   D. equine encephalitis

42. On ventral midline incision in the cow, how do you find the free margin of the omentum? 42.____
   A. Go anterior and pull the omentum posterior
   B. Go posterior and pull the omentum anterior
   C. Cut through the omentum
   D. Go to the left and pull to the right

43. Chagas disease is transmitted by the 43.____
   A. mosquito B. tsetse fly C. mite D. horse fly

44. The oxygen consumption or demand is reduced when 44.____
   A. $PCO_2$ *increases*
   B. metabolic activity *increases*
   C. metabolic activity *decreases*
   D. $PCO_2$ *decreases*

45. Distemper differs from ICH because 45.____
   A. foxes are NOT affected
   B. the virus is passed in the air
   C. the virus is passed in urine
   D. the virus CANNOT be passed via any media

46. When the vagus nerve is cut at the cervical area and the anterior end is stimulated 46.____
   A. the rumen contracts
   B. the esophogeal groove contracts
   C. ALL stomachs contract
   D. ALL sphincters contract

47. A complication of an open, draining tract in the axillary region is 47.____
   A. tetanus
   B. abscess formation
   C. emphysema in the surrounding tissue
   D. viral infection

48. The hormone that is MOST responsible for control of phosphate elimination in the kidney is 48.____
   A. vasopressin
   B. parathormone
   C. aldosterone
   D. FSH

49. The largest fluid filled compartment in the body is 49.____
A. intracellular B. interstitial
C. gastro-intestinal D. peritoneal

50. The innermost layer of muscle incised in the paralumbar fossa of cattle during surgery is the 50.____
A. external abdominal oblique
B. internal abdominal oblique
C. transversus
D. rectus abdomenus

---

# KEY (CORRECT ANSWERS)

| | | | | |
|---|---|---|---|---|
| 1. A | 11. A | 21. B | 31. D | 41. C |
| 2. B | 12. A | 22. A | 32. A | 42. B |
| 3. C | 13. B | 23. A | 33. C | 43. B |
| 4. A | 14. A | 24. C | 34. C | 44. C |
| 5. D | 15. B | 25. C | 35. A | 45. C |
| 6. C | 16. B | 26. C | 36. A | 46. C |
| 7. A | 17. A | 27. C | 37. A | 47. C |
| 8. C | 18. B | 28. D | 38. B | 48. B |
| 9. B | 19. D | 29. C | 39. B | 49. A |
| 10. C | 20. A | 30. C | 40. A | 50. C |

---

# EXAMINATION SECTION

## TEST 1

DIRECTIONS: Each question consists of a statement. You are to indicate whether the statement is TRUE (T) or FALSE (F). *PRINT THE LETTER OF THE CORRECT ANSWER IN THE SPACE AT THE RIGHT.*

1. Agglutination is a test for mycoplasma. 1. T

2. When an outbreak of scabies starts, the veterinarian can treat WITHOUT reporting it. 2. F

3. In cattle posterior pituitary hormone plays a role in causing contraction of udder alveoli and *increased* mammary pressure. 3. T

4. In Fe treatment, parenteral administration is better than oral. 4. F

5. In renal secondary hyperparathyroidism, blood and urine analyses reveal *increased* pH and *decreased* $Ca^{++}$. 5. X

6. Ganglionic blocking agents are used in treating pulmonary edema as they *decrease* the pulmonary blood volume. 6. F

7. Winter tetany is associated with a diet *low* in grain. 7. F

8. Palaxolone reduces bloat by reducing froth. 8. T

9. Foreleg paresis is a *primary* sign of cervical disc disease. 9. T

10. Adrenocorticoids cause protein conversion to glucose. 10. T

11. An affect of digitalis is compensation of the heart. 11. T

12. To perform colopexy, tack the bladder down to the abdominal wall. 12. F

13. The approach of castration in the dog is over each testicle. 13. F

14. The simple continuous suture pattern is the only type of pattern used to close the kidney after a nephrolithatomy. 14. F

15. Sterilization of non-steamable instruments can be done by ethylene oxide. 15. T

16. If histamine is injected IV, a sign that is seen is arterial BP. 16. T

17. Non-absorbable sutures should NOT be used for teat lacerations. 17. F

18. Cervical salivary cysts *usually* involve the parotid salivary gland. 18. X

19. The action of heparin is terminated by protamine sulfate. 19. T

20. Thrombin causes the conversion of fibrin to fibrinogen. 20. F

21. A cow with uncomplicated LDA shows signs of a drop in milk production, frequent acetonemia, and scant watery stool. 21. T

22. The disposition of a cow with extensive lesions of actinomycosis should be killed, tanked and condemned. 22. T

23. A method of early pregnancy testing in bovine is to slip the placenta. 23. F

24. The cause of inhalation pneumonia of cattle is dry and muddy feed. 24. F

25. A dog is under morphine and sodium pentobarbital anesthesia. Administration of $O_2$ causes depression of chemoreceptor response. 25. F

26. A cow that is NOT milked out and develops allergy to her own retained milk has a milk allergy. 26. F

27. Navicular disease is evidenced by bony changes on the anteriodistal border of the navicular. 27. F

28. Ectopic ureters are difficult to visualize by intravenous urography. 28. F

29. Perianal adenoma is BEST treated by castration, radiation, and surgery. 29. T

30. Thoraco-lumbar spinal fractures by decompression, reduction, and fixation. 30. T

31. Metabolic bone disorders CANNOT be differentiated from traumatic lesions by symmetrical distribution. 31. F

32. A cow with mastitis, a walled-off abscess in the udder, shedding of pus with yellow granules is suffering from botryomycosis. 32. F

33. Salmon poisoning in dogs and foxes is caused by spoiled salmon. 33. F

34. In a closed circuit anesthetic system, the vaporizer delivers the proper anesthetic concentration. 34. T

35. The BEST time to fix a hematoma on a bull's penis is after 5 to 7 days, when it is clotted. 35. T

36. Tumor removal is an indication for a pubic symphas-ectomy in a cow. 36. F

37. The *only* possible site of lympho in the cat is the kidney. 37.____

38. In elective gastro-intestinal surgery, the drug of *choice* to reduce the bacterial flora encountered would be streptomycin. 38.____

39. Saddle thrombus in the cat is located in the posterior aorta and iliac arteries. 39.____

40. Fracture of a bull's penis results from deviation of the anterior tip of the penis. 40.____

41. A colopexy is performed to tie the uterine body to the colon. 41.____

42. Post-surgical treatment of phosphate crystals in the bladder of a dog includes acidification of urine and antibiotic treatment. 42.____

43. The mechanism by which antihistamines work is stabilization of mast cells. 43.____

44. The lesions of rhinopneumonitis in the horse are characterized by focal necrosis of the liver with intranuclear inclusions in the mare. 44.____

45. Foot and mouth disease does NOT affect horses. 45.____

46. Amnionic plaques in the fetal membrane are caused by calcification. 46.____

47. To prevent excess $I_{131}$ contamination after heavy $I_{131}$ fallout, the BEST procedure would be to bring in cattle from the pasture and feed them stored feed. 47.____

48. Vascular disease in the horse is associated with strongylus vulgaris (larvae). 48.____

49. Ascarid eggs are NOT very resistant to environmental conditions and CANNOT withstand extremely cold temperatures. 49.____

50. In the dog, the flea is the internal host for diplydium caninum. 50.____

---

# KEY (CORRECT ANSWERS)

| | | | | |
|---|---|---|---|---|
| 1. T | 11. T | 21. T | 31. F | 41. F |
| 2. F | 12. F | 22. T | 32. F | 42. T |
| 3. T | 13. F | 23. T | 33. F | 43. F |
| 4. T | 14. F | 24. F | 34. T | 44. F |
| 5. F | 15. T | 25. T | 35. T | 45. T |
| 6. F | 16. F | 26. T | 36. F | 46. F |
| 7. F | 17. F | 27. T | 37. F | 47. T |
| 8. T | 18. F | 28. F | 38. F | 48. T |
| 9. T | 19. T | 29. T | 39. T | 49. F |
| 10. T | 20. F | 30. T | 40. T | 50. T |

# TEST 2

DIRECTIONS: Each question consists of a statement. You are to indicate whether the statement is TRUE (T) or FALSE (F). *PRINT THE LETTER OF THE CORRECT ANSWER IN THE SPACE AT THE RIGHT.*

1. The vagus causes MAJOR abomasal contractions. 1.____

2. Hypoglycemia is unrelated to hunger contractions. 2.____

3. An *increased* innervation ratio of muscles results in LESS delicate movements. 3.____

4. In fully developed ventricular fibrillation, the blood pressure falls quite low and there is little or no pulse. 4.____

5. The standing reflex is integrated at the spinal level. 5.____

6. The osmotic pressure in the plasma proteins in the filtrated blood and the presence of antidiuretic hormone produced by the posterior pituitary gland provides the stimulus for the reabsorption of water from the kidney tubules. 6.____

7. The function of Kupfer cells in the liver is to ingest particular matter, especially erythrocytes, and to act as macrophages for fighting infection in the body. 7.____

8. ALL animals have *sweat* as a mechanism for heat elimination. 8.____

9. Cholecystitis is inflammation of the gallbladder. 9.____

10. Hemangiomas and lymphangiomas are malignant. 10.____

11. Thrombin administered locally deters blood clotting. 11.____

12. Oxalic acid in low concentration destroys antithrombin. 12.____

13. Thyrotropic hormone is necessary for normal thyroid activity. 13.____

14. Skeletal muscle is non-striated and involuntary. 14.____

15. Lang's treatment is used for treatment of impaction in the horse. 15.____

16. If you suspect a case of glanders, you should use antimony or arsenical compounds. 16.____

17. Cutting the vagus nerve in the cranial region, and stimulating the peripheral end would slow the heart rate, constrict the bronchioles, contract the stomach and close the esophageal groove. 17.____

18. Bronchiolectasis is dilation of the bronchioles. 18. T

19. Capillary blood pressure as compared with blood pressure of the rest of the body is MORE on the venous and LESS on the arteriole end. 19. F

20. Viruses are classified by tissue predilection. 20. T

21. The method of removal of a papilloma or fibropapilloma from the penis of a bull is x-ray and surgery. 21. F

22. Lesions of viral diseases CANNOT be differentiated by animal inoculation . 22. F

23. As the pressure *increases* MORE atmospheric air is absorbed by the alveoli, and as the atmospheric pressure *decreases* there is LESS air absorbed. 23. T

24. Rotation of the heart, to the right during systole, causes a sudden *increase* in pressure against the chest wall, resulting in apex heart beat in the dog. 24. X T

25. The milky white substance absorbed by the lymphatics from the digestive tract is chyle. 25. T

26. In domestic animals, blood enters the lymph glands at the hilus. 26. T

27. The PRIMARY cause of canine pneumothorax is diaphragmatic hernia. 27. T

28. A neurectomy of the peroneal nerve cut above the line of demarcation between the long and lateral digital extensor m. is above the hock. 28. T

29. Intestinal obstruction rarely occurs at the pelvic flexure. 29. F

30. Strangles can be treated MORE effectively today than 25 years ago because of the discovery of penicillin. 30. T

31. Scrotal hernias in pigs are NOT hereditary. 31. F

32. Severing the superficial flexor in the horse causes the fetlock to be raised in relation to the ground. 32. X F

33. In axillary lacerations of thoracic punctures in the horse, emphysema of the surrounding tissue is a common complication. 33. X T

34. Lesion in the brain can cause prolonged gestation in guernsey cattle. 34. T

35. The humoral factor, renin, *decreases* the blood pressure. 35. F

36. The eggs of hens may contain capillaris helminth eggs. 36.____

37. In swine, leptospiruvia persists after clinical recovery for 3 months or LESS. 37.____

38. Tannic acid is used as an absorbent in the precipitate protein test. 38.____

39. Tissue anoxia stimulates erythrocyte production with vitamin $B_{12}$. 39.____

40. Cardiac abnormalities are impossible during general anesthesia because of the mechanism of anesthesia. 40.____

41. Wheezing is a sign of laryngeal hemiplegia. 41.____

42. Atropine is indicated in the treatment of glaucoma. 42.____

43. Insulin is part of the treatment of ketosis. 43.____

44. Anthrax usually cause hemolysis of blood agar. 44.____

45. Aortic thrombosis is LEAST common in the turkey. 45.____

46. The MAIN motor nerve innervation to the tongue is hypoglossal. 46.____

47. In the esophagus, parasitic infection is frequently followed by neoplasia. 47.____

48. Hippurid acid is absorbed by the kidneys. 48.____

49. Iodine forms a large alcohol-soluable molecule with the gentian violet which is removed from the gram negative bacteria, but retained by those which stain positive. 49.____

50. TB organisms are acid fast, nonmotile, nonencapsulated and aerobic. 50.____

---

# KEY (CORRECT ANSWERS)

| | | | | |
|---|---|---|---|---|
| 1. T | 11. F | 21. T | 31. F | 41. T |
| 2. F | 12. T | 22. F | 32. F | 42. F |
| 3. F | 13. T | 23. T | 33. T | 43. T |
| 4. T | 14. F | 24. T | 34. T | 44. F |
| 5. F | 15. T | 25. T | 35. F | 45. F |
| 6. T | 16. F | 26. T | 36. F | 46. T |
| 7. T | 17. T | 27. T | 37. F | 47. T |
| 8. F | 18. T | 28. T | 38. T | 48. F |
| 9. T | 19. F | 29. F | 39. F | 49. T |
| 10. F | 20. T | 30. T | 40. F | 50. T |

---

# EXAMINATION SECTION

## TEST 1

Questions 1-35.

DIRECTIONS: Fill in the blank space(s) the word (or words) which is (are) the correct answer(s) to the question.

1. On doing a necropsy of the chicken, one would find the syrinx at________.

2. In the dog apocrine sweat glands are found in ________.

3. Pathological penile deviation in a bull is due to an insufficiency of the ________.

4. The grounol substance of connective tissue is *mainly* composed of ________.

5. The superficial layer of the cornea is composed of ________.

6. Blood flow to the pelvic gland is routed *primarily* via the ________.

7. Filtration within the kidney is performed by the ________.

8. While the function of the posterior pituitary gland is to act as a starch release gland of hormones, it receives stimuli from the ________.

9. Repolarization of the action potential within the ventricular cell is *principally* due to ________.

10. Calcitomine is involved in the regulation of extracellular calcium.
    This hormone is *probably* produced in the ________.

11. The MOST common tumors in horses contain sarcoid tissue that recurs from excision.
    Such tumors are best described as ________.

12. A *common* sequela of esophageal obstruction in the horse is ________.

13. Two antibiotics that have been linked with gastro-intestinal disorders and diarrhea in horses are ________.

14. Pregnancy disease of ewes is MOST common in ________.

15. A jugular pulse in pericarditis, caused by hardware disease, is due to ________.

16. In cattle that are in shock, blood may pool in the abdominal viscera and be found in the intestinal lumen after death. This type of blood crossing is called ________.

17. Clencyzoonosis is a relatively rare disease of cats. The premonitory clinical signs are ________.

18. In addition to gastro-intestinal symptoms, panleukopenia is a disease that produces ________.

19. Pseudoacetaminophen and acetophenethodine are contraindicated in the treatment of saws because they are often associated with ________.

20. Tuberculosis in cats is *generally* caused by tuberculi bacilli type ________.

21. A common ear mite in cats is ________.

22. A moraxella bovis infection is transmitted between cattle *mainly* via ________.

23. Diagnosis of ascarid cramps is BEST made by ________.

24. Digitalis toxicity is potentiated by ________.

25. Halothane could trigger malignant ________ in an animal.

26. Chloramphenicol and erythromycin are *similar* in that both drugs are *primarily* ________.

27. Guaiaphenesin, a muscle relaxant, acts MOST specifically on ________.

28. The MOST probable cause of death in amoranthus poisoning, which causes perirenal edema, is ________.

29. The in vitro procedure of *choice* for confirming diagnosis of autoimmune thrombocytopenia in the dog is ________.

30. Excessive protein transport is associated with ________.

31. In a positive tuberculine test, antigenic specificity is provided by ________.

32. Schistosomiasis can occur in humans after swimming in waters containing ________.

33. The control of hydatid disease, and the elimination of its danger to humans, can be BEST obtained by ________.

34. The cause for bovine ringworm is ________.

35. The drug of *choice* for skin mycotic disease is ________.

Questions 36-50.

DIRECTIONS: Answer the following questions directly, briefly, and succinctly.

36. What is the LONGEST time that female ferrets may remain in estrus?

37. What is well known for its complicity in inducing activity of the liver's microsomal enzyme system, altering the biotransformation of other drugs?

38. What infection is MOST likely to occur concurrently with corynobacterium rhinopneumonia in a horse?

39. In the dog, what condition should be considered with cyanosis as a clinical finding?

40. Which one of the following breeds of dogs is MOST commonly affected with atopy?

41. Which gene of bacteria is MOST commonly isolated from the mammary glands of sows?

42. What muscle relaxant prevents the depolarization of the membrane at the myoneural junction by acetylcholine?

43. The antihistamine dibutamine, a beta one antagonist, would be expected to have what formacological aspects?

44. What drug is considered to cause CNS excitement in dogs?

45. On a farm, you observe a yellow-brown gas coming from a silo. In addition, you notice that 4 to 5 cows have died. What is this gas?

46. What plant is associated *primarily* with the production of teratogenic changes?

47. What cells synthetize antibodies?

48. What disease is disseminated by aerosols to humans?

49. What do you do when you discover vibriosis on a farm?

50. What must you do with a cow that shows TB lesions in its lymph nodes at slaughter?

# KEY (CORRECT ANSWERS)

1. located where the trunks originate from the trachea
2. ALL hairy areas
3. dorsal ligament
4. mucopolysaccharides
5. stratified squamous epithelium
6. femoral artery
7. glomerulol secretional layer of the Capsule of Bowman
8. hypothalamus
9. an increase in the $K^+$ conductance
10. parafollicular cells of the thyroid
11. infiltrative fibromas
12. esophageal stricture
13. tetracyclines and lyncomycin
14. older animals during the last two months of gestation
15. pressure from exudate in the pericardial sac
16. diapetesis
17. anemia, icterus, depression and fever
18. anemia and granulocytes
19. methemoglobinemia
20. bovine
21. otodectes cynotis
22. insect vector
23. observation of remission of signs following atropine sulfate therapy
24. serum levels of potassium ($K^+$)
25. hyperthemia

26. active inhibitors of protein synthesis at the ribosomal level
27. centrally acting skeletal muscles
28. hyperkalemia
29. a plate with factor-3 test
30. the aminoglobulin class
31. leukocytes
32. infected cercarial
33. the elimination of echinococcus granulosus infections in dogs
34. trichophyton verrucosum
35. griseofulvin
36. 4 months.
37. Phenobarbital.
38. Ulcerative colitis.
39. Tetralogy of Fallot.
40. Scottish terrier.
41. Klebsiella.
42. D-tubocurarine.
43. Increasing cardiac output.
44. Ethylene glycol.
45. Nitrous dioxide.
46. False ellebore (aflatoxins)
47. Plasma cells
48. Q-fever.
49. Institute sexual rest for 90 days.
50. Tank and condemn carcass.

# TEST 2

Questions 1-27.

DIRECTIONS: Fill in the blank space(s) the word (or words) which is (are) the correct answer(s) to the question.

1. Although leptospira canicula infections in dogs usually cause nephritis, they are not usually found in large numbers in the urine or sections of the kidney examined with specific fluorescent antibodies. This lack of numerous leptospira organisms is caused by ______.

2. The MOST common explanation for reactions to a TB test administered to TB infected cattle that show no visible lesions is that ______.

3. The interstate regulations regarding the production and sale of produce is under the authority of the ______.

4. Endoscopic examination of a horse suffering from dyspnea at rest reveals extreme dimpling and left displacement of the left arythenoid cartilage, causing obstruction of the larynx. The MOST likely diagnosis is ______.

5. In the horse, megalocitic hepathopaty is characteristic of ______.

6. A three year old thoroughbred was shipped from Florida to New York on rail. Following the trip, the animal is found to be depressed, anorectic, and reluctant to move. Auscultation of the thorax reveals absence of lung sounds ventral to the point of the shoulder.
   Your MOST definitive diagnostic procedure should next be ______.

7. In the acute stage of salt poisoning in swine, during the first 48 hours, the change in the cellular composition of the blood is ______.

8. The annual dose of radiation exposure of a professional radiologist is ______.

9. The normal glucose serum level in birds is ______.

10. A recently captured wild Robin is presented with severe dyspnea. Microscopic examination of droppings from the cage reveals numerous double operculated, oval-shaped ova.
    The MOST likely diagnosis is ______.

11. Feline scabies is a contagious parasitic disease of cats caused by Notoedres cat.
    Lesions are confined primarily to the ______.

12. Histopathological examination of multiple small raised tumors in the skin of a cat reveals a bunch of mononuclear cells. The MOST likely diagnosis is _mast_. cell tumor

13. A drug used in the treatment of canine atrial fibrillation is ______.

14. The treatment for Listeriosis in goats is ______.

15. After treatment for the adult heartworm, the clinical manifestations of pulmonary thromboembolism usually appear ______.

16. Canine hypothyroidism can best be treated with ______.

17. Adjusting the KV rather than MS on a twin lead x-ray machine is practical because it allows ______.

18. Pancreatic insulinoma symptoms include ______.

19. An example of a bacteriostatic antibiotic is ______.

20. A pair of antibiotics that should NOT be given to horses include ______.

21. ______ is an arthropod that transmits leukocytozoon in ducks.

22. Ascarus lumbricoides infections occur by ______.

23. Cryptococcus neoformans is an etiological agent which localizes in ______.

24. Pemphigus is a group of ______.

25. The *characteristic* feature of panleukopenia infections in kittens is _hydroceph_

26. Parakerotosis in swine is due to Zn deficiency as well as _vit A_.

27. Diarrhea in young pigs infected with rotavirus causes destruction of _villi_.

Questions 28-50.

DIRECTIONS: Answer the following questions directly, briefly, and succinctly.

28. Which equine skin disease is characterized by small patches of hair along the dorsum that are easily epilated, leaving a moist, oozing surface?

29. A shetland pony mare is presented to your clinic showing *inter alia,* hirsutism, and a glucose level of 225. Based on this information, what is the *probable* cause?

30. In what feline cardiac disease does non-selective venous-angiocautiography have the *greatest* applications?

31. What drug is MOST appropriate for sinus bradychordia in a dog?

32. What drug is MOST commonly used to manage functional pancreatic insulinoma with a piloric metastasis in the dog?

33. Pre-treated acid paper strip dipped into a beaker containing rumen contents is turned deep red within a few minutes. What causes this change in color?

34. What anthelmintic is contraindicated for removal of ascarids from a 6 months old horse who has never been wormed?

35. A dog that scratches over his ears, face, and legs is most likely to have which ectoparasite?

36. What is a horse who recovers from a respiratory disease most likely to acquire as a sequela?

37. Humans are MOST susceptible to TB from what animal?

38. What drug should be used on a cat with cardiomiopathy?

39. What is a breed of cat that has natural occurring nystagnus and strobism?

40. A horse with dysphagia *probably* has what illness?

41. What is the *difference* between the lungs of a horse and the lungs of other domestic animals?

42. Haemalopinus suis is an external parasite. In how many hosts does it have all of its stages?

43. What is the etiology of swine with a cough, a temperature of $105^{o}$-$107^{o}$, and pneumonia?

44. What occurs when there is a rupture of the gastrocnemus tendon of the cat?

45. What lesions are found in a necropsy of an animal with diabetes mellitus?

46. What is a neoplasia of badgesiers that produces lameness?

47. What muscle do you cut to relieve fibrosing hyopathy?

48. What medications do you give swine confined to concrete environment?

49. What is the treatment for transverse fractures of the splint bones in dogs?

50. What type of placenta is found in the dog?

---

# KEY (CORRECT ANSWERS)

1. the presence of antibodies in the blood and urine
2. the disease has not progressed sufficiently to be macroscopically evident
3. Secretary of Agriculture
4. left arythenoid chondritis
5. pyrrolizidine alkaloid toxicity
6. paracentesis
7. eosinopenia
8. 5000 millirems
9. 210 - 530
10. syngamus trachea
11. face, ears, feet and neck
12. mast cell tumor
13. digoxin
14. administration of oxytetracyclines
15. during the second week after treatment
16. L-thyroxin
17. the minimum exposure time to be utilized
18. hypoglycemia, convulsions, coma, death
19. chloramphenicol
20. tetracyclin and lincomycin
21. Simulium
22. ingestion of infected ovum

23. the CNS of cats

24. immune-mediated blistering diseases

25. cerebellar hypoplasia

26. an increase in Ca#

27. mature epithelium on the villastipa

28. Dermatophilosis.

29. Pituitary neoplasia.

30. Cardiomyopathy.

31. Atropine.

32. Diazoxide or proglycem.

33. Dextro-hydrogen cyanide.

34. Dichlorvos.

35. Sarcoptic mange.

36. Bronchopneumonia.

37. Monkeys.

38. Propanolol.

39. Siamese.

40. Guttural pouch infection.

41. In the horse, the lungs are not divided into lobes by fissures.

42. One.

43. Pasteurella multicida.

44. The cat will walk on the plantar surface of the metatarsus.

45. Fatty degeneration of the liver and pancreas atrophy.

46. Renal carcinoma.

47. Semitendineus.

48. Iron dextran.

49. Pin and tension bond

50. Endothelialchorial.

# TEST 3

Questions 1-12.

DIRECTIONS: Fill in the blank space(s) the word (or words) which is (are) the correct answer(s) to the question.

1. The BEST method of diagnosis for keratitis sicca is ______.

2. The MOST recent evidence of the cause of atrophic rhinitis in swine is ______.

3. The organ MOST likely to cause death in shock is the ______.

4. The most useful test for the diagnosis of leptospira is ______.

5. Clinical signs of feline asthma include ______.

6. The BEST drug for a dog in status epilepticus seizure is ______.

7. Amputation of the hind limb of a cat is performed at the ______.

8. The MOST common fracture of the intercarpal joints of the horse is at the ______.

9. The MOST common species of the pet population having the ability to transmit TB to humans by the ingestion of milk is ______.

10. When you inject an anesthetic into the artery of a horse, ______ occur.

11. Demodex canis is located in the ______ of the dog.

12. When there is mismating, ______ should be used to bring about an abortion.

Questions 13-50.

DIRECTIONS: Answer the following questions directly, briefly, and succinctly.

13. What breed of dog is most prevalent in Legg-Perthes disease?

14. When should bone grafts be used?

15. A cat with retinal detachment has been eating only dog food. What kind of deficiency does this cat have?

16. What is the gestation period of sheep?

17. How long is the estrous cycle of a sow?

18. How long is the estrous cycle of a ewe?

19. What percent of its body weight should a 4 day old cow receive of milk?

20. How many mg is ¼ grain of morphine?

21. Amoranthus poisoning causes what lesion?

22. A disease of swine (piglets) that causes vomiting, diarrhea, dehydration and death to 4-5 piglets has also affected some breeder pigs.
What is the diagnosis?

23. How does transmission of brucellosis in swine MOST commonly occur?

24. How do you determine the sex of budgeriens?

25. A child who plays with household kittens develops choroid retinitis.
What is the cause?

26. How is malignant edema acquired?

27. What hormone is contained in HCG?

28. Why do you give aspirin to cats with cardiomiopathy?

29. Which suture material is most apt to cause dehescence due to bacterial infiltrate?

30. How do you make a definite diagnosis of giardiasis?

31. What is an example of a drug *commonly* used to destroy giardiasis?

32. What wormer is contraindicated in a foal 6 months old that has never been wormed?

33. What is the percent of extracellular fluid in the body?

34. What species is the carrier of pseudorabies?

35. Where are the scent glands located on male goats?

36. What medication would you use to treat epileptic fits in cats?

37. What is the color of parrakeet's feces?

38. In the eye of a cat there are two rows of cilia. What are they called?

39. Comedones, popules and postules are found under a cat's chin. What is the diagnosis?

40. What drug would MOST effectively stabilize the estrus cycle?

41. What are the *prominent* clinical signs of equine purpura hemorragiea?

42. What anion is most commonly found in body fluids?

43. What is the largest organ involved in anaphylactic shock?

44. What should be done to a dog who has come in contact with a rabies positive animal?

45. A two day old foal develops profuse diarrhea. What is the MOST likely cause?

46. What is the MOST prominent clinical sign of enterotoxemia in swine?

47. What is the cause of a jugular pulse observed in a cow with traumatic pericarditis?

48. A goat refuses to let her kid nurse. You notice a nodule on one of the farmer's hands. What is the MOST likely cause?

49. What is the MOST common vector of conjunctive keratitis in cows?

50. At 60 days of gestation, how can you best determine if a cow is pregnant?

# KEY (CORRECT ANSWERS)

1. Schiumer's tear test
2. bordetella bronchiseptica
3. lung
4. hemagglutination lysistes
5. expiratory dyspnea and coughing
6. valium (diazepam)
7. distal third of the femur
8. third carpal
9. canine
10. convulsions
11. hair follicules
12. estrogen
13. Boston terrier.
14. When there is no contact between bones.
15. Taurine.
16. 145 days.
17. 21 days (16-24).
18. 16½ days (14-20)
19. 10%.
20. 15 mg.
21. Peri-renal edema.
22. T.G.E.
23. Infected boars.
24. Cere is blue in the male and brown in the female.
25. Toxoplasmosis.
26. Cl. septicum (ducking, castration, unsanitary vaccinations, parturition, shearing.
27. L.H.
28. It prevents blood clots.
29. Silk.
30. Direct smear.
31. Flagyl or atabrine.
32. Dichlorvos.
33. 30% (5% plasma and 25% intestinal).
34. Swine.
35. In the horns.
36. Phenobarbital or Valium.
37. It is green and white.
38. Distichiasis.
39. Feline acne.
40. Prostaglandins.
41. Sub. Q. edema in the muzzle, neutrophilia and a normal platelet count.
42. $K^+$ (potassium).
43. The liver.
44. The dog must be isolated for 6 months.
45. Salmonella.
46. Facial edema.
47. Large amounts of exudate which push against the jugular vein.
48. Contagious ectyma.
49. Mosquitoes.
50. Membrane slip.

# EXAMINATION SECTION

## TEST 1

Questions 1-14.

DIRECTIONS: Answer the following questions directly, briefly, and succinctly.

1. Paralysis of the extensor muscle (the elbow, carpus and digits) indicates injury to what nerve?
2. What hormone depresses FSH?
3. What do you submit to diagnose abortion from pig enterovirus?
4. What kind of tumor causes femininity in male dogs?
5. What connects the oral cavity and nasal cavity with the esophagus and larynx?
6. What are the excretory ducts of the kidneys?
7. Where does grit do the grinding of feed in the chicken?
8. Are hemangio-endotheliomas and lymphangio-endotheliomas malignant or benign?
9. What type of muscles are the non-striated, voluntary muscle layers within the walls of the intestine, blood vessels and uterus?
10. What type of muscle is the muscle of the tongue?
11. What hormone prepares the uterus for implantation?
12. Where are the sites of actinobacillosis lesions?
13. What is the etiology for oxalate formation in the kidney?
14. In canines used as show animals, what type of rabies vaccine is MOST usually recommended?

Questions 15-50.

DIRECTIONS: Fill in the blank space(s) the word (or words) which is (are) the correct answer(s) to the question.

15. The production of sperm is called ______.
16. The pre-anesthesia excitement stage in the dog is due to the release of ______.

17. The nerve supplying sensation to the plantar surface below the paw is the ______.

18. Parasympathetic supply to the rectum is via the ______.

19. The hormone that causes permeability of the collecting ducts is ______.

20. A cat with XXY chromosomes is showing ______.

21. The location of feline acne is under the ______.

22. The skin tumor that is LEAST sensitive to radiation treatment is the ______.

23. Steatitis in cats indicates a deficiency of vitamin ______.

24. The MOST common neoplasm in ALL species is the ______.

25. The pulmonary artery connects the heart to the ______.

26. The type of placentation in bovines is ______.

27. The nerve of the superficial digital flexor of the hind limb is the ______.

28. Fibers from the optic tract to the thalamus synapse is the ______.

29. The oxygen combining power of *Hb* depends on its content of ______.

30. A splenic hemangioma may be BEST treated by performing a ______.

31. The hormone that stimulates secretion by the adrenal cortex is ______.

32. The hormone that initiates lactation following mammary development is ______.

33. The science that deals with the function of the living organism and its parts is ______.

34. The fluid that circulates through the heart, arteries, veins, and capillaries carrying nutrients and oxygen to the body tissue is ______.

35. The hormones, secretin and pancreozymin, that govern pancreatic secretion originate from the ______.

36. The treatment for stringhalt involves removal of the ______.

37. In the chicken, the ureters empty into the ______.

38. The hormone that inhibits FSH is ______.

39. A functional beta cell tumor of the pancreas directly results in ______.

40. Immunizing agents made from dead organisms are generally called bacterins, while immunizing agents made from living organisms are called ______.

41. Antibodies to the toxins of microorganisms are called ______.

42. An organism is characterized as long, slender gram positive rods, 2 to 5 microns in length, with rounded ends. This organism is anaerobic, very resistant due to spores, and motile with peritrichous flagellae. This organism is ______.

43. The vessel affected in bleeding from the gutteral pouch is the ______.

44. The sinus opened to remove a piece of a bone between the canine tooth and zygomatic process of the frontal bone is the ______.

45. Malignant bone tumors start in the ______.

46. The primary control of colibacillosis in baby pigs is sanitation of the ______.

47. The species with MOST frequent gastric torsion is the ______.

48. The MOST potent glucocorticoid is ______.

49. T-cells are formed in the ______.

50. The normal leukocyte count in the canine is ______.

# KEY (CORRECT ANSWERS)

1. Radial nerve.
2. Progesterone.
3. Sow serum.
4. Sertoli cell tumor.
5. The pharynx.
6. The ureters.
7. Gizzard.
8. Malignant.
9. Smooth muscles.
10. Skeletal.
11. Progesterone.
12. Tongue.
13. Ethylene glycol.
14. Rabies modified live vaccines with annual booster injected intra-muscularly.
15. spermatogenesis
16. adrenalin
17. tibial nerve
18. pelvic nerve
19. ADH
20. Kleifelters syndrome
21. chin
22. melanoma
23. E
24. lymphosarcoma
25. lungs
26. cotyledonary
27. digital nerve
28. lateral geniculate body
29. Fe
30. splenectomy
31. adrenocorticotropic hormone (ACTH)
32. prolactin
33. physiology
34. blood
35. small intestine
36. lateral digital extensor
37. urodeum
38. LH
39. hypoglycemia
40. vaccines
41. antitoxins
42. tetanus
43. internal carotid
44. maxillary sinus
45. medullary cavity
46. udder
47. dog
48. dexamethason
49. thymus
50. 10,000-12,000

# TEST 2

Questions 1-27.

DIRECTIONS: Answer the following questions directly, briefly, and succinctly.

1. Why is it BEST to view an x-ray film *after* it has dried?
2. What is the optimum incubation temperature for a dermatophyte?
3. What is the BEST method of confirming lead poisoning?
4. What metabolic disorder occurs when the BUN is elevated over 50 mg/ml?
5. How long does it take barium to reach the colon?
6. What does not cause loss of contrast in an x-ray film?
7. What disease occurs when a horse gets edema after a respiratory infection?
8. What is the cause of elevated glucose levels, glucosurea, polydipsia and polyurea?
9. What causes a bilateral renal enlargement?
10. What is the BEST treatment for actino bacillosis?
11. What drug should be used when you have an arrythmia caused by an injection of thiamylol sodium?
12. When is the best time to administer cortisone to an animal?
13. What drug is indicated in a second or third degree AV heart block?
14. What condition is MOST commonly aggravated by the administration of thyroxine?
15. What is the BEST solution for IV administration in a keto-acidotic dog?
16. What is the treatment of choice for psittacine birds with psittacosis?
17. What is the simplest treatment of foals with weak flexors and extensors of the fetlock?
18. What is the *principal* difference between rickets and osteomalacia?
19. What is the MOST common abnormality in cancer patients?

20. Why is piroplasmosis found *principally* in southern states?

21. *How* is contagious equine metritis spread?

22. What is the normal gastric emptying time in the cat with a barium mix?

23. Feline cardiomyopathy is more common among members of which sex?

24. What is the cause of keratitis sicca in the dog?

25. The symptoms include a soft eyeball, inflammed conjunctiva, and injected sclera.
What is indicated?

26. Where is the site for a bovine traumatic pericarditis incision?

27. What is the BEST direction for a surgical approach to remove a tumor or vermin on the cerebellum?

Questions 28-50.

DIRECTIONS: Fill in the blank space(s) the word (or words) which is (are) the correct answer(s) to the question.

28. An example of a hepatic specific enzyme for large animals is ______.

29. Feline leukemia and leukemia are MOST often associated with ______.

30. The BEST diagnostic test to measure hypothyroidism is the ______.

31. The test used to determine feline leukemia is the ______.

32. A dog that scratches over its ears, face, and ventral abdomen is most likely to have ______.

33. Photophobia in a horse would MOST likely be caused by ______.

34. The MOST prominent side effect of dexamethasone administered to a near-term pregnant cow is a ______.

35. The two MAIN components of a complete nephron are the ______.

36. Panniculus adiposis is a layer of fat that develops in the ______.

37. The three main structures that compose the middle ear are the ______.

38. Blood vessels that supply nutrition to the skin are located in the ______.

39. The accessory lobe of the mammalian lung lies in the ______.

40. Coronary blood flow equals ______ percent of cardiac output.

41. Visceral smooth muscle contracts when stretched due to the ______.

42. The partial pressure of $CO_2$ is greatest in ______ blood.

43. In the upper abomasum, a drop in pH to 1.0 causes ______.

44. Ketosis in ruminants may occur because of a lack of ______ in the liver mitochondria.

45. Viral infections are *mainly* characterized by ______.

46. The PRIMARY metabolic disturbances in a horse with renal failure include ______.

47. Alopecia is a skin lesion inherited by Mendelian ______ genes.

48. Chronic obstructive pulmonary disease in the horse is MOST commonly associated with previous infections of ______.

49. Mycotic gutteral pouch infections are MOST commonly associated with ______.

50. ______ is the surgical treatment for canine and Cushing syndrome.

---

# KEY (CORRECT ANSWERS)

1. As the film dries, its emulsion shrinks, enhancing its detail.
2. 25$^{O}$C.
3. X-ray.
4. Hypoadrenocorticism.
5. 60 minutes.
6. Pneumoperitonium.
7. Purpura hemorrhageca.
8. Pituitary tumor.
9. Lymphosarcoma.
10. Sodium Iodide.
11. Lidocaine.
12. In the morning.
13. Atropine.
14. Congestive heart failure.
15. 0.45% NaCl.
16. Chlostetracycline.
17. Exercise and no support.
18. Rickets is a disease of the young.
19. Anemia.
20. The ticks are limited to that area.
21. By a contaminated stallion.
22. Less than 1 hour.
23. Males.
24. Administration of sulfasoxazole.
25. Ureal tract inflammation.
26. At the 5th or 6th rib on the left side.
27. Posterior dorsal occipital.

28. SDH
29. hypercalcemia
30. TSH response test
31. Fluorescent antibody test
32. sarcoptic mange
33. a corneal ulcer
34. retained placenta
35. renal corpuscle and the urine ferous tubule
36. subcutaneous skin layer
37. tympanic membrane, osseus bulla, and auditory ossicles
38. dermis (corium)
39. mediastinal recess
40. 5
41. myenteric reflex
42. venous
43. an increase in reticular motility
44. oxaloacetate
45. decreased leukocytes and neutrophils
46. hypophosphatencia, hypocalcemia, increased BUN and increased creatinine
47. recessive
48. influenza virus
49. dysphagia
50. bilateral adrenalectomy

# TEST 3

Questions 1-22.

DIRECTIONS: Answer the following questions directly, briefly, and succinctly.

1. In what order are the MAIN nerves blocked in a Peterson Eye Block?

2. What is a ranula?

3. What species of domestic animal has an accessory ligament that prevents a coxo-femoral luxation?

4. In what bone does non-union occur most frequently?

5. In a medial deviation of the carpus, repaired using a figure eight wire and plate with screws, where are the screws seated?

6. What is the BEST treatment of a hygroma of the carpus of a valuable cow?

7. How is the hip positioned in a cranio-dorsal, coxo-femoral luxation with an Ehrmis sling?

8. Cereal grains contain the MOST of what nutrient?

9. In the surgical management of a mammary adenocarcinoma, what is the MAIN difference between a dog and a cat?

10. What occurs following the consumption of acid-forming foods by the pig?

11. Where is a stallion ring placed?

12. What is the gestation period of guinea pigs?

13. In sheep, what occurs if the lateral wall of the hoof is not worn?

14. During what segment of surgery are malpractice claims MOST frequent?

15. Avian TB is considered important in domestic poultry and in what other species?

16. During what time of the year is tularemia epizootic in rabbits?

17. In what species are immunodeficiency of IgM defects congenital?

18. In what species do natural auto-immune thyroiditis occur?

19. What does Japanese Yew poison cause?

20. What is the appropriate therapy for filarae parasites infecting the ventral midline of cattle?

21. What antibiotic can produce respiratory failure due to neuromuscular blockage?

22. What is a *likely* complication of oral administration of multi-doses of neomycin?

Questions 23-50.

DIRECTIONS: Fill in the blank space(s) the word (or words) which is (are) the correct answer(s) to the question.

23. For surgery of the thoracic duct of a cat, the BEST approach is through the ______ space.

24. The location of a compression plate in the radius of a horse is ______.

25. Early weaned pigs are showing signs of diarrhea, weight loss and high mortality. These symptoms MOST likely indicate ______.

26. The most serious infertility problem in a dairy herd is ______.

27. The use of teat dips reduces gram positive organisms the next year by ______ percent.

28. The amount of colostrum necessary for sufficient antibodies IgG and IgA in calves is ______ liters in ______ hours.

29. In a closed building with slotted floors and manure pits, ______ percent of the air should be exhausted by pit fans.

30. The responsibility of a veterinarian who is acting as a bailee is to ______.

31. Actinomycosis in man is caused by ______.

32. Rocky Mountain spotted fever is most prevalent in ______.

33. Dissemination of large numbers of Rickettsias from placentas is *likely* to result in an increase of ______.

34. A cysticercus cellulosa infection results from ingestion of food and drink contaminated by ______.

35. An ante mortem inspection is essential for the detection of ______.

36. TGE vaccine administered ______ provides the highest titer.

37. Malignant edema is diagnostically differentiated from Blackleg by ______.

38. Local immunity against viral and bacteriological pathogens in the alimentary tract of neonatal pigs occurs by ______.

39. Immunity to IBR following intranasal vaccination occurs via ______.

40. Chronic lead poisoning in horses is *likely* to cause laryngeal ______.

41. The action of *lasix* occurs in ______.

42. Diabetes mellitus is an endocrine disorder causing hyperglycemia and glucosurea.
The cat can develop diabetes mellitus from the use of Ovaban, which can be treated with ______.

43. The hormone which causes bone marrow hypoplasia is ______.

44. ______ is an antagonist of morphine in the horse that has analgesic properties when administered alone.

45. Horses with chronic ventral midline dermatitis respond to oral ______.

46. Coccidiosis caused by eimeria tenella occurs in ______ only.

47. Dermatitis caused by bacterial hypersensitivity can be treated by ______.

48. Tetracycline and calcium are drugs which CANNOT be mixed prior to ______.

49. An effect of Carbachol following the use of atropine is a(n) ______ in blood pressure.

50. The actions of sulfa drugs is to completely inhibit the utilization of ______.

# KEY (CORRECT ANSWERS)

1. Optic, occulomotor, ophthalmic of trigeminal, and maxillary of trigeminal.
2. A salivary retention cyst.
3. The horse.
4. The radius.
5. On the meta and epicondyles of the medial surfaces.
6. Extirpation.
7. It is placed in adduction and internal rotation.
8. Phosphorus.
9. The lymphatics of the cat cross the midline.
10. There is an increase in the synthesis of $NH_3$ with conservation of body base.
11. It is placed around the stallion's penis.
12. 59-72 days.
13. It will grow long and fold under, necessitating trimming.
14. During anesthesia.
15. Swine.
16. During the late summer.
17. In the horse.
18. In dogs.
19. Acute death without lesions.
20. No treatment.
21. Gentamycin.
22. Super infection.
23. 8-10 left intercostal
24. cranial
25. improper ingredients in food rationing

26. post-service anestrus

27. 50

28. 2, 2

29. 50

30. isolate an animal with a contagious disease and protect the hospital patients

31. an organism that is a normal inhabitant of the mucus membranes of the mouth

32. the southeast

33. Q fever

34. feces of persons with taenea solium

35. CN disease

36. orally

37. bacteriologic procedures

38. the secretion of IgA antibodies in the milk of sows

39. T-cells, secretory IgA and serum IgG

40. hemiplegia

41. the loop of Henle

42. insulin

43. estradiol cygronate

44. pentazocine

45. diethylcarbamazine

46. chickens

47. antibiotics and steroids

48. IV administration

49. increase

50. PABA

# EXAMINATION SECTION

# TEST 1

Questions 1-16.

DIRECTIONS: Answer the following questions directly, briefly, and succinctly.

1. What is an example of a virus that can be found in bovine semen?
2. Where are the lesions of swine anthrax *principally* located?
3. What occurs to a swine that has recovered from Anjesky's disease?
4. What is the MAIN characteristic of Bracken fern poisoning?
5. To what *two* species is monensin MOST toxic?
6. What are the *two* MAIN toxins contained in the venom of snake poison?
7. What is the FASTEST acting mydriatic?
8. Which are the *two* MOST common bacteria cultured from the mare uterus with endometritis?
9. Where are the eggs of gasterophilus intestinalis placed in the horse?
10. What is the reason that atropine does NOT cause mydriasis in the avian species?
11. In what location does bone spavin involve the bones of the horse?
12. What kind of epithelial tissue lines the esophagus?
13. A snake is brought in to your office. She appears blind and she did NOT eat last night.
    What is occurring?
14. After how many days does implantation in the mare occur during pregnancy?
15. In a population of 50,000, 10 animals are infected monthly.
    What is the infective population?
16. Why is the technique used for the suture of the esophagus *different* from that used on the intestines?

Questions 17-50.

DIRECTIONS: Fill in the blank space(s) the word (or words) which is (are) the correct answer(s) to the question.

17. The incubation period of rabies is ______.

18. Canine infectious hepatitis is *principally* transmitted via ______.

19. The incubation period of staphylococci poisoning is ______.

20. An anammestic response is ______.

21. The MAIN effect of *increased* vitamin D absorption is ______.

22. In the therapy of a sulfonamide sensitive infection, the formation of sulfa-crystals is favored by ______.

23. The hormone of pregnant mare serum stimulates the release of ______.

24. An injection of 50 mg of rompun to a 1400 lb bovine causes ______.

25. For the treatment of feline idiopathic hypertrophic cardiomyopathy, the drug of *choice* is ______.

26. The causative agent of feline cardiomyopathy is ______.

27. The MAIN cause of the blister disease in snakes is ______.

28. The MOST recent evidence of the cause of atrophic rhinitis in swine is ______.

29. The pre-patent period of strongylus vulgaris is ______.

30. In the horse, the pathogenesis of a clostridium tetani infection is ______.

31. The MOST common sequel to the swine erysipelas infection is ______.

32. The MOST commonly found tumor of bovine is ______.

33. The *characteristic* sign of dypsnea in a horse with "heaves" is due to ______.

34. The MOST common ovarian tumor in the mare is the ______.

35. The *principal* reason for acetonemia in ovine is ______.

36. The *normal* respiratory rate of canines is ______.

37. An increase in the right atrial pressure *directly* results in ______.

38. In swine, the sparing action of niacin is due to ______.

39. The *final* maturation of spermatogenesis is controlled by ______.

40. The epithelial lining of the bladder of the newborn foal is composed of ______ tissue.

41. In a field case of ammonium toxicity, the treatment of *choice* would be ______.

42. The method of prevention of enterotoxemia in sheep is ______.

43. The MAIN procedure utilized to prevent losses due to malignant catarrhal fever is ______.

44. The cause of depigmentation of the haircoat in cattle is ______.

45. The *current* hypothesis on hypertrophic osteodystrophy is that it is associated with a metabolic disturbance of ______.

46. The *minimum* temperature necessary to perform cryosurgery is ______.

47. All cases of leukemia in bovine CANNOT be diagnosed by microscopic examination of the blood because ______.

48. The differential count of the normal horse and the normal cow reveals that ______.

49. Subcutaneous emphysema in bovine is MOST commonly associated with ______.

50. A visual ailment that occurs only in diabetic felines and not in normal cats is ______.

# KEY (CORRECT ANSWERS)

1. IBR, BVD, or Blue tongue.
2. Pharyngeal glands.
3. The swine will shed the virus whenever stressed.
4. Hemorrhages due to a reduction in the amount of blood platelets produced.
5. Equine porcine.
6. Neurotoxin and hemotoxin.
7. Tropicamide.
8. E-coli and streptococcus.
9. In the front position of the scapula and on the foreleg.
10. The iris is composed of skeletal muscle.
11. Tarsus.
12. Stratified squamous.
13. The snake is going to shed her skin.
14. 70-90 days.
15. 24/10,000.
16. The esophagus has a weak serasa and has a reduced blood supply.
17. 10-60 days
18. the urine
19. 2-6 hours
20. the prompt production of an antibody after the second injection of an antigen
21. soft tissue calcification
22. acid
23. FSH
24. a decrease in the CNS response and a reduction in blood pressure
25. propranolol

26. unknown

27. excessive moisture in the environment

28. bordetella bronchiseptica

29. 6 months

30. exotoxin

31. arthritis

32. benign paplomatosis of the skin

33. the horse trying to expel entrapped air from the lower respiratory tract

34. granulosa cell tumor

35. increased cortisol levels

36. 10-30/minute

37. an increase in cardiac output

38. tryptophan

39. androgens and FSH

40. transitional

41. acetic acid in order to neutralize toxins

42. vaccination

43. separating the sheep and cattle

44. copper deficiency

45. vitamin C

46. $-20^{o}$ C

47. in aleukemic leukemia, the total leukocyte count is normal and the periferal blood is devoid of neoplastic cells

48. the lymphocytes in the cow are equal to the neutrophyles in the horse

49. acute alveolar emphysema

50. cataracts

# TEST 2

Questions 1-15.

DIRECTIONS: Answer the following questions directly, briefly, and succinctly.

1. In performing a prostatectomy, where is the incision line?
2. What is the MOST common non-absorbable, non-capillary suture material?
3. Where do you perform a thoracocentesis in a horse?
4. When should a non-rebreathing inhalation anesthetic system be used?
5. What is the *primary* post mortem lesion of infectious canine hepatitis?
6. Where do you perform a trocarization of cecum in the zebra?
7. In what disease are the *largest* number of eosinophils found skin lesions?
8. What is found in a direct blood smear when examining anthrax?
9. What antibiotic is contraindicated in an open fracture?
10. What is affected in Wobbler disease of horses?
11. Where do you find the MARCUS PLICATUS?
12. What species has ovulation at the fossa?
13. What parasitic egg do eggs of Taenea resemble?
14. What is the recommended schedule for testing monkeys for TB?
15. Where do you hear the "tinkling" sound in displaced abomasum?

Questions 16-50.

DIRECTIONS: Fill in the blank space(s) the word (or words) which is (are) the correct answer(s) to the question.

16. The *principal* cause of salivary cysts is ______.
17. The prognosis when there is a fractured splint bone depends on ______.

18. The *primary* objective in the surgical treatment of suppurative atlantal bursitis in the horse is ______.

19. The MOST common complication in an ovario-hysterectomy of a feline with the use of ketamine HCl is ______.

20. In the horse, the *two* muscles which must be separated during a laryngeoplasty are the ______.

21. The *primary* sequela of swine endocarditis is ______.

22. In the horse, the *characteristic* sign of a short anterior stride in the hindleg, and a "snap" when it is returned to the ground indicates ______.

23. A *complete* spinal cord lesion at the 3rd cervical vertebrate causes ______.

24. An essential *difference* between digoxin therapy in cats and dogs is that ______.

25. An example of topical therapy for recurrent uveitis in the horse is ______.

26. ________ should be administered to a cow 60 days post partum with cystic follicules.

27. In snakes, the dosage interval for gentacin is ______.

28. The antibiotic of *choice* for erysipelas in turkeys is ______.

29. The function of prostaglandins in cows is to ______.

30. Radiography shows a cone shape in the intestines of a feline. The structure is ______.

31. The ability of an x-ray tube to achieve *repeated* x-ray output is limited because ______.

32. The type of non-metastizing tumor of head, legs and feet in the dog is ______.

33. The *primary* cause of abortions in sheep is ______, which can be prevented by vaccination.

34. The *characteristic* symptom of eripipelosis in swine is ______.

35. *Conclusive* evidence of congenital ventricular septal defect in the horse is ______.

36. A blood picture shows thrombocytopenia, non-regenative anemia, and granulocytopenia.
This indicates ______.

37. The *primary* pathopneumonic sign of peroneus tertions rupture is ______.

38. In the Ramstedt operation, the incision is *to* ______.

39. Measurement of the circumference of the scrotum of the bull indicates the bull's ______.

40. Tar on cat hair should be removed with ______.

41. The Hering-Beuer reflex exerts action on ______.

42. Unilateral paralysis of the lips indicates damage to the ______.

43. The BEST laboratory method providing a *definite* diagnosis for anaplasmosis is ______.

44. The eruption of the canine teeth in the feline occurs within ______.

45. In the horse, injury to the distal sesamoids causes ______.

46. The medication MOST commonly used in glaucoma is ______.

47. The treatment used on bovine with acetonemia is ______.

48. The medication that is contraindicated in a dog with heartworm infection is ______.

49. The lesion in kerato-conjunctivitis is ______.

50. The bulbo urethral glands are located caudal to the ______.

# KEY (CORRECT ANSWERS)

1. At the caudal paramedian.
2. Nylon.
3. At the 7th intercostal space dorsal to the lateral thoracic vein on the left side.
4. On all animals weighing less than 15 lbs.
5. Thickened walls of the bladder.
6. At the right upper flank.
7. Allergic dermatosis.
8. Chains of gram positive rods with no spores.
9. Erythromycin.
10. Both hind legs are affected.
11. It divides the stomach into glandular and non-glandular parts.
12. Equine.
13. Ancylostoma caninum.
14. Test, repeat in 30 days, and repeat annually.
15. In the last few intercostal spaces on-the left side.
16. stenosis of the duct
17. the degree of desmitis of the suspensory ligament
18. removal of the purulent portion of the ligament nuchae and the surrounding bursa
19. corneal ulceration
20. thyropharyngeal and cricopharyngeal
21. swine erysipelas
22. fibrosing myopathy
23. spastic tetraplegia
24. cats receive lower doses than dogs
25. gentamycin, glucocorticoid or atropine

26. luteolytic hormone
27. 72 hours
28. IM injection of penicillin
29. regress the corpus luteum
30. an intestinal tumor
31. heat is generated at the anode
32. histocytomas
33. vibrio
34. lameness from arthritis
35. increased $O_2$ tension in the pulmonary artery and right ventricular blood
36. myclopathosic anemia
37. flexion of the stifle without reciprocal flexion of the lockjoint
38. the mucosa
39. fertility
40. vegetable oil and shampoo
41. the lungs
42. facial nerve
43. a blood smear
44. 6 months
45. calcification of distal sesmoids
46. glycerol
47. glucose solution
48. dichlorvos.
49. corneal ulceration
50. ureter

# TEST 3

Questions 1-19.

DIRECTIONS: Answer the following questions directly, briefly, and succinctly.

1. What is the location of the adrenal glands in relation to the kidneys? cranial

2. After travelling 40 miles under a hot sun, a horse collapses, panting heavily.
   What is occurring? dehydration, dyspnea, acidosis, no E left

3. Does a veterinarian who performs duties for a state lose his accreditation if he falsifies a diagnosis? Yes

4. Does a state who wishes to enter a national program have to have veterinarians take an exam to get accreditation? ~~Yes~~ No

5. A cow who has shown a reaction to TB test shows no lesions at post mortem.
   What is the MOST likely reason for this? X react (too small)

6. A lack of what vitamins, other than vitamin D, causes rickets? Vit ? A

7. What *kind* of vessels contain the largest amount of blood? Veins

8. A veterinarian accidently gets a dose of rabies modified live vaccine. What should he do? Get shot booster

9. In eclampsia in the bitch, what type of reaction is seen? ~~type 3~~

10. What sound is heard during atrial contraction? ~~S4~~ None

11. What occurs when there is a fracture of the hyoid bone in equines? dysphagia

12. What is the MOST likely cause of extreme pain in foals two days after birth? ruptured bladder

13. Should an ovario-hysterectomy be indicated for a dog with mammary tumors? Yes

14. On examination of blood smears of young pigs, bodies are observed in the erythrocytes.
    What disease does this indicate? ~~Babesia, Anaplasmosis~~ Erysipel

15. How is breeding stock retained after brucellosis is discovered in swine? Testing

16. Two cows are TB reactors in a barn.
    What is your recommendation to the farmer? Get rid of 2 cows

17. In a good herd, what is the MOST common reason that calves are becoming ill?

18. What do you do with a *newborn* foal that has an inguinal hernia?

19. What tissue graft is MOST likely to be rejected?

Questions 20-50.

DIRECTIONS: Fill in the blank space(s) the word (or words) which is (are) the correct answer(s) to the question.

20. The MOST common lesions to the spinal cord of dogs occurs at the cervical vertebrae between ______.

21. The drug of *choice* to reduce edema in the brain region is ______.

22. The BEST treatment for atrial fibrillation is ______.

23. The urethral glands are located caudal to the ______.

24. When $pCO_2$ is elevated, the chloride shift is characterized by ______ and ______ ions moving in the *same* direction.

25. The use of prostaglandins in a cow 100 days pregnant causes ______.

26. The topical solution used on a cat with a superficial scratch on the iris is ______.

27. The portion or organ cranial to the opening of the uterus on the floor of the vagina is the ______.

28. ALL cystic calculi are caused *principally* by ______.

29. ______ tissue uses $CO_2$ as a source of energy.

30. ______ tissue is STRICTLY dependent on glucose as its source of energy.

31. Changes in the bacterial population of the rumen are MOST commonly due to ______.

32. Cystic stones are *principally* made up of ______.

33. The *greatest* amount of $CO_2$ is present in the ______ capillaries.

34. The percentage of $O_2$ in the hemoglobin is dependent on ______.

35. Response in the respiratory center of the brain is due to an *increase* in ______.

36. The period of estrus is *shortest* in the Cow.

37. In the cat, the treatment for a malignant portion of the pinna is excision.

38. The *two* MOST common drugs that prevent estrus are ~~DES~~ ovaban. milibo[illegible]

39. The urine specific gravity of a dog with diabetes insipidus is *fixed* at 1010.

40. The cause of sudden death in an untreated hepatectomized animal is ~~hemorrhage~~. ↓ Glu

41. The MOST sterile method of collecting urine for diagnosis in a cat is ~~catheter~~. cysto

42. The outcome of an animal with pseudorabies is death.

43. There is *less* botulism in the United States today *mainly* because of better. canning

44. The nerve blocked in diagnosing navicular disease is the palmar digital (post.)

45. The treatment for a chronic fistula is excision.

46. Urine dribbling from the umbilicus in newborn foal is termed patent urachus

47. The *primary* location of anesthesia in performing a rumenotomy is ~~epidural~~. T13 - L1 L2

48. A virus which crosses over and invades the tissues is classified as ______. an infection

49. The age for *maximum* protection in distemper vaccination is 16 wk.

50. The *newest* internal mycotic medication for internal mycotic infections is Ketaconazole.

Amphoterican ______

# KEY (CORRECT ANSWERS)

1. Anterior and medial.
2. Metabolic alkalosis.
3. Yes.
4. No.
5. The lesions are too small to be detected.
6. Vitamin A.
7. Veins.
8. Nothing.
9. Spontaneous with progression to coma and death if untreated.
10. None, as the sound is obscured by 1st heart sound.
11. The horse can not drink or swallow.
12. Meconiss.
13. No, as there is no significant extension of survival time.
14. Erysipelotrix.
15. After checking newborn females, reactors are eliminated and negatives are separated.
16. Destroy both and disinfect the entire barn.
17. The farmer places older and younger calves in the same pen.
18. Nothing.
19. Xenograft.
20. $C_2$ - $C_4$
21. mannitol
22. electric shock
23. cervix
24. Cl and Na
25. hemorrhage with abortion

26. atropine 1% and chloromycetin
27. vestibulary gland
28. bacterial infection
29. cardiac
30. brain
31. changes in diet
32. phosphates
33. pulmonary
34. $pO_2$
35. $pCO_2$
36. cow
37. surgical excision
38. ovaban and miliborne
39. 1.010
40. hypoglycemia
41. cystocentesis
42. coma and death
43. better canning methods
44. posterior digital nerve
45. surgical repair
46. urachus
47. $T_{13} - L_1L_2$
48. an infection
49. 9-12 weeks
50. amphotericin B.

# EXAMINATION SECTION

DIRECTIONS: Each question or incomplete statement is followed by several suggested answers or completions. Select the one that BEST answers the question or completes the statement. *PRINT THE LETTER OF THE CORRECT ANSWER IN THE SPACE AT THE RIGHT.*

1. Conception is *most likely* if the female is mated — 1. ___
   A. at the first sign of her heat cycle
   B. at the first appearance of a discharge
   C. during the first week of the heat cycle
   D. during the tenth to the fourteenth day of her heat cycle
   E. during the eighteenth to the twenty-first day of her heat cycle

2. All of the following are signs that a female is close to whelping EXCEPT: She — 2. ___
   A. pants and breathes heavily
   B. looks anxiously at her rear quarters
   C. frequently urinates
   D. refuses food
   E. exhibits extreme restlessness

3. During whelping, — 3. ___
   A. always remain a good distance from the female
   B. keep her alone in a dimly-lit room
   C. prevent her from eating the placenta
   D. keep a bowl of hot water nearby
   E. stay with her and be prepared to give assistance

4. The *largest* of the terrier family is the ______ Terrier. — 4. ___
   A. Airedale  B. American Staffordshire
   C. Cairn  D. Lakeland  E. Scottish

5. A dog with a very wiry coat and a characteristic "otter-like" head describes the __________ Terrier. — 5. ___
   A. Cairn  B. Bull  C. Irish  D. Skye
   E. Border

6. A toy dog covered from head to foot with a characteristic mantle of silky, white hair describes the — 6. ___
   A. Shih Tzu  B. Pekinese  C. Maltese
   D. Silky Terrier  E. Yorkshire Terrier

7. The *largest* and *tallest* of the galloping hounds is the — 7. ___
   A. Afghan Hound  B. Black and Tan Coonhound
   C. Irish Wolfhound  D. Basenji
   E. American Foxhound

8. An exotic expression, a long silky topnot, very prominent hip bones, and thick, silky hair describes the — 8. ___
   A. Borzoi  B. Saluki  C. Otter Hound
   D. Afghan Hound  E. Long-haired Dachshund

9. A short-legged dog, heavier in bone for its size than any other breed, describes the 9. ___
A. Beagle B. Dachshund C. Sealyham Terrier
D. Sussex Spaniel E. Basset Hound

10. The skin is thin to the touch and extremely loose, especially about the head and neck where it hangs in deep folds, describes the 10. ___
A. Bloodhound B. St. Bernard C. Black and Tan Coonhound
D. Vizsla E. Manchester Terrier

11. An extremely hardy hunting dog with a distinctive dense gray coat is the 11. ___
A. Irish Wolfhound B. Otter Hound
C. Rhodesian Ridgeback D. Scottish Deerhound
E. Norwegian Elkhound

12. A dog that hunts on both land and water with a rough double coat and webbed feet describes the 12. ___
A. Black and Tan Coonhound B. Otter Hound C. Basenji
D. Bloodhound E. English Foxhound

13. African Lion Hound is another name for the 13. ___
A. Rhodesian Ridgeback B. Chow Chow C. Akita
D. Bichon Frise E. Ibizan Hound

14. The royal dog of Egypt, bred for speed and endurance to kill quarry over deep sand and rocky mountains, is the 14. ___
A. Schipperke B. Samoyed C. Vizsla
D. Puli E. Saluki

15. Distinguished by a grayish-white face with either cap-like or mask-like markings and "snowshoe"-type feet aptly describes the 15. ___
A. Samoyed B. Great Pyrenees C. Akita
D. Alaskan Malamute E. Bernese Mountain Dog

16. A tog dog, distinguished by beautiful, erect butterfly-like ears, is the 16. ___
A. Papillon B. Shih-tzu C. Pomeranian
D. Yorkshire Terrier E. Japanese Spaniel

17. The *best* way to administer liquid medicine is to pour it 17. ___
A. down the back of the dog's throat
B. under his tongue
C. into his water bowl
D. on the wide, flat part of the tongue
E. into the funnel-like pounch of the bottom lip

18. All of the following are used in sled-work *except* the 18. ___
A. Kuvasz B. Great Pyrenees C. Alaskan Malamute
D. Samoyed E. Siberian Husky

19. Stripping is a term signifying removal of 19. ___
A. matted hair B. dead hair C. all hair
D. some hair for appearance E. tangled hair

20. A hound glove is used to 20. ___
A. give a hunting dog the scent
B. handle game
C. polish the coat of short-haired dogs
D. separate tangles of long-haired dogs
E. shape thick, curly-coated hair

21. Pure-bred puppies are produced by all of the following EXCEPT: 21. ___
A. Any mating between identical dogs of the same breed
B. Out-breeding
C. Cross-breeding
D. Line-breeding
E. In-breeding

22. The *best* time to mate a female for the *first* time is ______ of age. 22. ___
A. at six months B. one year C. eighteen months
D. three years E. five years

23. If a puppy has not begun to breathe after birth, 23. C
A. place the puppy on the mother's nipple
B. keep the puppy warm
C. clear the puppy's mouth of mucus
D. follow the rules for artificial respiration
E. there is nothing that can be done

24. *How many* teeth does an adult dog have? 24. ___
A. Twenty B. Twenty-two C. Thirty-two
D. Thirty-six E. Forty-two

25. The *first* secretion in the female's nipples essential to new-born puppies is 25. ___
A. lactogen B. colostrum C. proestrum
D. anestrum E. metestrum

26. The *average* length of the female heat cycle is 26. C
A. one week B. ten days C. twenty-one days
D. one month E. six months

27. All of the following are true of new-born puppies EXCEPT: They 27. ___
A. cannot see B. do not have the instinct for elimination
C. are born without hair D. are born without teeth
E. cannot hear

28. A pregnant female needs *more* 28. ___
A. egg whites B. yeast C. mulk and meat
D. milk and oil E. salt

29. A puppy does not completely control his bladder and anus until he is 29. ___
A. weaned B. removed from the mother
C. eight weeks old D. four months old E. six months old

30. Sarcoptic mange mites cause a disease called 30. ___
A. bubonic plague B. scabies C. coccidiosis
D. leptospirosis E. acne

31. Severe anemia can be caused by 31. ___
A. fleas B. whipworms C. mites
D. hookworms E. tapeworms

32. The larvae of tapeworms is carried by 32. ___
A. flies B. mosquitoes C. ticks
D. mites E. fleas

33. Heartworm is transmitted directly to the dog by an infected 33. ___
A. tick B. mosquito C. mite D. rat E. fly

34. A human should not let his skin come into contact with a dog infected with 34. ___
A. ringworm B. tapeworm C. eczema
D. whip E. heartworm

35. Leptospirosis is a dangerous disease because of the damage it does to the 35. ___
A. liver B. heart C. kidneys D. nervous system
E. reproductive organs

36. Leptospirosis is a bacterial disease carried by 36. ___
A. ticks B. lice C. flies D. mosquitoes
E. rats

37. The normal body temperature of a dog is 37. ___
A. 96.8° B. 101.5° C. 98.6° D. 99.2° E. 103°

38. The *first* symptom of progressive retinal atrophy is 38. ___
A. opacity of the lens B. corneal opacity
C. inturned lids D. night blindness
E. excessive blinking

39. The viral disease that can infect *both* humans and dogs is 39. ___
A. canine herpesvirus B. canine infectious hepatitis
C. distemper D. canine tracheobronchitis
E. rabies

40. Brandy is useful 40. ___
A. to calm a dog involved in an accident
B. after a heart attack
C. to warm an older dog
D. after a fainting spell
E. after a fit

41. All of the following are reasons why you should *not* attempt to worm a dog with a commercial medication EXCEPT: 41. ___
A. Worms may not be the trouble and indiscriminate worming will do further harm
B. A normal dose given to a sick or run-down dog may be lethal
C. The type of worm must be identified for the treatment to be effective
D. When the worms are not killed but only stunned enough to be passed out in the stool, they endanger other animals
E. Some dogs require preliminary measures such as blood transfusions before worming is begun

42. An *important* point to remember in beginning a heartworm prevention program is 42. ___

A. to begin after the last frost in spring and continue through to the first frost of autumn
B. to make certain through a blood test that the dog is not already infected with heartworm
C. that the dog must have a transfusion before treatment is begun
D. to give the dog an enema to clear the intestines of other internal parasites
E. to make certain through microscoptic examination of a stool sample that the dog is not already infected with heartworm

43. Luxation of the matella or dislocation of the knee cap is *more common* 43. ___

A. in hunting dogs
B. among racing dogs
C. in larger breeds
D. in miniature and toy dogs
E. among older dogs

44. Distemper virus is *most commonly* spread by 44. ___

A. contact with an infected dog's saliva
B. inhalation of infected air
C. contact with an infected dog's stool
D. drinking infected water
E. contact with an infected dog's urine

45. The *best* emergency treatment for a dog that is bleeding profusely is to 45. ___

A. apply a pressure bandage
B. locate the source and elevate that part of the dog
C. give aspirin to relieve the pain
D. tie a rope below the wound
E. keep the dog quiet and cover him with a blanket

46. A harness is preferable to a collar 46. ___

A. during a training session
B. with the larger breeds such as the Great Danes
C. with miniature breeds
D. with toy breeds
E. with neckless dogs such as the Pugs

47. The *best* way to hold a dog that might bite is to 47. ___

A. grasp the neck-folds, one hand on each side to control the head
B. grab the fur on the chest with one hand and the back of the neck with the other
C. encircle the neck with both hands
D. hold the dog's mouth shut
E. force the dog down and place a foot on his shoulder to immobilize him

48. *Which* of the following statements is(are) TRUE? 48. ___

I. A mongrel dog is more trainable than a pure-bred.
II. A mongrel dog is more resistant to disease than the pure-bred.
III. The mongrel is more intelligent than the pure-bred.
IV. The mongrel is more affectionate than the pure-bred.

The CORRECT answer is:
A. II *only* B. I,II C. I,IV D. I,II,III,IV
E. None of the above

49. An *easy* and *effective* way to deskunk a dog is to douse him with 49. ___
A. alcohol B. kerosene C. gasoline
D. tomato juice E. milk

50. The *most important* aspect of punishment is 50. ___
A. method B. tone of voice C. who punishes the dog
D. surprise E. timing

---

# KEY (CORRECT ANSWERS)

| | | | | | | | | | |
|---|---|---|---|---|---|---|---|---|---|
| 1. | D | 11. | E | 21. | C | 31. | D | 41. | D |
| 2. | C | 12. | B | 22. | C | 32. | E | 42. | B |
| 3. | E | 13. | A | 23. | D | 33. | B | 43. | D |
| 4. | A | 14. | E | 24. | E | 34. | A | 44. | B |
| 5. | E | 15. | D | 25. | B | 35. | C | 45. | A |
| 6. | C | 16. | A | 26. | C | 36. | E | 46. | E |
| 7. | C | 17. | E | 27. | C | 37. | B | 47. | A |
| 8. | D | 18. | A | 28. | C | 38. | D | 48. | E |
| 9. | E | 19. | B | 29. | D | 39. | E | 49. | D |
| 10. | A | 20. | C | 30. | B | 40. | C | 50. | E |

---

# EXAMINATION SECTION

DIRECTIONS: Each question or incomplete statement is followed by several suggested answers or completions. Select the one that BEST answers the question or completes the statement. *PRINT THE LETTER OF THE CORRECT ANSWER IN THE SPACE AT THE RIGHT.*

1. *What* is the *most common* symptom of intestinal disorders? 1. ___
   A. Diarrhea B. Vomiting C. Fever
   D. Bloody stools E. Loss of appetite

2. Effective treatment of Coprophagy includes: 2. ___
   I. Avoid long periods of confinement
   II. Arrange for regular exercise
   III. Remove feces from the premises daily
   IV. Prevent access to cat litter boxes
   V. Sprinkle meat tenderizer on the food

   The CORRECT answer is:
   A. I,II B. III,IV C. I,IV D. I,II,III,IV
   E. All of the above

3. *What* condition *rarely* appears in dogs under the age of five years? 3. ___
   A. Inflammation within the bones (Canine Panosteitis)
   B. Colitis
   C. Warts
   D. Gingival hypertrophy
   E. Rickets

4. *Which* condition is *most frequently* seen in large breeds of dogs? 4. ___
   A. Avascular Necrosis (Legg-Perthes Disease)
   B. Elbow Dysplasia
   C. Patellar Luxation
   D. Congenital Heart Disease
   E. Heat Stroke

5. Unpigmented nose skin is often subject to sunburn. *How* can this be prevented? 5. ___
   A. Coat the nose with sun tan lotion
   B. Coat the nose with a sun blocker lotion
   C. Coat the nose with petroleum jelly
   D. Administer daily dosages of Vitamin E
   E. Color the skin with a felt-tipped marking pencil

6. *Which* of the following is TRUE of debarking (devocalizing) the dog? 6. ___
   A. There are psychological effects
   B. The dog is unable to make any sound
   C. The dog can cry but not bark
   D. A gradual return of the dog's ability to bark is to be expected
   E. The procedure is inhumane and should never be done

7. *What* is the incubation time of Tetanus? 7. ___
A. 1 week B. 4-20 days C. 10-30 days D. 48-72 hours
E. 1-2 weeks

8. *What* type of tumor is *most common* in the female dog? _______ tumor. 8. ___
A. Uterus B. Breast C. Sertoli Cell
D. Vaginal E. Vulva

9. *Which* of the following statements is TRUE? 9. ___
A. Steak bones are the only type of bone that should ever be given to the dog.
B. All-meat diets provide good nutrition.
C. Hard suet is an acceptable fat supplement.
D. Table scraps are not nutritionally correct for the dog's diet.
E. Gelatin is not beneficial in the dog's diet.

10. All of the following are acceptable food additives EXCEPT 10. ___
A. sugar B. honey C. lemon D. vinegar E. garlic

11. *What* is *essential* to a self-feeding program? 11. ___
A. Canned dog food or meat supplements are supervised feedings
B. Regular meals are discontinued
C. Clean fresh water is available at all times
D. Only dry food is provided
E. The dog is not confined to the house

12. Pregnancy can *usually* be confirmed 12. ___
A. with a blood test two weeks after breeding
B. with a urine test ten days after breeding
C. by feeling for uterus enlargement a month after breeding
D. by x-ray examination three weeks after breeding
E. by taking the female's temperature twenty-four hours after breeding

13. *Which* of the following is TRUE of commercial canned dog food? 13. ___
A. Approximately three pounds of canned dog food is the equivalent of one pound of dry dog food
B. Canned dog food is less expensive than dry dog food
C. Water must be available at all times for a dog on a canned dog food diet
D. Canned dog food is used for dogs on self-feeding programs
E. Canned dog food provides more energy than dry dog food because of its high fat content

14 Dogs are MOST responsive to 14. ___
A. the scent of their masters B. food odors
C. the scent of strangers D. odors of animal origin
E. environmental odors

15. *What* is the BEST way to handle a puppy crying at night? 15. ___
A. Soothe him and then leave him alone
B. Scold him and then leave him alone
C. Hold him until he falls asleep and then put him back in his bed
D. Punish him
E. Ignore him

16. *What* skeletal differences are there between different breeds? 16. ___
I. Tail length
II. Presence and number of dew claws
III. Brain case size
IV. Bone size
V. Bone length

The CORRECT answer is:
A. IV,V
B. I,II,IV,V
C. III,IV,V
D. I,III,IV,V
E. All of the above

17. *Which* breed is the LARGEST member of the Spaniel family? 17. ___
______________ Spaniel.
A. Sussex
B. Irish Water
C. Field
D. English Springer
E. English Cocker

18. The Puli looks very much like a miniature version of the 18. ___
A. Briard
B. Newfoundland
C. Kuvasz
D. Giant Schnauzer
E. Bouvier des Flanders

19. *What* breed is considered the "King of the World's Shepherd Dogs?" 19. ___
A. Belgian Malinois
B. Belgian Sheepdog
C. Komondor
D. Belgian Tervuren
E. Bernese Mountain Dog

20. *What* breed has been nicknamed "the Hungarian Pointer?" 20. ___
A. Schipperke
B. Puli
C. Komondor
D. Kuvasz
E. Vizsla

21. *Which* of the following can be caused by eating indigestible material? 21. ___
I. Acute Gastritis
II. Acute Pancreatitis
III. Gastroenteritis
IV. Enteritis
V. Chronic Pancreatitis

The CORRECT answer is:
A. I,II,III
B. I,II,IV
C. I,III,IV,V
D. All of the above
E. None of the above

22. *Which* tooth is MOST frequently diseased due to its three very long roots? The 22. ___
A. first molar of the upper jaw
B. last molar of the upper jaw
C. incisors of the upper jaw
D. last premolar of the upper jaw
E. last molar of the lower jaw

23. All of the following can be transmitted to other dogs EXCEPT 23. ___
A. warts B. ringworm C. sarcoptic mange
D. canine brucellosis E. acral pruritic dermatitis

24. The presence of disease is *most often* detected by 24. ___
A. the condition of the dog's coat and skin
B. the clearness of the dog's eyes
C. an increase or decrease of the dog's appetite
D. mood changes
E. by changes in the dog's elimination patterns

25. *What* breed of dog is *most likely* to suffer from a sunburned nose? 25. ___
A. Briard B. German Shepherd C. Dachshund
D. Collie E. Great Dane

26. Oviarohysterectomy is recommended for all the following EXCEPT 26. ___
A. to prevent the female from having heat periods
B. to discourage the female from straying
C. to correct some skin diseases
D. to remove a severely infected uterus
E. when tumors or cysts are present

27. All of the following might be responsible for the presence of arthritis EXCEPT 27. ___
A. an inherited defect B. a congenital weakness
C. an injury D. an infection E. aging

28. Epilepsy occurs in 28. ___
A. mostly toy and miniature breeds
B. mostly the giant breeds
C. mostly mixed breeds
D. mostly the working breeds
E. all breeds

29. *What* food supplements can be used during weaning? 29. ___
I. Human baby cereal
II. Human baby canned meat and vegetables
III. Prescription diets (P/D)
IV. Commercial puppy chows
V. Ground beef

The CORRECT answer is:
A. III,IV B. I,II,IV C. II,III,IV,V
D. I,II,III,IV E. All of the above

30. The diet for a dog with gastrointestinal disorders may include: 30. ___
I. Cooked eggs II. Milk III. Cottage cheese
IV. Cooked rice V. Cooked vegetables

The CORRECT answer is:
A. II,III B. I,IV,V C. I,III,IV
D. I,II,III,IV E. All of the above

31. *What* is the *most common* eye disorder? 31. ___
A. Disease B. Inflammation C. Cataracts
D. Inturned lashes E. Cysts

32. The *next* heat period of the pregnant bitch will occur 32. ___
A. approximately six months after whelping
B. approximately six months after weaning
C. a year after the last period
D. six months after the last period
E. at any time after weaning

33. Frequent brushing 33. ___
A. irritates the skin B. reduces the need for a bath
C. produces dandruff D. may cause hair loss
E. may dull the coat

34. *Which* of the following statements is FALSE? The dog 34. ___
A. may hear higher tones than man
B. can estimate the distance over which a sound has travelled
C. can hear fainter sounds than man
D. is more adept than man at localizing the source of sounds
E. is more adept than man at determining the spatial location of sounds

35. A dog learns in all the following ways EXCEPT by 35. ___
A. mental images of past experiences
B. repeating the same action over and over again
C. imitating the behavior of another dog
D. fear of punishment
E. his eagerness to please

36. *Which* of the following is TRUE? 36. ___
A. A good hunting dog's offspring will also be good hunters
B. Once a female whelps a mongrel litter, subsequent litters will give evidence of it
C. Only in-bred, line-bred, and out-bred dogs are pure-blooded
D. Pregnant bitches can influence their puppies' development by maternal impressioning
E. During the cold months of the year, more males are conceived than females

37. *What* breed has been described as having the coloring of a Foxhound, the head of a Bloodhound, the running gear of a Dachshund, and a long, heavy body? 37. ___
A. Puli B. Welsh Corgi, Pembroke C. Bassett Hound
D. Australian Terrier E. French Bulldog

38. *What* breed is thought to be the BEST known worldwide because of its service to man? 38. ___
A. German Shepherd B. Doberman Pinscher
C. Collie D. Golden Retriever
E. Old English Sheepdog

39. *What* breed resembles the Doberman Pinscher but is heavier and slower? 39. ___

A. Manchester Terrier B. Great Dane
C. Rottweiler D. Smooth Collie
E. Pharoah Hound

40. The organ that causes the MOST problems for older dogs is the 40. ___

A. liver B. pancreas C. esophagus D. intestine
E. kidney

41. *What* condition is initially treated by withholding food and water? 41. ___

A. Acute pancreatitis B. Acute gastritis
C. Chronic gastritis D. Chronic pancreatitis
E. Diarrhea

42. All of the following are possible effects of dental tartar EXCEPT 42. ___

A. inflammation of the gums
B. recession of the gum tissue
C. small open sores on the inner lips
D. odorous breath
E. infection

43. *What* is the LARGEST gland in the male dog's body? The 43. ___

A. adrenal B. liver C. spleen D. prostate
E. testes

44. A *regular* grooming program should include: 44. ___

I. Brushing thd dog's teeth II. Emptying the anal sacs
III. Trimming the nails IV. Bathing
V. Removal of mats

The CORRECT answer is:
A. III,IV,V B. I,III,V C. I,III,IV,V
D. I,IV,V E. All of the above

45. Isolation is recommended during the initial stages of all the following EXCEPT 45. ___

A. canine brucellosis B. distemper
C. hepatitis D. tracheobronchitis
E. rabies

46. *What* is the *key* symptom of low blood sugar in a dog with Diabetes Mellitus? 46. ___

A. Lethargy B. Frenzy C. Depression
D. Trembling and shaking E. Sharp,frequent mood changes

47. *Which* of the following are *basic* principles of fracture cure? 47. ___

I. Placing the broken ends together
II. Fastening the fragments in place
III. Reattachment and anchoring the fragments
IV. Keeping the parts motionless
V. Suture repair

The CORRECT answer is:
A. I,IV B. I,III,IV C. I,II,IV
D. I,II,IV,V E. I,III,IV,V

48. *What* is the purpose of epilepsy medication? To 48. ___
A. cure the disease
B. limit the duration of the seizures
C. eliminate all disease symptoms
D. prolong life
E. control the disease

49. *What* room temperature should be maintained for newborn orphaned puppies? 49. ___
A. 75°F B. 70°F C. 80°F D. 85°F E. 95°F

50. *What* is the *most important* nutritional consideration in the treatment of a kidney problem? 50. ___
A. Providing adequate mineral supplements
B. Providing adequate vitamin supplements
C. Regulating fat in-take
D. Restriction of carbohydrates
E. Management of protein in-take

## KEY (CORRECT ANSWERS)

| | | | | | | | | | |
|---|---|---|---|---|---|---|---|---|---|
| 1. | A | 11. | C | 21. | C | 31. | D | 41. | A |
| 2. | E | 12. | C | 22. | D | 32. | D | 42. | C |
| 3. | D | 13. | A | 23. | E | 33. | B | 43. | B |
| 4. | D | 14. | D | 24. | A | 34. | B | 44. | B |
| 5. | E | 15. | E | 25. | D | 35. | A | 45. | E |
| 6. | D | 16. | B | 26. | B | 36. | E | 46. | D |
| 7. | B | 17. | B | 27. | A | 37. | C | 47. | B |
| 8. | B | 18. | A | 28. | E | 38. | A | 48. | E |
| 9. | D | 19. | C | 29. | E | 39. | C | 49. | D |
| 10. | A | 20. | E | 30. | C | 40. | E | 50. | E |

# EXAMINATION SECTION

DIRECTIONS: Each question or incomplete statement is followed by several suggested answers or completions. Select the one that BEST answers the question or completes the statement. *PRINT THE LETTER OF THE CORRECT ANSWER IN THE SPACE AT THE RIGHT.*

1. To become accredited, a graduate Veterinarian MUST 1.____
   A. receive approval of the State Veterinary Medical Association
   B. be licensed in the state, be a graduate of a college of veterinary medicine, pass the accreditation examination, and request accreditation by contacting state and federal animal health officials
   C. have had one year of experience since graduation
   D. hold a current license in at LEAST two states

2. The cooperative state-federal brucellosis eradication program is 2.____
   A. conducted under authority of state and federal laws and regulations using the recommended Uniform Methods and Rules of the USAHA as a guide
   B. Conducted under regulations of the United States Animal Health Association (USAHA)
   C. conducted under federal regulations
   D. conducted under state regulations

3. The U.S. Department of Agriculture administers Public Law 89-544 (The Laboratory Animal Welfare Act) which governs the humane care and treatment of 3.____
   A. horses, cows, swine, rabbits, guinea pigs, and rodents used for research
   B. all warmblooded vertebrate animals used for research
   C. dogs, cats, rabbits, guinea pigs, hamsters and monkeys used for research
   D. rabbits, rats, guinea pigs, hamsters, gerbils and mice used for research

4. Which of the following is a responsibility of veterinarians conducting the tuberculin test? 4.____
   A. Consider and record all deviations from normal
   B. Require animals to be restrained when infecting tuberculin
   C. Use technical skill in application and interpretation of the test
   D. All of the above

5. Cattle intended for export from the United States MUST 5.____
   A. be tuberculin and brucellosis tested irrespective of circumstances
   B. leave the country through the nearest port of export

C. be vaccinated for shipping fever according to regulations
D. be accompanied to port of embarkation by a properly issued and endorsed health certificate

6. Amendments to the federal regulations which deal with animal disease control and eradication activities are 6.____
A. formulated by the Association of State Department of Agriculture
B. acted upon by Congress
C. published in all local newspapers to meet legal requirements
D. promulgated by the Animal Health Division, ARS, and U.S. Department of Agriculture

7. One of the stated purposes of the Laboratory Animal Welfare Act is to 7.____
A. have government control of animals used during actual research
B. protect owners of dogs and cats from theft of such animals
C. prevent the unnecessary use of animals for research
D. promote a MORE efficient usage of the animals covered by the Act

8. The person responsible for familiarizing the accredited veterinarian with state and federal requirements relative to hog cholera regulations for shipping swine is the 8.____
A. accredited veterinarian himself
B. area veterinarian
C. president of the veterinarian's state association
D. ANH veterinarian in charge

9. The standards as required by the Laboratory Animal Welfare Act and as developed by USDA cover 9.____
A. maximum requirements to attain humane care and handling of the involved species of animals
B. maximum requirements for housing, feeding, watering, sanitation, ventilation, shelter, separation of species, and veterinary care
C. minimum requirements for housing, feeding, watering, sanitation, ventilation, shelter, separation of species, and veterinary care
D. the development of protocol for conducting research on the involved species of animals

10. The accredited veterinarian should 10.____
A. become well versed in his/her responsibilities to the state-federal hog cholera eradication program
B. see that swine with hog cholera are shipped immediately for slaughter
C. understand all phases of the state-federal hog cholera eradication program
D. be able to carry out both A. and C.

11. A carload of aged female cattle is being shipped to Canada for slaughter purposes only. To satisfy our export requirements, they MUST be inspected and 11.____
   A. exported through a designated port
   B. tested negative to tuberculosis alone
   C. shipped by rail only
   D. tested negative to tuberculosis and brucellosis

12. Outbreaks of domestic and suspected foreign poultry diseases should be reported by accredited veterinarians to 12.____
   A. public health officials
   B. local news media
   C. the appropriate state or federal animal health officials
   D. county sheriff

13. Official interstate health certificates may be issued only by 13.____
   A. accredited veterinarians and livestock inspectors
   B. graduate veterinarians
   C. accredited veterinarians and state or federal employees who are veterinarians
   D. licensed veterinarians

14. When identifying cattle with eartags for any official reason, the veterinarian should 14.____
   A. place an official tag in every animal
   B. place an official tag in every animal and in addition record the numbers of other tags already in the animals
   C. place official tags in untagged animals and record the numbers of other tags already in the animals
   D. leave the eartags with the owner

15. Responsibility for obtaining information concerning the health requirements of the country of destination including a prior permit rests primarily with the 15.____
   A. accredited veterinarian   B. state official
   C. carrier   D. exporter

16. Specimens from suspected vesicular and foreign diseases should 16.____
   A. not be shipped anywhere until shipment is approved
   B. be shipped immediately to the state-federal official in the state
   C. be shipped immediately to the Plum Island Laboratory
   D. be shipped immediately to the State Diagnostic Laboratory nearest the suspected outbreak

17. The primary responsibility for the control of interstate movements of animals lies with the 17.____
   A. Animal Health Division, USDA
   B. U.S. Animal Health Association

C. Animal Health officials of the State of destination
D. Interstate Commerce Commission

18. The state-federal Emergency Animal Disease Eradication Organization has been established in each state to handle 18.____
A. rabies in domestic animals
B. investigate cases of scrapie in sheep
C. outbreaks of exotic foreign animal diseases
D. all livestock diseases

19. A mink breeder requests for export shipment of two breeding mink to Canada, the issuance of a health certificate by an accredited veterinarian and an endorsement of the certificate by an ANH Division veterinarian authorized to perform that service. 19.____
A. The regulations of the Department require the issuance and endorsement of health certificates for the export shipment of mink
B. The accredited veterinarian CANNOT issue a health certificate for the export shipment of mink because there are no applicable regulations for such animals
C. The ANH Division has no objection to the issuance and endorsement of health certificates for the export shipment of mink if only accurate and true statements are made thereon
D. None of the statements is correct

20. The use of diagnostic facilities at the National Animal Disease Laboratory, Ames, Iowa are available 20.____
A. to accredited veterinarians only after clearance with their veterinarian in charge of the ANH Division
B. for the identification of certain disease organisms
C. to accredited veterinarians with no local diagnostic facilities
D. to all accredited veterinarians wishing to identify or confirm suspected disease conditions

21. An importer offers for entry into the United States at the Port of New York a dozen live adult partridges from Germany. These birds to be eligible for entry must: 21.____
I. be quarantined for a specific minimum period
II. be accompanied by a prior permit from the Hyattsville office of the ANH Division
III. be accompanied by a health certificate issued by a salaried veterinarian of the German Government
The correct answer is
A. all three statements are correct
B. only statements I and III are correct
C. only statement II is correct
D. none of the statements are correct

22. The responsibility of an accredited veterinarian when confronted with possible screwworm infestations is to 22.____
A. identify any specimens found and report the identification to state or federal authorities
B. treat infested wounds and spray the entire herd

C. collect specimens, treat the wound, and submit the specimens to state or federal animal disease officials for identification
D. treat the infested animals

23. John Doe wishes to import a prize Hereford bull directly to the United States from a country infected with foot and mouth disease, subsequent to quarantine at the Department's quarantine station at the Port of New York. He 23.____
A. MUST make arrangements for quarantine of the animal for 60 days
B. CANNOT do so because the movement which he proposes is presently prohibited by law
C. MUST have the bull tested
D. MUST first obtain a prior permit from the ANH Division in Hyattsville and MUST see that properly completed test charts and a health certificate accompany the animal

24. The Uniform Methods and Rules for Tuberculosis Eradication are changed 24.____
A. when found necessary be a meeting of state veterinarians
B. locally, when a state cannot get the required number of cattle tested
C. when infection has been reduced to the vanishing point
D. when recommended by the United States Animal Health Association and approved by the Animal Health Division of the U.S. Department of Agriculture

25. The cervical tuberculin test is used in known infected herds 25.____
A. because it NEVER fails to detect all of the tuberculosis infections in the herd
B. because it is an easier place to inject
C. because it appears more professional to the owner
D. when directed by local/state and federal officials

26. Vesicular conditions and other animal diseases NOT readily recognized or easily diagnosed should be reported to state and federal animal health officials promptly and without fail because 26.____
A. only domestic diseases are considered of importance
B. it is necessary to test the efficiency of state-federal emergency disease eradication organizations
C. *increased* world traffic by air and surface routes is multiplying the danger of foreign animal diseases entering the country
D. indemnity money may be available

27. When scrapie is suspected, the MOST important procedure to follow is to 27.____
    A. recommend immediate slaughter of affected animals
    B. report it immediately to state or federal animal health officials
    C. cull and ship for slaughter
    D. treat the sheep symptomatically

28. Frozen beef from foot and mouth disease infected countries is permitted entry into the U.S. 28.____
    A. if the shipment is transported under seal
    B. if upon inspection at the port of entry the shipment is accompanied by a proper certificate
    C. if the meat is packed in substantial tight leak-proof containers
    D. all of the above are INCORRECT

29. In reporting the history of a group of sheep suspected of having scrapie to the animal health official, which factor do you consider the MOST important? 29.____
    A. Whether the sheep are managed as a range band or farm flock
    B. Prevalence of sucking insects
    C. Purchases and sales in the past three to four years
    D. Quality of feed and general sanitation

30. Beef products may be imported into the U.S. from a country where foot and mouth disease exists WITHOUT restriction if 30.____
    A. effective and acceptable processing has been done in the country of origin
    B. the animals from which product is derived are vaccinated
    C. the shipment is moved *directly* to the port of entry
    D. the product is in tight containers

31. Anaplasmosis, an infectious and transmissible disease of cattle characterized by destruction of the erythrocytes 31.____
    A. is an example of another livestock disease that has been eradicated from the United States by the efforts of accredited veterinarians and cooperating state and federal regulatory officials
    B. has shown NO response to broad-spectrum antibiotic treatment
    C. has been reported in a majority of the states and movement of infected animals is subject to state and federal restrictions
    D. has been kept out of the United States by prompt application of control measures in the Hawaiian Islands in 1955

32. What does RESTRICTED ENTRY of animal by-products mean? 32.____
    A. Inspection of cargo at dockside
    B. Supervision of handling
    C. Release only to previously approved establishments
    D. All of the above

33. Which of the following possible courses of action by an accredited veterinarian in scabies work is NOT acceptable? 33.____
   A. Treat known cases WITHOUT reporting to animal health officials
   B. Acquire information relative to origin and possible spread of infestation
   C. Issue certificates for scabies-free sheep to move interstate
   D. Report ALL suspected cases to animal health officials

34. Before importing cultures of animal disease causing organisms, a scientist MUST obtain a permit from the USDA for the importation of 34.____
   A. ALL such cultures
   B. those organisms NOT present in the United States
   C. those organisms which will be used in studies involving animal inoculation
   D. those cultures originating in countries infected with foot and mouth disease or rinderpest

35. In the control and eradication of scabies in sheep or cattle, the accredited veterinarian should 35.____
   A. issue the permit for slaughter of affected sheep or cattle
   B. spray the infected animals
   C. arrange for dipping in chlordane
   D. do NONE of the above

# KEY (CORRECT ANSWERS)

| | | | |
|---|---|---|---|
| 1. B | 11. A | 21. A | 31. C |
| 2. A | 12. C | 22. C | 32. D |
| 3. C | 13. C | 23. B | 33. A |
| 4. D | 14. B | 24. D | 34. A |
| 5. D | 15. D | 25. D | 35. D |
| 6. D | 16. A | 26. C | |
| 7. B | 17. A | 27. B | |
| 8. A | 18. C | 28. D | |
| 9. C | 19. C | 29. C | |
| 10. D | 20. A | 30. A | |

# EXAMINATION SECTION

DIRECTIONS: Each question or incomplete statement is followed by several suggested answers or completions. Select the one that BEST answers the question or completes the statement. *PRINT THE LETTER OF THE CORRECT ANSWER IN THE SPACE AT THE RIGHT.*

1. Which of the following possible courses of action by an accredited veterinarian in scabies work is NOT acceptable? 1.____
   A. Report ALL suspected cases to livestock sanitary official
   B. Issue certificates for scabies-free sheep to move interstate
   C. Acquire information relative to origin and possible spread of infestation
   D. Treat known cases WITHOUT reporting to livestock sanitary officials

2. Dr. John Doe is an accredited veterinarian practicing in an area along the United States-Mexican border. He has a client living in Mexico who had an animal die from unknown causes. Dr. Doe performed a necropsy on the animal and brought (carefully packaged) tissue specimens into the United States for laboratory analysis. 2.____
   A. Dr. Doe should be commended for trying to determine the nature of an unknown disease in animals adjacent to our border
   B. Dr. Doe should not have brought the material into this country
   C. Under these circumstances, Dr. Doe was NOT required to obtain a permit from the Washington office of the AIQ Division
   D. only A. and C. are correct

3. In the control and eradication of scabies, the accredited veterinarian should 3.____
   A. treat the denuded area
   B. spray the affected sheep
   C. arrange for supervised dipping of all sheep in the flock
   D. advise immediate sale

4. There are accredited veterinarians in 60 major stockyards and thousands of local auctions to 4.____
   A. determine disease trends in interstate and intrastate travel
   B. prevent violation of law
   C. prevent diseased animals from entering the market
   D. test all animals for disease

5. Vesicular stomatitis is 5.____
   A. clinically distinguishable from foot and mouth disease
   B. of little importance
   C. a vesicular condition that should be reported promptly
   D. clinically distinguishable from vesicular exanthema

6. One of the stated purposes of the Laboratory Animal Welfare Act is to 6.____
   A. have government control of animals during actual research
   B. protect owners of dogs and cats from theft of such animals
   C. prevent the unnecessary use of animals for research
   D. promote MORE efficient usage of the animals covered by the Act

7. The Lab Animal Welfare Act regulations are the 7.____
   A. *maximum* requirements for human care and feeding of animals
   B. *maximum* requirements for feeding, housing, testing, and health care
   C. *minimum* requirements for feeding, housing, testing, and health care
   D. protocol for handling animals in research covered by the Act

8. What is the responsibility of the veterinarian in the hog cholera eradication program? 8.____
   A. Inform and educate campaigns concerning the disease and its eradication
   B. Permit shipment to slaughter hogs with hog cholera
   C. Know about ALL phases of the eradication program
   D. BOTH A. and C.

9. To become accredited, a graduate veterinarian must 9.____
   A. have had one year of experience since graduation
   B. receive approval of the State Veterinary Medical Association
   C. be licensed in the state, be a graduate of an approved veterinary college, and request accreditation by contacting state and federal livestock sanitary authorities
   D. hold a current license in AT LEAST two states

10. All states are referred to as being MODIFIED ACCREDITED for tuberculosis. This means that 10.____
   A. tuberculosis in cattle has been eradicated in that state
   B. there is *less than* 0.5 percent infection in the cattle in the state
   C. there is *less than* 0.5 percent infection in the cattle and poultry in the state
   D. ALL dairy herds are free of disease

11. The cooperative state-federal brucellosis eradication program is conducted under 11.____
   A. state regulations
   B. federal regulations
   C. regulation of the United States Livestock Sanitary Association (USLSA)
   D. authority of state and federal laws and regulations using the recommended Uniform Methods and Rules of the USLSA as a guide

12. Provisional accreditation, prior to a State Board Examination, may be 12.____
   A. obtained by submitting the names of three accredited veterinarians as references
   B. granted by the State Livestock Sanitary official and the Federal Veterinarian in charge of the state
   C. obtained by submitting a copy of the application to take the State Board Examination
   D. automatic, provided sufficient bond is posted

13. USDA export regulations administered by the Animal Inspection and Quarantine Division, are designed 13.____
   I. to insure that only healthy animals are exported
   II. to enable foreign countries to receive only high quality animals from the United States

   The CORRECT answer is
   A. *only* I is the correct answer
   B. *only* II is the correct answer
   C. *both* I and II are correct
   D. *neither* of the statements are correct

14. The primary purpose of accreditation of graduate veterinarians is to 14.____
   A. obtain a list of qualified veterinarians
   B. insure adequate animal disease control by authorized competent individuals acting in behalf of the livestock owners and the livestock industry as a whole, in the BEST interests of the public
   C. restrict the privilege of cooperation in livestock disease control and eradication activities to those individuals who are willing to carry out current policies
   D. instill in graduate veterinarians an idealistic sense of duty to the livestock industry

15. The export regulations of the U.S. Department of Agriculture are 15.____
   A. applicable to all animals and poultry
   B. the same as the import requirements of countries of destination
   C. minimum requirements and take precedence over the import regulations of other countries which may be less restrictive
   D. necessary to control the numbers and kinds of animals leaving the country

16. Equine piroplasmosis was FIRST diagnosed in the United States in 16.____
    A. 1910 B. 1937 C. 1956 D. 1961

17. Cattle intended for export from the United States MUST 17.____
    A. be accompanied to the port of embarkation by a properly issued and endorsed health certificate
    B. be vaccinated for shipping fever according to regulations
    C. leave the country through the *nearest* port of export
    D. be tuberculin and brucellosis tested irrespective of circumstances

18. Amendments to the federal regulations which deal with animal disease control and eradication activities are 18.____
    A. acted upon by Congress
    B. published in ALL local newspapers to meet legal requirements
    C. promulgated by the U.S. Department of Agriculture
    D. formulated by the Association of State Departments of Agriculture

19. Tuberculosis and brucellosis tests of cattle for export MUST be completed within ______ of the date of movement from the premises of origin. 19.____
    A. 60 days B. 3 months C. 3 weeks D. 30 days

20. Uniform Methods and Rules for Tuberculosis Eradication are changed 20.____
    A. when infection has been reduced to the vanising point
    B. locally, when a state CANNOT get the required number of cattle tested
    C. when recommended by United States livestock sanitary officials
    D. when found necessary by a meeting of state veterinarians

21. The cooperative state-federal brucellosis eradication program began as a drought relief program in 21.____
    A. 1904 B. Nebraska C. 1934 D. 15 states

22. Federal regulations concerning the hog cholera eradication program 22.____
    A. permit interstate shipment of hogs fed raw garbage
    B. permit interstate shipment of slaughter hogs affected with hog cholera if the hogs are consigned to a slaughtering establishment operating under federal inspection
    C. establish inspection and vaccination procedures for health, unexposed feeding and breeding swine moving interstate
    D. restrict intrastate movement of hogs

23. A two year old Holstein female, officially vaccinated against brucellosis at 7 months of age in a tuberculosis accredited and brucellosis certified free herd, is offered for export. 23.____
In order to meet AIQ export regulations, she MUST be
A. negative to tuberculin and brucellosis tests within 60 days
B. negative to the tuberculin test within 30 days
C. negative to the brucellosis test within 3 weeks
D. accompanied by a health certificate only

24. Outbreaks of domestic and suspected foreign poultry diseases should be reported by accredited veterinarians to 24.____
A. public health officials
B. the appropriate state livestock sanitary officials
C. local news media
D. county sheriff

25. The state-federal cooperative tuberculosis eradication program was started in 25.____
A. 1939 B. 1903 C. 1923 D. 1917

26. The responsibility for obtaining information concerning the health requirements of the country of destination, including a prior permit, rests primarily with the 27.____
A. carrier
B. owner or exporter
C. accredited veterinarian
D. state official

27. Specimens from suspected vesicular and foreign diseases should 28.____
A. be shipped immediately to the State Diagnostic Laboratory nearest the suspected outbreak
B. be shipped immediately to the Plum Island Laboratory
C. be shipped immediately to the state-federal official in the state
D. should NOT be shipped anywhere

28. The agency that has the primary responsibility for the control of interstate movements of animals is the 28.____
A. Animal Inspection and Quarantine Division (USDA)
B. livestock sanitary authority of state and destination
C. United States Livestock Sanitary Association
D. Animal Disease Eradication Division (USDA)

29. Official interstate health certificates may be issued only by 29.____
A. licensed veterinarians
B. accredited veterinarians and livestock inspectors
C. graduate veterinarians
D. accredited veterinarians and state and federal employees who are veterinarians

30. The State-Federal Emergency Disease Eradication Organization has been established in each state to handle 30.____
   A. rabies in domestic animals
   B. outbreaks of foreign animal diseases
   C. cases of scrapie in sheep
   D. cases of dourine or glanders

31. The National Council on Interstate Shipment of Milk has adopted an abnormal milk policy allowing for a leukocyte count of *less than* ______ per ml. 31.____
   A. 250,000 B. 500,000 C. 1,000,000 D. 2,000,000

32. Some states and municipalities require a permit for milk producing animals (physical examination) before they are allowed to produce milk for pasteurization. How many animals are allowed before one needs to file a permit with the issuing agency? 32.____
   A. 7 B. 10 C. 14 D. 21

33. You have a client who says he is flying to Canada to purchase 10 ampoules of bull semen. He will have a health certificate but wants to know what else is necessary to permit him to fly back with the semen. The client 33.____
   A. MUST get a prior permit from the ANH Division in Hyattsville, Maryland
   B. MUST have a health certificate and statement that the semen will be shipped frozen
   C. CANNOT fly back with the animal semen
   D. has NO further requirements

34. After being accredited in one state, a veterinarian seeking accreditation in another state MUST 34.____
   A. write the State Board of Examiners
   B. practice fulltime in the other state
   C. do nothing, since his accreditation is automatic for all states
   D. be licensed in the other state and request accreditation by contacting state and federal animal health officials in that state

35. Accreditation grants the veterinarian the privilege of representing the state and federal governments. Violations of the Standards of Accreditation could lead to 35.____
   A. revocation of accreditation
   B. serious charges by the livestock industry
   C. states receiving diseased livestock in interstate movement
   D. ANY or ALL of the above

# KEY (CORRECT ANSWERS)

1. D
2. B
3. C
4. C
5. C

6. B
7. C
8. D
9. C
10. B

11. D
12. B
13. A
14. B
15. C

16. D
17. A
18. C
19. D
20. C

21. C
22. C
23. B
24. B
25. D

26. B
27. D
28. B
29. D
30. B

31. D
32. B
33. A
34. D
35. D

# VETERINARY PRACTICE ACTS

## CONTENTS


| | Page |
|---|---|
| Alabama ...... Connecticut | 1 |
| Delaware ......Idaho | 2 |
| Illinois ......Kentucky | 3 |
| Louisiana ...... Michigan | 4 |
| Minnesota ...... Nebraska | 5 |
| Nevada ...... North Carolina | 6 |
| North Dakota ...... Rhode Island | 7 |
| South Carolina ...... Virginia | 8 |
| Washington ...... Puerto Rico | 9 |
| Virgin Islands ...... Nova Scotia | 10 |
| Ontario ...... Saskatchewan | 11 |

# Digests of Veterinary Practice Acts

For complete information on the requirements of any practice act, and inquiry should be addressed to the Executive Officer of the Board.

## Alabama

(From Alabama General Law, Regular Session 1915, Enacted March 17, 1915; revised September 13, 1951.)

EXAMINATIONS – at least two examinations each year, and more as may be deemed necessary, will be held at such times and places as the Board designates. Special examinations may be held anywhere in the state at the direction of the Board.

CREDENTIALS – Must be a graduate of school of veterinary medicine accredited by the Council on Education of the AVMA and supply proof of good moral character. Internship of three months under a qualified veterinarian, special limited permit being granted until examinations are given the Board.

FEE – $15.00 for certificate of qualification.

REGISTRATION – State registration of license required; annual fee $10.00. Initial registration of license required by county; fee, $1.00.

RECIPROCITY – Board does not reciprocate with any other state, but allows limited practice in counties of the state of Alabama which adjoin the county of residence of a practitioner in the adjoining state.

CITIZENSHIP – Must be a citizen of the United States.

EXECUTIVE OFFICER OF BOARD – Dr. Ray Ashwander, Secretary-Treasurer, Alabama State Board of Veterinary Medical Examiners, P. O. Box 1767, Decatur, AL 35601.

## Alaska

(Revised March 27, 1968.)

EXAMINATIONS – Examinations are held in November of each year.

FEES – Examination fee $25.00; Initial license fee $25.00; Biennial renewal $50.00; Temporary license $10.00.

EXECUTIVE OFFICER OF THE BOARD – Dr. James C. Beckley, 1521 Stacia St., Fairbanks, AK 99701.

## Arizona

(Practice law first enacted in 1923; revised March 27, 1947 and March 28, 1953. Revised June 12, 1967.)

EXAMINATIONS – Examinations shall be held in December and June of each year, and on such other dates as the Board may determine.

CREDENTIALS – Graduation from a recognized veterinary college and certificates of good moral character.

FEE – $100.00.

REGISTRATION – State registration of license required: annual fee fixed by law $25.00.

RECIPROCITY – None.

CITIZENSHIP – U. S. Citizen

EXECUTIVE OFFICER OF BOARD – Ms. Paula Jacobson, Executive Secretary, 1688 W. Adams, Rm. 319, Phoenix, AZ 85007.

## Arkansas

(Act 171 of 1963 created a new Veterinary Examining Board; amended by Act 217 of 1971; last revision and amendments were created by Act 650 of 1975).

EXAMINATIONS – Annually, usually in June each year and shall be held in the City of Little Rock.

CREDENTIALS – Diploma from an accredited college. Foreign graduates are required to have a certificate issued by the Education Commission for Foreign Veterinary Graduates (ECFVG). Applications must be filed 30 days prior to exam.

FEE – Examination $50.00; Reciprocity $100.00

REGISTRATION – State registration of license required; annual fee due March 31 each year $40.00. Participation in a Continuous Educational Program is required each year to renew license. The fee for inactive license renewal is $20.00; this applies to veterinarians not practicing in the state of Arkansas, or those persons who do not derive their livelihood from the practice of veterinary medicine.

RECIPROCITY – At discretion of the Board. (1) The Board may grant reciprocity to licensees who have practiced continuously for five years or more immediately before application and holds proof of license in that state which has license requirements substantially equivalent to the requirements of this state. (2) Within the next 3 years prior to filing his application successfully completed the examination conducted by the National Board of Veterinary Examiners.

CITIZENSHIP – Citizen of the United States or an applicant for citizenship.

EXECUTIVE OFFICER OF BOARD – Dr. Robert J. VanPatter, Secretary-Treasurer, Arkansas Veterinary Medical Examining Board, 2915 South Pine, Little Rock, AR 72204.

## California

(From Business and Professions Code, Chapter 933 of the Statues of 1937; Practice Law first enacted in 1893; last revised June, 1965.)

EXAMINATIONS – Semiannually, at School of Veterinary Medicine, University of California, Davis.

CREDENTIALS – Diploma from recognized veterinary school. Application must be filed thirty days before examination with board secretary.

FEE – $50.00 for Practical; $45.00 for National.

REGISTRATION – State registration of license required; biennial fee (2 years), $65.00; delinquent fee, $8.00.

RECIPROCITY – Practical examination required of all. Written examination may be waived under certain regulated circumstances.

EXECUTIVE BOARD OFFICER – Mr. Gary K. Hill, Executive Secretary, Board of Examiners in Veterinary Medicine, 1020 N. St., Rm. 419, Sacramento, CA 95814.

## Colorado

(Practice Act approval April 24, 1909; last amended July 1, 1973).

EXAMINATIONS – At such time and places as are designated by the Board and in mid-December; usually at Fort Collins following graduation of each veterinary class from Colorado State University.

CREDENTIALS – Diploma from a school or college of veterinary medicine, recognized by the AVMA or the holder of a Certificate of Competence issued by the Educational Commission for Foreign Veterinary Graduates and satisfactory evidence of having attained 21 years of age and being of good character.

FEE – $60.00 to be paid in advance of examination by applicant.

REGISTRATION – Annual renewal of license required before November 30, of each year. All licenses expire on December 31, of each year unless renewed. Renewal fee, $5.00, 16 hours continuing education required for renewal each year. Each licensee must notify the secretary of the Board immediately of any change in address.

RECIPROCITY – At the discretion of the Board with states whose standards equal those of Colorado.

CITIZENSHIP – Must be a United States citizen or have applied for citizenship.

EXECUTIVE OFFICER OF BOARD – Dr. Duane T. Albrecht, Secretary, Colorado Veterinary Medical Examining Board, 119 State Services Bldg., 1525 Sherman St., Denver, CO 80203.

## Connecticut

(From Chapter 384, General Statutes, Revision of 1959 Practice Law first enacted in 1905; revised in 1930, 1941, 1947, 1957 and 1959.)

EXAMINATIONS – The second Tuesday in January and July of each year at such places as the Board may designate and at such other times and places as it shall determine.

CREDENTIALS – The applicant will present, at the time of the examination, a photostat or original of his diploma and, likewise, a certificate of good moral character signed by two reputable citizens.

* Consult local board for latest fee and registration information

FEE – $150.00.

REGISTRATION – State registration of license required; annual fee, $150.00.

RECIPROCITY – Reciprocity may be granted, following satisfactory practical examination, to veterinarians who have been duly licensed and in practice in another state for five consecutive years or more preceding application, provided said state has at least equal requirements and also extends reciprocity to Connecticut licensees desiring same; reciprocity fee, $150.00.

CITIZENSHIP – No requirements.

EXECUTIVE OFFICER OF BOARD – Dr. Lewis I. Case, President, Connecticut State Board of Veterinary Registration and Examination, State Office Bldg., Room 279, Hartford, CT 06115.

## Delaware

(From Chapter 24 - No. 736, Section 1 through Section 8 of No. 743 of the Revised Code of Delaware 1935).

EXAMINATIONS – Annually, time designated by the Board, usually in June or June National Board common regional date.

CREDENTIALS – Diploma from a recognized veterinary school. One year Internship for foreign students; transcript of veterinary school grades.

FEE – $75.00 if National is not taken in Delaware. $100.00 if National is taken in Delaware.

REGISTRATION – $10.00 annual registration fee, plus $50.00 license fee, plus .003 license tax on gross income.

RECIPROCITY – None.

EXECUTIVE OFFICER OF BOARD – Dr. Donald A. Gooss, Secretary-Treasurer, Delaware State Board of Veterinary Medical Examiners, 307 N. du Pont Hwy., Georgetown, DE 19947.

## District of Columbia

(From the United States Statutes at Large, Vol. 34, Part 1, Public Laws, pages 870-873, 59th Congress, 2nd Session - Public No. 48, Senate No. 5989, Revised July 25, 1956).

EXAMINATIONS – To be given once a year. (Deadline to file is May 1st of each year.)

CREDENTIALS – Diploma from a veterinary school approved by the AVMA Council on Education. Graduates of foreign schools of veterinary medicine (except England and Canada) must submit a notarized copy of the examination certificate issued by the Educational Council on Foreign Veterinary Graduates (ECFVG).

FEE – Application $10.00, Examination $30.00, License $10.00.

REGISTRATION – No annual registration of license required.

RECIPROCITY – Possible only when a formal written agreement exists between jurisdictions.

CITIZENSHIP – No requirements.

EXECUTIVE OFFICER OF BOARD – District of Columbia Board of Examiners in Veterinary Medicine, Occupational & Professional Licensing Division, 614 H St., N.W., Washington, D.C. 20001.

## Florida

(From Chapter 474, approved name changed to Veterinary Medical Practice Act.)

EXAMINATIONS – At least once each year at time and place designated by the president of the Board. Applications & forms supplied by the Board to be filed with secretary at least 30 days prior to the examination.

CREDENTIALS – Proof of graduation from a recognized veterinary college.

FEE – $25.00

ANNUAL RENEWAL FEE – $20.00.

RECIPROCITY – None.

TEMPORARY PERMITS – If licensed in another state of the United States, may be issued at any time. If not licensed in another state of the United States, can only be issued ninety (90) days before the next examination. Must be associated and limited to the practice of a licensed doctor of veterinary medicine.

CITIZENSHIP – Must be a citizen of the United States.

EXECUTIVE OFFICER OF BOARD – Dr. Malcolm T. Barksdale, Secretary-Treasurer, Florida Board of Veterinary Medicine, 1601 Lee Road, Winter Park, FL 32789.

## Georgia

(From Sections 84-1501 through 84-1525 of Georgia Code Annotated. Practice Law enacted in 1908; amended in 1973).

EXAMINATIONS – Annually in June and December at the State Capitol, Atlanta. Applications must be made on forms supplied by Joint Secretary, State Examining Boards, 166 Pryor St., S.W., Atlanta.

CREDENTIALS – Must be graduate of approved school, and be of good moral character, and pass examination in required subjects.

FEE – $25.00, to accompany application form.

REGISTRATION – $5.00 annual registration fee if paid before December 31, of each year; $10.00 reinstatement fee if paid after that date.

RECIPROCITY – The Georgia Board does not reciprocate with any state at this time. Registration by examination only.

CITIZENSHIP – Required (By statute) or an application for citizenship.

EXECUTIVE OFFICER OF BOARD – James E. Skrine, Acting Joint Secretary, State Examining Boards, 166 Pryor St., S.W., Atlanta, GA 30303.

## Hawaii

(Veterinary Practice Act last revised in 1973.)

EXAMINATIONS – Examinations shall be given by the Board in April and September of each year. They shall be composed of written and oral questions and practical demonstrations. Applications shall be filed in such form as shall be prescribed by the Board by March 1 for the April examination and by August 1 for the September examination.

CREDENTIALS – Applicant must be a graduate of veterinary college meeting all the standards established by the AVMA.

FEE – $100.00.

REGISTRATION – Biennial registration of license in each even numbered year required; fee $30.00 on or before June 30 of each even numbered year.

CITIZENSHIP – No requirement.

EXECUTIVE OFFICER OF BOARD – Mrs. Maybelle Clark, Executive Secretary, Board of Veterinary Examiners, Box 3469, Honolulu, HI 96801.

## Idaho

The Idaho State Board of Veterinary Examiners have new laws as a result of legislation which became effective July 1, 1974: (From Idaho Code, Title 54, Chapter 21 and Title 67, Chapter 26.)

EXAMINATIONS – Examination for licensure shall be held once each year; the time and place being announced by the secretary-treasurer at least one hundred twenty (120) days prior to the date set for the examination. Applications to take the examination must be on file with Occupational License Bureau at least sixty (60) days prior to the date of the examination. The objective type of examination by the National Board of Veterinary Medical Examiners may be used, plus oral interviews and practical demonstrations.

CREDENTIALS – Graduate of a veterinary school.

FEES – As established by the Board.

REGISTRATION – State registration of license required; annual renewal fee, $20.00.

RECIPROCITY – May be granted to a veterinary graduate who: 1) has been practicing as a licensed veterinarian in a locality whose requirements at the time he was first licensed were equal to Idaho's for five (5) years previous to making application in Idaho; 2) has successfully completed the National Board Examination within the five (5) years prior to making application in Idaho; or 3) has a license in a locality which has requirements equal to Idaho's had has extended like privileges to applicants licensed in Idaho. The Board may orally or practically examine a reciprocity applicant.

CITIZENSHIP – U. S. citizenship or an applicant for U.S. citizenship required.

PERSON TO CONTACT FOR INFORMATION – M. D. Gregersen, Chief, Occupational LIcense Bureau, 2404 Bank Drive, Room 312, Boise, ID 83705.

### Illinois

(From the Illinois Veterinary Medicine and Surgery Act, approved April 24, 1899, last amended 1974.)

EXAMINATIONS – Semiannually in June and December, on dates set by the Department, June examination to be conducted at the University of Illinois, Champaign, Illinois, December examination, open.

CREDENTIALS – Application must be made on forms supplied by Department and accompanied by diploma from veterinary college and affidavit of graduation; supplemental application showing two years preveterinary collegiate training; application must be filed twenty days prior to examination with Department of Registration and Education, Springfield, IL.

FEE – $50.00 to accompany application.

REGISTRATION – The Department may reciprocate with other states in the interstate recognition and exchange of licenses upon a basis of equality of educational standard and mutual recognition, which standard shall not be lower than the requirements of this Act. An application from a person who desires to secure a license, by reciprocity, from the Department to practice veterinary medicine and surgery in the State shall be accompanied by a satisfactory proof that the applicant so applying for a license has been engaged in the actual and lawful practice of veterinary medicine and surgery in some other state for 2 consecutive years immediately prior to such application.

CITIZENSHIP – Citizenship or who has made a declaration of intention to become a citizen.

PERSON TO CONTACT – Mr. Ronald E. Stackler, Director, Department of Registration and Education, 628 E. Adams St., Springfield, IL 62706.

### Indiana

(Chapter 387, Acts of the Indiana General Assembly, 1959; Amended 1961, 1965, 1975.)

EXAMINATIONS – Board required by statute to hold one regular meeting annually at Indianapolis, Indiana and any special meeting which may be deemed necessary at a place fixed by the Board. The Board shall designate by regulation the day or days on which the regular meeting is to be held.

CREDENTIALS – List of recognized schools, colleges and universities established by Regulation Three. Affidavit of good moral character and loyalty oath required, tax statement required and such other statements or matter of proof as the Board may specify.

FEE – For the examination or re-examination of an applicant for a license to practice as a veterinarian, seventy dollars ($70.00). - For the granting of licenses by reciprocity, seventy dollars ($70.00). - For the granting of duplicate licenses, five dollars ($5.00). - For the issuance of a license to practice as a veterinarian, five dollars ($5.00). - For renewal of a certificate of registration to practice as a veterinarian, ten dollars ($10.00) per annum, payable biennially in advance. - For restoration of an expired certificate of registration to practice as a veterinarian, five dollars ($5.00) for up to one year of delinquency, plus the renewal fees required above. After one year, the fee for restoration of an expired certificate of registration is twenty-five dollars ($25.00) plus the renewal fees required above.

REGISTRATION – Ten dollars ($10.00) per annum, payable biennially in advance.

RECIPROCITY – Reciprocity now exists with the State of Ohio.

CITIZENSHIP – Proof of citizenship required if born outside of the United States. Aliens may be granted license at the discretion of the Board and subject to such conditions as the Board may see fit to impose.

EXECUTIVE OFFICER OF BOARD – Dr. Lowell W. Hinchman, State Veterinarian, Secretary of Examining Board, 801 State Office Bldg., 100 N. Senate Avenue, Indianapolis, IN 46204.

### Iowa

(From Chapter 169, Code of Iowa 1962. Practice Law first enacted in 1900, last revised 1965.)

EXAMINATIONS – At such times as designated by the Board, at the State House, Des Moines.

CREDENTIALS – Applications furnished by Department of Agriculture must be filed fifteen days prior to examination date with Division of Animal Industry and accompanied by license fee ($25.00) and proof of graduation from recognized school of veterinary medicine. Application for Professional Examination Service examination, fee $45.00, filed twenty-one days prior.

FEE – Total of $70.00 required for the two examinations (State and National).

REGISTRATION – State registration of license required; annual fee, $5.00.

RECIPROCITY – Subject to review by Board.

CITIZENSHIP – No requirement.

EXECUTIVE OFFICER OF BOARD – Dr. E. A. Butler, Secretary, Iowa State Veterinary Examining Board, State House, Des Moines, IA 50319.

### Kansas

(From Chapter 37, Laws of 1933 and Chapter 74, Article 25, General Statutes of 1935. Practice law first enacted in 1907, revised in 1935 and 1959, new law July 1, 1969.)

EXAMINATIONS – Held at Kansas State University, Manhattan, near end of school year, as set each year by Board, P.E.S. and practical exams used.

CREDENTIALS – Applicants must be citizens of the United States; a graduate of a recognized school of veterinary medicine and must furnish evidence of good moral character. Application in writing must be filed with board secretary prior to examination.

FEE – To be set.

REGISTRATION – State registration of license required; annual fee, $10.00.

RECIPROCITY – With any state having equal standards and will return reciprocity at the discretion of the board.

CITIZENSHIP – Required.

EXECUTIVE OFFICER OF BOARD – Dr. L. D. Jernigan, Secretary, Kansas State Board of Veterinary Examiners, R.R. 3, Council Grove, KS 66846.

### Kentucky

(From an Act of the Regular session of the Legislature in 1948 and approved by the Governor, March 29, 1948. Amended by an act of the Legislature, Regular Session, 1962 signed by Governor.)

EXAMINATIONS – At such times and places as scheduled by the Board.

CREDENTIALS – Must be a graduate of a school approved by the AVMA and by this board.

FEE – $25.00 application fee plus the amount charged by the Professional Examination Service for each examination.

REGISTRATION – State registration of license required; annual fee, $10.00

RECIPROCITY – With states accepting Kentucky licenses.

CITIZENSHIP – No requirements.

EXECUTIVE OFFICER OF BOARD – Mr. William E. Johnson, Executive Secretary and Legal Counsel, 326 W. Main St., P.O. Box 192, Frankfort, Ky. 40601.
Juanita M. Toole, Adm. Sec'y., 109 Spruce Drive, Frankfort, KY 40601.

## Louisiana

(Practice Law first enacted July 8, 1908; New Practice Act effective July 1, 1967.)

EXAMINATIONS – Held annually; notice of the examination published 120 days prior to examination date. The Louisiana Board of Veterinary Medicine shall meet annually but special meetings may be called by the president and secretary.

CREDENTIALS – Applicant must be a graduate of a veterinary college and approved by the Board. Each applicant must submit notarized application, examination fee and evidence of good character to the Board at least 30 days prior to the examination date.

FEE – Current Examination Fee $40.00; Original Registration Fee $10.00.

REGISTRATION – Annual registration of license, current fee $20.00.

RECIPROCITY – None.

CITIZENSHIP – Required.

EXECUTIVE OFFICER OF BOARD – Dr. Joe M. Dixon, Executive Secretary, Louisiana Board of Veterinary Medicine, P.O. Box 18460-B, Baton Rouge, LA 70803.

## Maine

(From Chapter 71-A, Maine Veterinary Practice Act of 1975. Practice Law first enacted May 19, 1905).

EXAMINATIONS – The oral-practical part of the examination is held in Augusta, Maine, near the end of the school year at a time designated by the Board.

The National Board part of the examination is held at the end of the school year, on a common date as designated by the Professional Examination Service and selected by the Board.

CITIZENSHIP – Applicants must be citizens of the United States or Canada.

CREDENTIALS – Applications must be made in writing on blanks provided for that purpose, accompanied by the current fee, a photostatic copy of the applicant's diploma from a veterinary college maintaining standards approved by the AVMA and the Maine Board, and a letter from the office of the dean stating the applicant's position in class.

Applications must be received at least 60 days before the date of the examination.

FEE – At discretion of the Board to reflect current Professional Examination Service fees.

RECIPROCITY – None.

REGISTRATION – Annual renewal of license required at a fee established by the Board.

EXECUTIVE OFFICER OF THE BOARD – Dr. Barry Fossett, 235 Hospital St., Augusta, ME 04330.

## Maryland

(Practice Law first enacted in 1895; revised by Acts of the Legislature in 1949, 1955 and 1972.)

EXAMINATIONS – Twice a year.

CREDENTIALS – Proof of graduation from a veterinary school approved by the AVMA and proof of completion of the course of study prescribed by such AVMA accredited school.

FEE – $50.00.

REGISTRATION – Annual registration required; fee $25.00.

RECIPROCITY – None.

CITIZENSHIP – Required, or E.C.F.V.G. dated after December 31, 1972.

EXECUTIVE OFFICER OF BOARD – Dr. E. Edgar Ruebush, Secretary-Treasurer, State Board of Veterinary Medical Examiners, 7979 Georgia Ave., Silver Spring, MD 20910.

## Massachusetts

(Practice Law first enacted in 1903; last revised August, 1974.)

EXAMINATIONS – Held January and June of each year.

CREDENTIALS – Birth certificate as proof applicant is 21 years of age or over; certification from dean of school which is approved by Board for Colleges, Universities and Schools of Veterinary Medicine, stating that applicant has attended for four years of at least 32 weeks each and has received degree of Doctor of Veterinary Medicine. Two passport pictures must accompany application which must be filed with board secretary at least one month before examination.

FEE – First examination $50.00 and thereafter $50.00 for each examination.

REGISTRATION – State registration of license required; annual fee, $15.00 payable prior to March 1st of each year.

RECIPROCITY – Any person who is a licensed or registered veterinarian in another state and who has been engaged in the practice of veterinary medicine for at least five consecutive years, and who presents to the board a copy of his certificate of registration or license, certified or attested under seal by the board of examiners or like board of any other state in which the requirements for registration are, in the opinion of the board, equivalent to the requirements of this commonwealth, may, upon application, accompanied by a fee of seventy-five dollars ($75.00) be given a practical examination, without examination on the theory of veterinary medicine, by the board, and if he demonstrates to said board his fitness to practice veterinary medicine, be registered as a veterinarian, and shall receive a certificate thereof; provided, that the applicant intends to remove to and reside in this commonwealth; and provided further, that such other state accords similar privilege to veterinarians registered under the laws of this commonwealth and removing to such other state.

CITIZENSHIP – Not required.

EXECUTIVE OFFICER OF BOARD – Dr. Burton D. Whitestone, Chairman, Board of Registration in Veterinary Medicine, Room 1514, Leverett Saltonstall Bldg., 100 Cambridge Street, Boston, MA 02202.

## Michigan

(Practice Law first enacted in 1907; new Practice Act enacted in 1956; amended by Act 33 of Public Acts of 1958, Act 33 of Public Acts of 1963 and Act No. 187, Public Acts of 1966; Act 182 of Public Acts of 1974)

EXAMINATIONS – Regular annual meeting of Board and examinations at Lansing. Dates to be announced. Meetings to conduct examinations or for purposes other than examinations may be held as often as the Board deems necessary. There will be at least one examination at the end of the spring term at Michigan State University, usually following graduation.

CREDENTIALS – Application setting forth length and terms of study, and diploma or certificate from a college registrar showing applicant possesses diploma from an approved veterinary college. Applications and credentials must be filed with secretary of Board at least thirty days prior to examination, except in the case of students, graduating less than thirty days before the examination.

FEE – Examination – $75.00 – Reciprocity – $100.00

REGISTRATION – Annual renewal of license required. An annual renewal fee of $10.00 shall be payable by each licensee on January 1 of each year. A license on which the annual renewal fee has not been paid by February 15 of the year in which the renewal fee is payable is delinquent and may be reinstated by the payment of an additional delinquent penalty fee of $10.00.

RECIPROCITY – The board may issue a license to practice veterinary medicine to an applicant by examination by the board who has been actively engaged in the profession in some other state, territory, or the District of Columbia for the preceding 2 years or has graduated from an approved school in the preceding 2 years upon the certificate of the proper licensing authority of that state, territory, or the District of Columbia, certifying that the applicant is duly licensed, that the license was never suspended or revoked, and that, so far as records of that authority are concerned, the applicant is entitled to its endorsement.

ADMINISTRATIVE OFFICER OF BOARD – Mrs. Shirley L. Smith, Administrative Secretary, Michigan State Board of Veterinary Examiners, Department of Licensing and Regulation, 1116 South Washington Avenue, Lansing, MI 48926.

### Minnesota

(From Minnesota statutes 1961, sections 156.01 through 156.14 as amended by Minnesota session laws 1965 chapter 204. Practice Law first enacted in 1896; last revised in 1965.)

EXAMINATIONS – Twice each year at a time and place prescribed by the Board.

CREDENTIALS – Application shall be made in writing to the Veterinary Examining Board upon a form furnished by the board, accompanied by satisfactory evidence that the applicant is at least 21 years of age, is of good moral character, and has received a diploma conferring the degree of doctor of veterinary school or its equivalent from a reputable veterinary school approved by the board. The application shall be filed with the secretary of the board at least 30 days before the date of examination. Every application shall contain the following information and meterial: 1) A fee of $50.00 in the form of check or money order payable to the state treasurer. 2) A certificate from the dean or secretary of an approved college of veterinary medicine showing the time spent in such school and the date of graduation. 3) Affidavits of at least two veterinarians and three other adults to enable the board to determine the moral character of applicant. 4) If the applicant has served in the Armed Forces he shall furnish a copy of his discharge.

FEE – $50.00.

REGISTRATION – State registration of license required; annual fee not to exceed $10.00, delinquent fee, $10.00.

RECIPROCITY – With qualifications, and such other tests the board considers proper. Reciprocity fee, $100.00. Contact examining board for additional information.

CITIZENSHIP – U. S. Citizenship not required.

EXECUTIVE OFFICER OF BOARD – Dr. Glen H. Nelson, Executive Secretary, Board of Veterinary Examiners, 2476 Sheldon St., St. Paul, MN 55113.

### Mississippi

(Practice Law first enacted in 1914; revised in 1916 and 1946. Amended 1971.)

EXAMINATIONS – On the third Tuesday in June of each year at Jackson, at a location selected by Board of Examiners. Applications must be filed with secretary of Board at least 30 days prior to examination.

CREDENTIALS – Applicants must be graduates of colleges recognized and approved by the AVMA and Bureau of Animal Industry.

FEE – $50.00.

REGISTRATION – $10.00 annual renewal fee. Require continuing education for renewal.

RECIPROCITY – None.

CITIZENSHIP – Applicant must be citizen of the United States.

EXECUTIVE OFFICER OF BOARD – Dr. R. E. Arline, Secretary-Treasurer, Mississippi Board of Veterinary Examiners, P. O. Box 1138, Greenwood, MS 38931.

### Missouri

(Original practice act enacted in 1905. Present Act enacted in 1963.)

EXAMINATIONS – At least once each year, at time and place selected by the Veterinary Medical Board. National Board Exam grades from other states acceptable in lieu of written portion of Missouri examination.

CREDENTIALS – Must be graduate of veterinary college having standards and requirements equal to the standards and requirements as may be adopted by the AVMA from time to time, or hold a certificate from AVMA Educational Commission for Foreign Veterinary Graduates.

FEE – $25.00, both examination and reciprocity.

REGISTRATION – Annual registration of licenses required, registration fee set by Veterinary Medical Board, but not to exceed $25.00.

RECIPROCITY – Reciprocity with states have comparable practice acts and who agree to reciprocate with the state of Missouri.

EXECUTIVE OFFICER OF BOARD – Dr. E. R. Price, Secretary, Missouri Veterinary Medical Board, P.O. Box 633, Jefferson City, MO 65101.

### Montana

(From Revised Codes of Montana, 1947. Practical Law first enacted in 1913; amended in 1965.)

EXAMINATIONS – Held in January and June of each year at a time and place specified by the Board.

CREDENTIALS – Applicants must furnish satisfactory evidence of good moral character, present a photostatic copy of the diploma as evidence of having graduated in and received a degree from a legally authorized veterinary medical school having educational standards equal to those approved by the AVMA. Applications must be made on forms furnished by the Board. Application must be submitted 14 days prior to examination date.

FEE – $25.00, to accompany application.

REGISTRATION – State registration of license required; annual registration fee, $10.00

RECIPROCITY – None.

CITIZENSHIP – Required.

EXECUTIVE OFFICER OF BOARD – Dr. W. W. Hawkins, Secretary-Treasurer, State Board of Veterinarians, Box 1253, Dillon, MT 59725.

### Nebraska

(Practice Law first enacted about 1905; last revised in 1927, 1959, 1967, 1969 and in 1971.)

EXAMINATIONS – At such times and places as designated by the Board of Examiners, usually at Lincoln.

CREDENTIALS – Evidence that applicant is at least 21 years of age and of good moral character. Proof of graduation from an accredited school of veterinary medicine and surgery, approved by the Department of Health upon the recommendation of the Board of Examiners and recognized by the AVMA.

FEE – $50.00.

RENEWAL – State renewal of license required; annual fee, $15.00.

RECIPROCITY – At discretion of the Department of Health and the Board. Oral examination by the Board required. Such examination to be given at the time of regular board meetings; or as required, fee $50.00.

EXECUTIVE OFFICER OF BOARD – Mr. Rex C. Higley, Director, Bureau of Examining Boards, 1003 "O" St., Lincoln, NE 68508.

### Nevada

(Practice Law first enacted in 1919: Last revised in 1975, Present Act as described in 1975, Nevada Revised Statutes.)

EXAMINATIONS – Annual, June, in Reno or Las Vegas.

CREDENTIALS – Diploma from veterinary school recognized by the American Veterinary Medical Association. Foreign veterinary graduates - E.C.F.V.G. Certificate dated after December 31, 1972 required.

FEE – $100.00, plus Professional Examination Service fee if National Board is taken in Nevada.

REGISTRATION – Annual registration of license. Registration fee, $15.00

RECIPROCITY – None.

CITIZENSHIP – Must be a citizen of the United States or has filed a declaration of intention to become a citizen.

EXECUTIVE OFFICER OF BOARD – Dr. John L. O'Harra, Secretary-Treasurer, Board of Veterinary Medical Examiners, P.O. Box 11100, Reno, NV 89510.

### New Hampshire

(From New Hampshire Session Laws of 1901, Chapter 57. Practice Law first enacted in 1901. Repealed and substituted Session Laws of 1907, Chapter 36. Amended Session Laws of 1947. Amended in 1955, and last amended in 1971 as RSA Chapter 328.)

EXAMINATIONS – On date specified by the Board during second Thursday of July each year, at the State House, Concord.

CREDENTIALS – Applicants must show proof of graduation from an accredited veterinary college acceptable to the AVMA. Applications must be filed on or before June 20 with the secretary. Temporary eligibility for examination and lfcense approved on condition.

FEE – $50.00.

REGISTRATION – State registration of license is required; annual fee, $10.00

RECIPROCITY – United States citizenship is not required.

EXECUTIVE OFFICER OF BOARD – Dr. Thomas J. Lockridge, Secretary-Treasurer, 1153 Hanover St., Manchester, NH 03104.

### New Jersey

(From Revised Statutes of New Jersey, 1937, as revised and amended. Practice Law first enacted in 1902; last revised in 1965.)

EXAMINATIONS – June and December each year in Trenton, exact date and place to be announced.

CREDENTIALS – Applications must be filed with secretary at least 30 days prior to the date of examination, accompanied by a passport photo, proof of graduation from a school approved by the Board, proof of approved preveterinary education. Applicants must be at least 21 years of age and of good moral character. Graduates of Foreign Veterinary Schools are first required to have satisfactorily passed a qualifying examination given by AVMA before applying for examination for licensure in New Jersey.

FEE – Application $10.00; National Boards $45.00; Oral & Written Practical $30.00.

REGISTRATION – State registration of license required; annual fee not to exceed $15.00.

RECIPROCITY – None. National Board scores converted to New Jersey standards acceptable.

EXECUTIVE OFFICER OF BOARD – Dr. George E. Boyle, Secretary-Treasurer, P.O. Box 214, Middletown, NJ 07748.

### New Mexico

(Enacted by the New Mexico Twenty Eighth Legislature, Chapter 62, Veterinary Practice Act, effective July 1, 1967, to regulate the Practice Act, effective July 1, 1967, to regulate the Practice of Veterinary Medicine and repealing first Act of 1931 and Amendments.)

EXAMINATIONS – January 12, 13, 1976, Airport Marina Hotel, Albuquerque, N.M. Dates set by the Board of Examiners. Application, furnished by the Board, must be filed two (2) weeks prior to examination.

CREDENTIALS – Diploma and proof of graduation from accredited Veterinary School, approved by the AVMA, two letters of recommendation, a recent photograph. Applicant must be at least 21 years of age, a United States citizen of applicant for citizenship, and of good moral character. A fee of $50.00 must accompany application and certification or satisfactory proof of licenses held in other states.

FEE – $50.00 must accompany application.

REGISTRATION – Annual fee set by Board, $20.00.

RECIPROCITY – Board may, at its discretion, waiver the written examination, providing the applicant meets the following requirements: 1) For 5 years, next, prior to filing his application been a practicing Veterinarian and licensed in a State, Territory or District of the United States, having license requirements at the time applicant was first licensed, which were substantially equivalent to the requirements of the Veterinary Practice Act. 2) Within the three years prior to filing his application, successfully completed the examination conducted by the National Board of Veterinary Examiners. 3) Successfully complete a Practical and Oral Examination given by the Board.

CITIZENSHIP – United States or applicant for United States Citizenship.

EXECUTIVE OFFICER OF BOARD – Dr. Charles Webster, Jr., Secretary, Board of Veterinary Examiners, P.O. Box 4596, Santa Fe, NM 87502.

### New York

(From Education Law as amended to 1971.)

EXAMINATIONS – The licensing examination shall be both practical and written and shall be held at times and places to be determined by the Commissioner. Original application for examination shall be filed with the Department not less than sixty days before the examination.

CREDENTIALS – Applications must be filed with the Director, Division of Professional Licensing Services, 1818 Twin Towers, 99 Washington Ave., Albany, N.Y. 12230. Applicants must submit satisfactory evidence of age (more than twenty-one), good moral character, required preliminary education, completion of satisfactory veterinary course and degree from a veterinary medical school registered with the department.

FEE – $$55.00.

REGISTRATION – Biennial registration of license with State Education Department required; fee $15.00.

COUNTY REGISTRATION – No longer required.

RECIPROCITY – Endorsement of basis of equivalent education, licensure, examination and 5 years of practice.

CITIZENSHIP – Required.

EXECUTIVE OFFICER OF BOARD – Dr. Kenneth T. Stringer, Secretary, New York State Board of Veterinary Medical Examiners, Rm. 1841, Twin Towers, 99 Washington Ave., Albany, NY 12210.

### North Carolina

(Practice Law first enacted in 1903; revised April 3, 1974.)

EXAMINATIONS – During the first or second week in June at North Carolina State University, Raleigh, North Carolina. National Board score required and professional board examination given on common date. Oral, practical and written examination given.

CREDENTIALS – Applicant must be 18 years of age and of good moral character. Must present notarized application for examination with satisfactory evidence of being a graduate of accredited veterinary school, approved by the AVMA. Must also furnish transcript of grades and must furnish photograph.

FEE – $25.00 plus fee charged by Professional Examination Service for professional examination.

REGISTRATION – Annual registration of license is required by January 1 of each year.

RECIPROCITY – May at the discretion of the Examining Board.

CITIZENSHIP – Must be native born or naturalized citizen.

EXECUTIVE OFFICER OF BOARD – Dr. C. R. Swearingen, Secretary-Treasurer, North Carolina Veterinary Medical Board, P.O. Box 425, Smithfield, NC 27577.

## North Dakota

(Enacted by the Forty-third Legislative Assembly of the State of North Dakota, 1973.)

EXAMINATION – Will be given at the State Capitol Building at 9 a.m. local time on the second Wednesday and Thursday in May and October.

CREDENTIALS – No person shall practice, or hold himself out as a practitioner in veterinary medicine, surgery, or dentistry, or any department thereof, unless he is a graduate of the veterinary course offered in a veterinary school or in a college or university recognized by the board, nor unless he possesses a certificate or permit issued by the state board of veterinary medical examiners which is in full force and effect.

FEE – $50.00 paid prior to examination.

REGISTRATION – Annual $10.00 renewal fee.

RECIPROCITY – At the discretion of the State Board.

CITIZENSHIP – No requirements.

EXECUTIVE SECRETARY OF BOARD – Dr. Dean E. Flagg, Executive Secretary, North Dakota Veterinary Medical Examining Board, c/o North Dakota Livestock Sanitary Board, Box 2056, Bismarck, ND 58505.

## Ohio

(Practice Law first enacted in 1895; last revised in 1961.)

EXAMINATIONS – The examination will be given on the Common Dates established by the Association of American State Boards of Examiners in Veterinary Medicine at a place in Columbus designated by the Board. Applications for examination shall be made at least thirty days prior to date of the examination.

CREDENTIALS – Proof of graduation from a recognized veterinary college verified by photostatic copy of college record, including dates in attendance, classes completed, grades received and diplomas issued.

FEE – $100.00.

RECIPROCITY – With Michigan, Indiana, Texas, West Virginia, Kentucky, Kansas, Missouri, Connecticut, Massachusetts, Washington, and District of Columbia.

CITIZENSHIP – Must be a citizen of United States or show proof of application therefor.

EXECUTIVE OFFICER OF BOARD – Dr. Harry E. Goldstein, Executive Secretary of Veterinary Medical Board, Ohio Department of Agriculture Laboratories, Reynoldsburg, OH 43068.

## Oklahoma

(Practice Law first enacted in 1937; revised in 1953 and May, 1971.)

EXAMINATIONS – Once a year at time and place designated by the Board. Applications for examinations must be on file 30 days prior to examination.

CREDENTIALS – Must be a graduate of a school approved by the AVMA, Bureau of Animal Industry and the Board.

FEE – Examination $70.00.

REGISTRATION – State registration of license required; $20.00 active license renewal fee if actively engaged in practice in Oklahoma; in-active license renewal $10.00. Due on or before the 2nd day of July.

RECIPROCITY – Board may, at its discretion, grant licenses to graduates licensed in those states which will grant reciprocity to graduates holding Oklahoma licenses; fee $70.00.

CITIZENSHIP – Must be a citizen of the United States.

EXECUTIVE OFFICER OF BOARD – Mrs. Bonnie Jean Neuffer, Executive Secretary, 4321 S. Lee St., Oklahoma City, OK 73109.

## Oregon

(Practice Law first enacted in 1903; revised in 1947; last revised in 1975.)

EXAMINATIONS – Annually during June at such time and place (usually Portland) as designated by the Board.

CREDENTIALS – Diploma from a school approved by the Oregon State Veterinary Medical Examining Board. Board demands minimum of six months internship in practice, or other qualifying service, before granting permanent license. Applications for examination must be submitted to the secretary at least one month prior to date of examination.

FEE – $35.00.

REGISTRATION – State registration of license required; annual fee, $20.00.

RECIPROCITY – None.

CITIZENSHIP – Citizen of the United States or has declared intention to become a citizen within 2 years after being licensed.

EXECUTIVE OFFICER OF BOARD – Dr. Clarke C. Brown, Executive Secretary, Oregon State Veterinary Medical Examining Board, 580 State Street, Salem, OR 97301.

## Pennsylvania

(From act of April 27, 1945, P.L. No. 141, as amended. Practice Law first enacted in 1915; not revised since 1945.)

EXAMINATIONS – In June of each year at the School of Veterinary Medicine, University of Pennsylvania, Philadelphia.

CREDENTIALS – Applications must be filed 60 days prior to examination, with State Board of Veterinary Medical Examiner, Harrisburg. Diploma from a recognized veterinary college. Foreign graduates are required to have AVMA Certification dated after December 31, 1972.

FEE – $50.00.

REGISTRATION – State registration of license required; biennial fee, $10.00

CITIZENSHIP – None Required.

EXECUTIVE OFFICER OF BOARD – Dr. Lillian A. Giuliani, Secretary, State Board of Veterinary Medical Examiners, Box 2649, 279 Boas St., Harrisburg, PA 17120.

## Rhode Island

(Title 5, Chapter 25, General Laws 1956, revised in 1969.)

EXAMINATIONS – In June or July of each year, once only, at a time and place designated by the Board. Application must be in by May 15th.

CREDENTIALS – Proof of graduation (Diploma) from a recognized veterinary college.

FEE – $35.00.

REGISTRATION – No annual renewal fee required.

RECIPROCITY – Board may grant reciprocity, following satisfactory practical and oral examination to veterinarians who have been duly licensed and in practice in another state for five consecutive years or more preceding application, provided said state has at least equal requirements and also extends reciprocity to Rhode Island licensees on the same basis. Must show proof of graduation from a recognized veterinary college.

CITIZENSHIP – No requirements.

EXECUTIVE OFFICER OF BOARD – Dr. Richard M. Mello, Secretary, State Board of Veterinarians, 581 Metacom Ave., Warren, RI 02885.

### South Carolina

(Practice Law first enacted in 1920; not revised since July 9, 1974.)

EXAMINATIONS – Examinations are given in June each year at Columbia.

CREDENTIALS – Applications on forms furnished by the Board must be filed with the secretary at least two weeks prior to examination together with fee.

FEE – $50.00.

REGISTRATION – State registration of license required; annual fee, $10.00.

RECIPROCITY – None.

CITIZENSHIP – Required.

EXECUTIVE OFFICER OF BOARD – Dr. H. L. Sutherland, Secretary-Treasurer, South Carolina State Board of Veterinary Examiners, P.O. Box 87, Union, SC 29379.

### South Dakota

(Practice Law first enacted in 1909; last revised in 1961.)

EXAMINATIONS – Applications must be received by May 15, examinations held in June.

CREDENTIALS – Twenty-one years of age. Citizen of the United-States, and graduate of approved school of veterinary medicines.

FEE – $25.00.

REGISTRATION – Annual fee, $25.00.

RECIPROCITY – Board may, in its descretion, grant license to graduate licensed in those states which reciprocate with South Dakota. In addition, an oral examination is required of all applicants.

CITIZENSHIP – Citizen of the United States.

EXECUTIVE OFFICER OF BOARD – Dr. Paul Wittenberg, Secretary-Treasurer, South Dakota Veterinary Examining Board, Box 113, Star Rt., Hot Springs, SD 57747.

### Tennessee

(Practice Law first enacted in 1905; revised in 1949; last revised in 1971.)

EXAMINATIONS – To be decided by the State Board.

CREDENTIALS – Application must be made in writing on blanks provided for that purpose, accompanied by $25.00 fee, and photostatic copy of diploma. Applications must be in 21 days before examination.

FEE – $25.00 examination fee.

REGISTRATION – Renewal fee $10.00 per year. Participation in a Continuous Education Program required each year to renew license.

RECIPROCITY – None.

CITIZENSHIP – Required.

EXECUTIVE OFFICER OF BOARD – Dr. Daniel Fitzpatrick, Secretary, State Board of Veterinary Medical Examiners, 3926 Nolensville Rd., Nashville, TN 37211.

### Texas

(From Vernon's Revised Civil Statutes of Texas Article 7465 (a), 1953 as amended. Practice Act enacted in 1911, revised in 1920, 1953, 1957, 1959; last revised in 1967.)

EXAMINATIONS – Examinations will be held twice yearly at such times and places as the Board deems convenient for applicants for examinations.

CREDENTIALS – Applicant must be of good moral character, be a citizen of the United States, be at least 21 years of age, and a graduate of a reputable school or college of veterinary medicine as approved by the Board.

FEE – Applicants for examination shall pay $50.00; applicants for license under reciprocal provisions, $100.00.

REGISTRATION – State registration of licenses is required annually at a fee of not less than $5.00 and not in excess of $30.00, as determined by the Board.

RECIPROCITY – Established with Michigan, North Dakota, South Dakota, Kansas, Missouri, Ohio, Oklahoma and Washington.

CITIZENSHIP – Must be a citizen of the United States.

EXECUTIVE OFFICER OF BOARD – T. D. Weaver, Executive Secretary, Board of Veterinary Medical Examiners of Texas, 603 Capital National Bank Bldg., Austin, TX 78701.

### Utah

(Practice Law first enacted in 1911; last revised in 1961.)

EXAMINATIONS – Usually in June or July of each year at State of Utah Business Regulation, Department of Registration, 330 East 4th South, Salt Lake City, Utah, at time designated by the Board.

CREDENTIALS – Diploma from a recognized veterinary college, and two letters of recommendation. Application must be filed fifteen days before examination.

FEE – $50.00.

RECIPROCITY – With Idaho and Washington.

CITIZENSHIP – United States citizenship required.

EXECUTIVE OFFICER OF BOARD – Dr. Glenn N. Taylor, Chairman of the Utah State Veterinary Board, University of Utah, Salt Lake City, UT 84132.

### Vermont

(From Chapter 35, Title 26, VSA 2351-2435 Vermont General Laws. Practice Law first enacted in 1912.)

EXAMINATIONS – Given at State House in Montpelier, January and June.

CREDENTIALS – Diploma from an American Veterinary Medical Association approved college. Applications must be filed fifteen days prior to examination with the secretary of the Board.

FEE – $20.00.

REGISTRATION – State registration of license required; annual fee, $5.00.

RECIPROCITY – May reciprocate with other States and Provinces in an interstate requisition and exchange of licenses, upon the basis of equality of educational standard and requisite, which standard shall not be lower than that required by the provision of this Chapter.

CITIZENSHIP – No requirement.

EXECUTIVE OFFICER OF BOARD – Dr. Robert Lunna, Secretary-Treasurer of Veterinary Registration and Examination, Swanton, VT 05488.

### Virginia

(From Chapter 19 of the Code of Virginia, 1950 Sections 54-776 through 54-788. Last amended, 1974. Practice Law first enacted in 1895.)

EXAMINATIONS – All examinations by the Board shall be both theoretical and practical and shall embrace such subjects as the Board shall from time to time prescribe and shall be both written and oral. The Board shall hold at least one examination annually. The date of the examination shall be announced by the Board at least six months prior to the date of the examination. The Board may elect to prepare its own examination or, if it so chooses, may use the examination prepared by the National Board of Veterinary Medical Examiners.

CREDENTIALS – Must have a diploma from a veterinary college approved by the Board.

FEE – $50.00.

REGISTRATION – State registration of license required; $20.00.

RECIPROCITY – Waiver of Written Examination. The Board, in its discretion, may waive the written part of the examination provided an applicant for such examination meets the following requirements:

(a) In the opinion of the Board, the applicant has met all of the requirements provided for in § 54-788.1 of the Code of Virginia; (b) The applicant has filed the required application as provided for in these rules and regulations; (c) The applicant has been issued a certificate to practice veterinary medicine and surgery in another state; (d) The applicant has taken the written examination prepared by the National Board of Veterinary Medical Examiners given by a duly constituted Board of Veterinary Examiners of another state and the grade assigned thereto is judged to be a passing grade by the Board in accordance with the formula adopted by the Board in the year such examination was given; (e) The applicant furnishes to the Board a certification of the grades made on the aforementioned examination at the time he submits an application to sit for the Virginia examination; (f) The applicant is endorsed by boards or other appropriate authorities of other states, territories, counties and the District of Columbia with which reciprocal relations have not been established to receive a certificate as provided for in these rules and regulations.

EXECUTIVE OFFICER OF BOARD – Mrs. Ruth J. Herrink, Director, Virginia State Board of Veterinary Examiners, P O. Box 1-X. Richmond, VA 23202.

## Washington

(From Chapter 71, Laws of 1941. Practice Law first enacted in 1907; last revised in 1974.)

EXAMINATIONS – Held at least once each year at such times and places as the director may authorize.

CREDENTIALS – Signed, sworn application filed thirty days prior to date of examination. Diploma from some legally chartered veterinary College recognized by the AVMA, offering at least four academic years of thirty-two to thirty-six weeks each. Applicant must be at least 21 years of age and of good moral character.

FEE – Application and examination, National Board, $50.00, Oral and Practical, $50.00; License renewal, $15.00.

REGISTRATION – State registration of license required; annual fee, $10.00.

RECIPROCITY – Board may grant reciprocity to licensees who have practiced continuously for two years or more immediately before application and who file attested certificate of license and registration in any of the following states: Arkansas, Idaho, Illinois, Kansas, Massachusetts, Michigan, Minnesota, Missouri, North Dakota, Ohio, South Dakota, Texas, Utah, Vermont; Fee, $100.00.

CITIZENSHIP – No requirements.

EXECUTIVE OFFICER OF BOARD – Mr. Loren D. Ford, Secretary, P.O. Box 962, Bellevue, WA 98009.

## West Virginia

(Practice Law first enacted in 1915; revised in 1931, 1959 and 1974.)

EXAMINATIONS – The second or third Monday in June, Charleston, W.V.

CREDENTIALS – Diploma from an AVMA approved veterinary college. Applications must be filed with secretary of Board at least 30 days prior to examination.

FEE – $55.00.

REGISTRATION – Renewal of license each year, $5.00 at discretion of the Board.

RECIPROCITY – Ohio.

CITIZENSHIP – Citizen of the United States or filed citizenship papers.

EXECUTIVE OFFICER OF BOARD – Dr. Joe B. Jolliffe, Secretary, The West Virginia Board of Veterinary Medicine, Kingwood, WV 26537.

## Wisconsin

(Practice Law enacted in 1961.)

EXAMINATIONS – One examination annually, usually in June.

CREDENTIALS – Applicant must be a graduate of a veterinary college approved by the board, and must be 18 years of age.

FEE – $65.00 for State Board examination.

REGISTRATION – State registration of license required; annual fee, $15.00.

RECIPROCITY – None.

CITIZENSHIP – No requirements.

EXECUTIVE OFFICER OF BOARD – Chairman, Wisconsin Veterinary Examining Board, 201 E. Washington Ave., Madison, WI 53702.

## Wyoming

(New Practice Act, Chapter 37, Session Laws of Wyoming 1967.)

EXAMINATIONS – June of each year at State Office Bldg., Cheyenne, Wy. or at such time and place as designated by President of the Board.

CREDENTIALS – Diploma of recognized college of veterinary medicine, 21 years old, 2 letters of recommendation and photo.

FEE – $25.00.

REGISTRATION – State registration of license required, annual fee, $10.00.

CITIZENSHIP – Citizen of the United States or an applicant for citizenship.

EXECUTIVE OFFICER OF BOARD – Dr. N. R. Swanson, State Veterinarian and Secretary-Treasurer, Wyoming Board of Veterinary Medicine, State Office Bldg., East Cheyenne, WY 82002.

## Puerto Rico

(Law 59. Providing for the organization of a Board of Veterinary Examiners, approved April 13, 1916; last amended 1933.)

EXAMINATIONS – The first Tuesday in January and August at San Juan, Puerto Rico, and at such other times as the Board may deem necessary.

CREDENTIALS – Application in writing must be filed with Board accompanied by proof (diploma) and veterinary college transcript that the applicant is a graduate from veterinary college or institution that maintains a standard satisfying the requirements of the Bureau of Animal Industry, USDA and the AVMA.

FEE – $15.00 to accompany application. Candidate is entitled to a second examination within the next six months without having to pay another fee in case he fails to pass the first examination.

REGISTRATION – License must be registered by applicant at the Department of Health within sixty days after date of issue; fee, $1.00. Annual registration not required.

RECIPROCITY – No reciprocity, all aspirants for a license must sit for examination.

CITIZENSHIP – No requirement.

ADMINISTRATIVE OFFICER OF BOARD – Mr. Justino Valles, Board of Veterinary Examiners of Puerto Rico, P.O. Box 3271, San Juan, PR

## Virgin Islands

(Includes the three (3) U. S. Virgin Island - St. Croix, St John and St Thomas. Practice Law first enacted in 1952, revised in 1957 and 1958.)

EXAMINATIONS – On the second Wednesday of June and November each year.

CREDENTIALS – Applicants must be graduates of colleges recognized and approved by the American Veterinary Medical Association, over 21 years of age and of good moral character.

FEE – $100.00 due with application.

REGISTRATION – Annual registration of license is required; annual fee, $100.00.

RECIPROCITY – Applicants are required to take an examination.

CITIZENSHIP – Residence in the U. S. Virgin Islands for six (6) consecutive months immediately preceding filing of application.

EXECUTIVE OFFICER OF BOARD – Dr. Andrew Williamson, Chairman, Box 384, Charlotte Amalie, St. Thomas, VI 00801.

## Alberta

(Veterinary Practice Law first enacted in 1906; revised in 1921; replaced by Veterinary Surgeon's Acts in 1953 with amendments in 1960 and 1964.)

EXAMINATIONS – Not required if applicant's qualifications are acceptable to General Faculty Council of University of Alberta. Generally, foreign graduates are required to take examinations, held twice yearly, spring and fall. Apply to Registrar, University of Alberta, Edmonton, Alta.

CREDENTIALS – Degree from recognized veterinary college plus Certificate of Qualification from National Examining Board.

REGISTRATION – $100.00. Annual dues effective January 1. Membership subject to approval by admission committee.

RECIPROCITY – None.

EXECUTIVE OFFICER OF COUNCIL – Dr. J. P. Best, Secretary-Treasurer, and Registrar, Alberta Veterinary Medical Association, 7904-148th St., Edmonton, AB

## British Columbia

((Veterinary Practice Law first enacted in 1911.)

EXAMINATIONS – Twice annually in early May and November at Vancouver. Applications must be filed with secretary sixty days before examination or at the discretion of the Council.

CREDENTIALS – Veterinary graduates of all Colleges, other than Canadian, must first be processed by the C.V.M.A. National Examining Board, 360 Bronson Ave., Ottawa KIR 6J3, Ontario, Can., before they will be allowed to sit for Provincial Boards. Phone: 613-236-1162.

FEE – $75.00. Special examinations may be arranged at other dates if requested. Fee is $150.00.

REGISTRATION – Provincial registration and license required; annual fee, $175.00.

RECIPROCITY – None.

CITIZENSHIP – None specified.

EXECUTIVE OFFICER OF COUNCIL – Dr. W. G. Thomson, Secretary-Treasurer and Registrar, British Columbia Veterinary Medical Association, Rm. 210, 1070 W. Broadway, Vancouver, V6H 1E7. Phone: 604-733-9312.

## Manitoba

(Veterinary Practice Law first enacted in 1881; revised in 1899; further revised and cited as "The Veterinary Medical Association Act of Manitoba;" assented to March 29, 1957; further revised and cited as "The Veterinary Medical Act"; assented to June 10, 1974.)

EXAMINATIONS – As prescribed by and at such times as designated by the Veterinary Medical Board of Manitoba. Application may be made at any time through the Secretary-Treasurer of the Association and the Registrar of the Board.

CREDENTIALS – Diploma from a veterinary college "accredited" by the National Examining Board of the Canadian Veterinary Medical Association; or a positive assessment of credentials of a graduate of a college "Recognized" by the National Examining Board.

REGISTRATION – Annual registration of membership with Secretary-Treasurer of the Manitoba Veterinary Medical Association required; fee $100 per annum.

REGISTRATION – Annual registration of license with registrar of the Veterinary Medical Board of Manitoba required; fee $10.00 per annum.

RECIPROCITY – None.

EXECUTIVE OFFICER OF COUNCIL – Dr. Ross Fitzpatrick, Secretary, MVHA, Box 1646, Winnipeg, Manitoba, R3C 0K0.

EXECUTIVE OFFICER OF BOARD – Dr. Jay M. Isa, Registrar, The Veterinary Medical Board of Manitoba, Agricultural Services Complex, University Cres. and S. Dyke Road, Winnipeg, Manitoba, R3T 2N2.

## New Brunswick

(New Brunswick Veterinary Medical Association Act passed April 3, 1965.)

EXAMINATIONS – Canadian Veterinary Medical Association Examining Board.

CREDENTIALS – Must be a graduate of a recognized school or college on the approved list issued by the Canadian Veterinary Medical Association.

FEE – $50.00 plus any additional expenses entailed.

REGISTRATION – Annual registration of license required, the fee, as established by the N.B.V.M.A.

RECIPROCITY – With provinces that grant like priviliges to licentiates of New Brunswick.

EXECUTIVE OFFICER – Dr. D. M. DuPlessis, Secretary-Treasurer and Registrar, New Brunswick Veterinary Medical Association, P.O. Box 338, Moncton, NB

## Nova Scotia

(Practice Law first enacted in 1913; amended in 1923, 1958 and 1975.)

EXAMINATIONS – As set by the National Examining Board of the C.V.M.A., at such times and places as designated by the Board.

CREDENTIALS – Graduation from recognized veterinary college.

ADMISSION FEE – $25.00.

REGISTRATION – Annual provincial registration of license required; fee $70.00.

CITIZENSHIP – No requirement.

EXECUTIVE OFFICER OF BOARD – Dr. R. M. Phillips, Secretary, Registrar, c/o N.S.A.C., Truro, NS B2N 5E3.

## Ontario

(The Veterinarians Act 1958.)

EXAMINATIONS – Spring and Fall at Guelph.

CREDENTIALS – Proof of academic certification from National Examining Board, c/o C.V.M.A., 360 Bronson Ave., Ottawa, ON. KIR 6J3, or graduation from a Canadian Veterinary College.

FEE – $140.00.

REGISTRATION – Membership in Ontario Veterinary Association required to practice. Annual fee, $140.00.

RECIPROCITY – None.

CITIZENSHIP – No requirement.

EXECUTIVE OFFICER OF BOARD – Mr. M. H. Hudspeth, Secretary-Registrar, Ontario Veterinary Association, 33 Cork St., W., Guelph, ON NIH 6N9.

## Prince Edward Island

(Veterinary Practice Law first enacted in 1920; last revised in 1957, and in 1970.)

EXAMINATIONS – Any person, residing in another province who wishes to practice in Prince Edward Island, may have to pass an examination set by the Board of Examiners of the Canadian Veterinary Medical Association.

CREDENTIALS – Applicant must be a graduate of a recognized veterinary college and his application must first be approved by the P.E.I. Veterinary Medical Association.

FEE – $35.00.

REGISTRATION – Annual registration, required with registrar of Council of P.E.I. Veterinary Association; fee, $35.00.

CITIZENSHIP – Must be a citizen of Canada.

EXECUTIVE OFFICER OF COUNCIL – Dr. James I. Higgins, P.O. Box 3000, Charlottetown, PE

## Quebec

(The Law constituting the "Corporation of Veterinarians of the Province of Quebec" was enacted in 1902, and revised in February, 1956 and July, 1973.)

EXAMINATIONS – By the Bureau of the order of Medical Veterinarians of Quebec.

ADMISSIBILITY – Certificate of Qualification from the Canadian Veterinary Medical Association; Certificate of Proficiency in the French language, issued by the Department of Immigration of the Government of Quebec.

FEES – Minimum rate is $55.00.

RECIPROCITY – None.

CITIZENSHIP – Not required.

SECRETARY'S OFFICE – Dr. Henri-Paul Girouard, Secretary General, 250 Est Boulevard St-Joseph-Ste 505, Montreal, Quebec

## Saskatchewan

(Veterinary Practice Law first enacted in 1908; revised in 1912, 1960 and last revision 1971.)

EXAMINATIONS – Set by National Examining Board. Canadian Veterinary Medical Association, Applications for examinations made to Chairman, National Examining Board C.V.M.A.. 360 Bronson Ave., Ottawa, K1R 6J3 Ontario.

CREDENTIALS – Academic qualifications and credentials subject to examination and approval of National Examining Board.

REGISTRATION – Annual registration of license to practice required with registrar of Saskatchewan Veterinary Medical Association; fee, $50.00.

RECIPROCITY – All non Canadian graduates must meet the requirements of the National Examining Board of the C.V.M.A. and be in possession of the Certificate of Qualification issued by that Board.

CITIZENSHIP – Not required.

EXECUTIVE OFFICER OF BOARD – Dr. E. E. Carlson, Secretary-Treasurer and Registrar, 15 Hawthorne Crescent, Regina, Sk S4S 4Y1.

# ANSWER SHEET

TEST NO. ______ PART ______ TITLE OF POSITION ______
(AS GIVEN IN EXAMINATION ANNOUNCEMENT - INCLUDE OPTION, IF ANY)

PLACE OF EXAMINATION ______ (CITY OR TOWN) ______ (STATE) DATE ______

| RATING |
|---|
| |

USE THE SPECIAL PENCIL. MAKE GLOSSY BLACK MARKS.

| | | | | | | | | | |
|---|---|---|---|---|---|---|---|---|---|
| 1 | A B C D E | 26 | A B C D E | 51 | A B C D E | 76 | A B C D E | 101 | A B C D E |
| 2 | A B C D E | 27 | A B C D E | 52 | A B C D E | 77 | A B C D E | 102 | A B C D E |
| 3 | A B C D E | 28 | A B C D E | 53 | A B C D E | 78 | A B C D E | 103 | A B C D E |
| 4 | A B C D E | 29 | A B C D E | 54 | A B C D E | 79 | A B C D E | 104 | A B C D E |
| 5 | A B C D E | 30 | A B C D E | 55 | A B C D E | 80 | A B C D E | 105 | A B C D E |
| 6 | A B C D E | 31 | A B C D E | 56 | A B C D E | 81 | A B C D E | 106 | A B C D E |
| 7 | A B C D E | 32 | A B C D E | 57 | A B C D E | 82 | A B C D E | 107 | A B C D E |
| 8 | A B C D E | 33 | A B C D E | 58 | A B C D E | 83 | A B C D E | 108 | A B C D E |
| 9 | A B C D E | 34 | A B C D E | 59 | A B C D E | 84 | A B C D E | 109 | A B C D E |
| 10 | A B C D E | 35 | A B C D E | 60 | A B C D E | 85 | A B C D E | 110 | A B C D E |

Make only ONE mark for each answer. Additional and stray marks may be counted as mistakes. In making corrections, erase errors COMPLETELY.

| | | | | | | | | | |
|---|---|---|---|---|---|---|---|---|---|
| 11 | A B C D E | 36 | A B C D E | 61 | A B C D E | 86 | A B C D E | 111 | A B C D E |
| 12 | A B C D E | 37 | A B C D E | 62 | A B C D E | 87 | A B C D E | 112 | A B C D E |
| 13 | A B C D E | 38 | A B C D E | 63 | A B C D E | 88 | A B C D E | 113 | A B C D E |
| 14 | A B C D E | 39 | A B C D E | 64 | A B C D E | 89 | A B C D E | 114 | A B C D E |
| 15 | A B C D E | 40 | A B C D E | 65 | A B C D E | 90 | A B C D E | 115 | A B C D E |
| 16 | A B C D E | 41 | A B C D E | 66 | A B C D E | 91 | A B C D E | 116 | A B C D E |
| 17 | A B C D E | 42 | A B C D E | 67 | A B C D E | 92 | A B C D E | 117 | A B C D E |
| 18 | A B C D E | 43 | A B C D E | 68 | A B C D E | 93 | A B C D E | 118 | A B C D E |
| 19 | A B C D E | 44 | A B C D E | 69 | A B C D E | 94 | A B C D E | 119 | A B C D E |
| 20 | A B C D E | 45 | A B C D E | 70 | A B C D E | 95 | A B C D E | 120 | A B C D E |
| 21 | A B C D E | 46 | A B C D E | 71 | A B C D E | 96 | A B C D E | 121 | A B C D E |
| 22 | A B C D E | 47 | A B C D E | 72 | A B C D E | 97 | A B C D E | 122 | A B C D E |
| 23 | A B C D E | 48 | A B C D E | 73 | A B C D E | 98 | A B C D E | 123 | A B C D E |
| 24 | A B C D E | 49 | A B C D E | 74 | A B C D E | 99 | A B C D E | 124 | A B C D E |
| 25 | A B C D E | 50 | A B C D E | 75 | A B C D E | 100 | A B C D E | 125 | A B C D E |

# ANSWER SHEET

TEST NO. ______________ PART ______ TITLE OF POSITION ______________________________
(AS GIVEN IN EXAMINATION ANNOUNCEMENT - INCLUDE OPTION, IF ANY)

PLACE OF EXAMINATION ______________________ (CITY OR TOWN) ______________ (STATE) DATE ______________

| RATING |
|---|
| |

USE THE SPECIAL PENCIL. MAKE GLOSSY BLACK MARKS.

| | | | | |
|---|---|---|---|---|
| 1 A B C D E | 26 A B C D E | 51 A B C D E | 76 A B C D E | 101 A B C D E |
| 2 A B C D E | 27 A B C D E | 52 A B C D E | 77 A B C D E | 102 A B C D E |
| 3 A B C D E | 28 A B C D E | 53 A B C D E | 78 A B C D E | 103 A B C D E |
| 4 A B C D E | 29 A B C D E | 54 A B C D E | 79 A B C D E | 104 A B C D E |
| 5 A B C D E | 30 A B C D E | 55 A B C D E | 80 A B C D E | 105 A B C D E |
| 6 A B C D E | 31 A B C D E | 56 A B C D E | 81 A B C D E | 106 A B C D E |
| 7 A B C D E | 32 A B C D E | 57 A B C D E | 82 A B C D E | 107 A B C D E |
| 8 A B C D E | 33 A B C D E | 58 A B C D E | 83 A B C D E | 108 A B C D E |
| 9 A B C D E | 34 A B C D E | 59 A B C D E | 84 A B C D E | 109 A B C D E |
| 10 A B C D E | 35 A B C D E | 60 A B C D E | 85 A B C D E | 110 A B C D E |

Make only ONE mark for each answer. Additional and stray marks may be counted as mistakes. In making corrections, erase errors COMPLETELY.

| | | | | |
|---|---|---|---|---|
| 11 A B C D E | 36 A B C D E | 61 A B C D E | 86 A B C D E | 111 A B C D E |
| 12 A B C D E | 37 A B C D E | 62 A B C D E | 87 A B C D E | 112 A B C D E |
| 13 A B C D E | 38 A B C D E | 63 A B C D E | 88 A B C D E | 113 A B C D E |
| 14 A B C D E | 39 A B C D E | 64 A B C D E | 89 A B C D E | 114 A B C D E |
| 15 A B C D E | 40 A B C D E | 65 A B C D E | 90 A B C D E | 115 A B C D E |
| 16 A B C D E | 41 A B C D E | 66 A B C D E | 91 A B C D E | 116 A B C D E |
| 17 A B C D E | 42 A B C D E | 67 A B C D E | 92 A B C D E | 117 A B C D E |
| 18 A B C D E | 43 A B C D E | 68 A B C D E | 93 A B C D E | 118 A B C D E |
| 19 A B C D E | 44 A B C D E | 69 A B C D E | 94 A B C D E | 119 A B C D E |
| 20 A B C D E | 45 A B C D E | 70 A B C D E | 95 A B C D E | 120 A B C D E |
| 21 A B C D E | 46 A B C D E | 71 A B C D E | 96 A B C D E | 121 A B C D E |
| 22 A B C D E | 47 A B C D E | 72 A B C D E | 97 A B C D E | 122 A B C D E |
| 23 A B C D E | 48 A B C D E | 73 A B C D E | 98 A B C D E | 123 A B C D E |
| 24 A B C D E | 49 A B C D E | 74 A B C D E | 99 A B C D E | 124 A B C D E |
| 25 A B C D E | 50 A B C D E | 75 A B C D E | 100 A B C D E | 125 A B C D E |